Cognitive Biology

Vienna Series in Theoretical Biology

Gerd B. Müller, Günter P. Wagner, and Werner Callebaut, editors

Cognitive Biology
Evolutionary and Developmental Perspectives on Mind, Brain and Behavior

edited by Luca Tommasi, Mary A. Peterson and Lynn Nadel

The MIT Press
Cambridge, Massachusetts
London, England

MIT Press books may be purchased at special quantity discounts for business or sales promotional use. For information, please email special_sales@mitpress.mit.edu or write to Special Sales Department, The MIT Press, 55 Hayward Street, Cambridge, MA 02142.

This book was set in Times Roman 10/13pt by SNP Best-set Typesetter Ltd., Hong Kong. Printed and bound in the United States of America.

Library of Congress Cataloging-in-Publication Data

Cognitive biology : evolutionary and developmental perspectives on mind, brain, and behavior / edited by Luca Tommasi, Mary A. Peterson, and Lynn Nadel.
    p. ; cm.—(Vienna series in theoretical biology)
  Includes bibliographical references and index.
  ISBN-13: 978-0-262-01293-5 (hardcover : alk. paper)
  ISBN-10: 0-262-01293-6 (hardcover : alk. paper) 1. Brain–Evolution. 2. Cognitive science. I. Tommasi, Luca, 1970–. II. Peterson, Mary A., 1950–. III. Nadel, Lynn. IV. Series.
  [DNLM: 1. Adaptation, Physiological. 2. Cognition–physiology. 3. Evolution. QT 140 C676 2009]
  QL933.C64 2009
  153–dc22
                                                                                        2008035962

10 9 8 7 6 5 4 3 2 1

Contents

Series Foreword

Biology is becoming the leading science in this century. As in all other sciences, progress in biology depends on interactions between empirical research, theory building, and modeling. But whereas the techniques and methods of descriptive and experimental biology have dramatically evolved in recent years, generating a flood of highly detailed empirical data, the integration of these results into useful theoretical frameworks has lagged behind. Driven largely by pragmatic and technical considerations, research in biology continues to be less guided by theory than seems indicated.

By promoting the formulation and discussion of new theoretical concepts in the biosciences, this series intends to help fill the gaps in our understanding of some of the major open questions of biology, such as the origin and organization of organismal form, the relationship between development and evolution, and the biological bases of cognition and mind.

Theoretical biology has important roots in the experimental biology movement of early-twentieth-century Vienna. Paul Weiss and Ludwig von Bertalanffy were among the first to use the term *theoretical biology* in a modern scientific context. In their understanding the subject was not limited to mathematical formalization, as is often the case today, but extended to the conceptual problems and foundations of biology. It is this commitment to a comprehensive, cross-disciplinary integration of theoretical concepts that the present series intends to emphasize. Today theoretical biology has genetic, developmental, and evolutionary components, the central connective themes in modern biology, but also includes relevant aspects of computational biology, semiotics, and cognition research, and extends to the naturalistic philosophy of sciences.

The "Vienna Series" grew out of theory-oriented workshops organized by the Konrad Lorenz Institute for Evolution and Cognition Research (KLI), an international center for advanced study closely associated with the University of Vienna. The KLI fosters research projects, workshops, archives, book projects, and the journal *Biological Theory*, all devoted to aspects of theoretical biology, with an emphasis on integrating the developmental, evolutionary, and cognitive sciences. The series editors welcome suggestions for book projects in these fields.

Gerd B. Müller, University of Vienna and KLI
Günter P. Wagner, Yale University and KLI
Werner Callebaut, Hasselt University and KLI

Preface

In the tradition of the Vienna Series in Theoretical Biology, this book represents the outcome of a complex and creative enterprise, whose first step is that of bringing together representatives from a number of disciplines to discuss and exchange ideas around a main topic that is defined well in advance by half a handful of organizers.

Such first step was accomplished during a three-day workshop that took place in June 2006 at the beautiful mansion of the Konrad Lorenz family, in Altenberg, near Vienna, a location that now hosts the Konrad Lorenz Institute for Evolution and Cognition Research. Here, the convened participants had the hard task of presenting their research and confronting their ideas about the emerging directions that see the cognitive sciences as deeply involved in what looks like an epistemic revolution, more or less fifty years after their official birth. The workshop had in fact been entitled "The New Cognitive Sciences" because it was felt that in the last two decades, many sources of inspiration in the multidisciplinary field of the cognitive sciences were coming from some subfields of the "founding disciplines" more than others.

Whereas the cognitive sciences were strongly dominated by the computational metaphor during a first stage of their existence, and by brain research during a second stage, we felt that, still fully recognizing the relevance of these sources for the flow of fresh ideas into the boiling pot, many other ingredients were being added to the ongoing recipe in a more recent stage. These derive mostly from research at the intersection of psychology and not simply neuroscience, but biology in its wider sense. Results and insights from comparative, developmental and cross-cultural psychology (i.e. from subfields of psychology that have been less relevant for some decades in the cognitive sciences) have recently engendered questions and provided evidence that have become spicy ingredients for the research carried out in the cognitive neurosciences (both theoretical and experimental; i.e. electrophysiology, neuroimaging, and computational neuroscience) but also in harbors of the life sciences that not necessarily are pleasant sanctuaries to many a cognitive scientist, such as genetics, ecology, developmental and evolutionary biology. The aim of the workshop was thus that of providing an overview and engendering discussion on the cross-disciplinary integration between evolutionary and developmental approaches to cognition in the light of contributions from the life sciences that are not limited to neuroscience.

The second step of the enterprise was that of organizing this book. However, the undertaking of this step was initiated at the end of the first step, under a lucky star: on the last day of the workshop the participants agreed, before getting involved in an adventurous cruise along the Danube, that the content of the book that would grow from their meeting could be explicit from its very outset, that is the title. "Cognitive Biology" sounded like a potential candidate to capture the merging of the cognitive and the life sciences that the workshop aimed at representing with a number of isolated (and fascinating) examples: we believe that this title reflects those examples as well as the bigger picture, and we hope that the book will increase the awareness that this change of attitude shared by a large number of scholars worldwide is, in fact, a serious enterprise reflecting a new understanding of mind, brain and behavior.

The book is structured into four main parts, which probably echo too much our own inclinations for the "hot topics." This is something we feel responsible for, humbly apologizing to those topics that might have been included but have not. The four parts feature chapters devoted, respectively, to spatial cognition (part II, Space), to the relationship among attention, perception and learning (part III, Qualities and Objects), to representations of numbers and economic value (part IV, Numbers and Probability), and to social cognition (part V, Social Entities), all issues central to the contemporary cognitive sciences.

We thank the staff of the KLI for their marvelous hospitality in an unrivalled setting, and for the continuous support provided before, during and after the workshop. As science is nowadays a tough business, it is tremendously reassuring to know that there are still scientific institutions offering so much space to the main ingredient that should enter the boiling pot: ideas.

I INTRODUCTION

1 Cognitive Biology: The New Cognitive Sciences

Luca Tommasi, Lynn Nadel, and Mary A. Peterson

Most who have written about the history of the cognitive sciences have conceived of the field as an interdisciplinary gathering of psychology, philosophy, computer science, linguistics, neuroscience, and anthropology. For the last fifty years it has been expected that pooling information from these disciplines would unveil the hidden secrets of the mind. Many introductory, advanced, and encyclopedic accounts of the history of the cognitive sciences have portrayed the field as a large alliance of disciplines studying cognitive phenomena in their natural and artificial manifestations, a field that is strongly interdisciplinary in nature and that pursues both basic and applied research (Gardner 1985; Bechtel et al. 1998; Nadel and Piattelli Palmarini 2003; Boden 2006).

In the past decade cognitive science has undergone a transformation that, although tangible in the everyday practice of cognitive scientists, has not yet been integrated into the definition of the field. This transition took place when the fields of developmental psychology, comparative psychology, and the neurosciences began to share and compare data obtained using similar methodologies in animals and humans, and at different stages of developmental change. As a consequence, many cognitive abilities have now been explored in a wide range of organisms and developmental stages.

Results have revealed the nature and origin of the understanding of numbers, places, values, objects, identity of other individuals, causal events, agency, intentionality, and many other instances of the cognitive life of organisms. In a growing number of cases these results have passed a "comparative check" and a "developmental check" before being further explored at the level of the nervous system. Indeed, the possibilities offered by genetics, ecology, and the neurosciences for elucidating the small- and large-scale biological mechanisms underlying these domains have greatly helped in renewing the whole field. In this introduction we intend to give a schematic but realistic portrait of these sources of change in the cognitive sciences and provide a basis for what we have chosen to call cognitive biology.

A Good Time for a Change in the Definition of Cognitive Science

In his famous book dedicated to the praiseworthy aim of advising young researchers, *Advice for a Young Investigator,* Santiago Ramón y Cajal, one of the founding fathers of the neurosciences, wrote, "It is a wonderful and fortunate thing for a scientist to be born during one of these great decisive moments in the history of ideas, when much of what has been done in the past is invalidated. Under these circumstances, it could not be easier to choose a fertile area of investigation" (Ramón y Cajal 1899, p. 14).

The cognitive sciences currently represent such an example, attracting the interest of armies of young investigators from established disciplines who are bringing their expertise and efforts to solving the conundrum of the mind. This happened in at least three waves over almost fifty years. The first wave, in the 1950s, overtook behaviorism and established the field; the crucial keyword of this wave was *information*. The second wave brought matter and energy to the fore in the 1970s; the crucial keyword of this wave was "*brain.*" The third wave, the one contributing to the picture this book plans to portray, brought in evolutionary theory and developmental issues: the crucial keyword of this wave is "*change.*"

Precursors of the Cognitive Sciences

Interest in the functions of the mind and its relation to the natural sciences was already in place by the time of Greek classic philosophy, and has been a matter of constant speculation, reappearing in many forms throughout the history of scientific and philosophical thinking, from Descartes to Darwin. The so-called sciences of the "three Ps," philosophy, physiology, and psychology, went through a complex reshaping process in the nineteenth century that strongly revolved around the need for an interdisciplinary approach to the study of the mind. Moreover, since the eventual birth of experimental psychology by the end of the nineteenth century, a number of general theories provided their own integrated accounts of the mind, some of them breaking interdisciplinary boundaries, at least on theoretical grounds (for example, Gestalt theory, genetic epistemology, and other theories such as those of William James and Donald Hebb).

Classical Cognitive Sciences

Cognitive science has always been by definition a hybrid field. Nonetheless, it has a quite precise manifesto: the explicit assumption that the mind can be the subject of scientific investigation that merges experimental, theoretical, and applied practices. This original manifesto, in the broadest of forms, comprised a number of disciplines, including psychology, artificial intelligence, neuroscience, philosophy, linguistics, and anthropology.

Beginning in the mid-1950s, in the cultural milieu of recently introduced ideas (such as information theory and Noam Chomsky's universal grammar), the field was initially a group of established disciplines sharing the common currency of an interest in cognition.

By the mid-1960s, the limits inherent in carrying out research that neglected the results of one or more of the other disciplines were becoming obvious. As a result of this inter-disciplinary turn, new disciplines achieved an autonomous status, a striking example being cognitive neuroscience, which fruitfully exploited new techniques (neuroimaging, multiple cell recording, fast computerized processing of complex signals, and so forth) in order to understand old problems concerning the mind-brain relationship.

The New Cognitive Sciences

What has become clear in recent decades is that the cognitive sciences cannot ignore the dynamics of cognition. Such a stance is compelled by both ontogenetic and phylogenetic reasons, stemming from empirical evidence, theoretical considerations, and changes in the overall scenario of science. Cognition is the set of representations and processes crucial for dealing with the physical and biosocial world. Any organism must deal with space, time, number, objects, events, and other organisms. Therefore, developmental and evolutionary constraints must have played a role in the implementation of their cognitive counterparts, just as they played a role in determining the shape and function of a lung or a fin. Representations and processes that take place in the minds of animals depend crucially on the tuning of brain structures during specific time courses, and ultimately on the genetic instructions that code for the building of these brain structures. Genetics and developmental biology are providing compelling evidence that cognitive functions are constrained by the timing of molecular events that produce their effects at different time scales, from the protracted establishment of the "protomap" that shapes the regional anatomy of the mammalian neocortex in separated modules during corticogenesis to the rapid molecular cascades triggered by a single learning experience during hippocampal long-term potentiation.

The State of Affairs

Cognition

It might sound trivial to affirm the importance of the study of cognition in contemporary science. Cognition has become an integrated aspect of many disciplines, not only those usually associated with "cognitive sciences" or "cognitive studies." From sociology and political studies to ethnology and archaeology, medicine, and economics, the ubiquitous reference to cognition suggests the incorporation, in the scientific understanding of many complex phenomena, of explanations ascribed to the processes taking place in the mind. Methodological advances in contemporary cognitive science frequently derive from the necessity of acquiring knowledge in indirect ways, through ingenious experimentation, the invention of sophisticated statistical tools, and a strong appeal to theoretical modeling. The current state of affairs in psychology suggests an inevitable merging of the discipline with neuroscience. The convergence of methods devised to grasp the workings of mental facts with experimental rigor, together with techniques developed to show the functions of the brain, has moved forward so fast in recent decades that nowadays it is not really possible to speak about cognition without referring to the brain. Cognitive neuroscience, the investigation of the neural correlates of the mind, is a field witnessing enormous success, reflected by the ever-increasing popularization of themes connected to the mind and the brain in the mass media and in popular culture. The related field of social neuroscience—bringing the methods of cognitive neuroscience to the study of the social life of organisms—has more recently shown the same explosive growth (see, for example, Cacioppo and Berntson 2002). Although this success is fully deserved, and insights into the understanding of mental phenomena have come from brain imaging studies (and the other way around), the mind-brain coupling is subject to serious temptations: the standard cognitive neuroscience formula (mental phenomenon + imaging = fabulous discovery) has been applied quite liberally, and often incautiously, to the brain correlates of justice, beauty, and truth, to name but a few examples. Neuroimaging incursions in the most fundamental corners of human cultural complexity are literally flourishing: labels such as "neuroethics," "neuroaesthetics," "neuropolitics," or "neurotheology" increasingly populate scientific journals and academic publications, and one has the feeling that belief in the explanatory power of human neuroscience may exceed the genuine knowledge being returned by these disciplinary joint ventures. Weisberg and colleagues (2008) have recently shown that nonexperts judge explanations of psychological phenomena as more satisfying when they include neuroscientific information, even when that information is logically irrelevant. Most worrisome is the striking ability of neuroscientific information to mask bad explanations. Notwithstanding this trend, we believe that many fundamental problems will be tackled and solved by the progressive accumulation of evidence from research at the border of psychology and neuroscience (Christensen and Tommasi 2006). Moreover, one should not forget that imaging tools can be fancy toys for basic scientists, but they are also precious equipment in the hands of clinicians whose main preoccupation is human health rather than pure knowledge.

On the "applied side," it must be added that the construction of theoretical or biologically inspired models of the mind in artificial intelligence and cognitive engineering has seldom proved able to offer answers to relevant, let alone fundamental, questions about cognition. The liveliest debates generated from such endeavors, which should have constituted the core subject for interaction chiefly among psychology, neuroscience, and information science and engineering, have come from philosophers focused on research about the representational, computational, and emergent properties of the mind-brain. It is also true that cognitive engineering has successfully profited from knowledge in psychology and the neurosciences to implement intelligent systems, but apart from the recurrent inspirational reference to mental and neural functions (and their overwhelming complexity), modeling and theoretical research have involved simulation of well-known facts rather than discovery of new ones. At any rate, out of the huge territory that once delimited artificial intelligence, the fields of computational cognitive neuroscience and neuroinformatics are among the few domains likely to survive.

Evolution

Those engaged in the cognitive sciences in recent decades are quite familiar with the idea that cognitive abilities evolve and with the proposal that the study of cognitive evolution deserves special attention. The idea of evolution of cognitive abilities, suggested long ago by Charles Darwin and William James, has been at the forefront of renewed approaches to psychology and the neurosciences. The field of evolutionary cognitive neuroscience reflects a biologically oriented approach to the themes of evolutionary psychology, focusing on the evolutionary bases of the neural underpinnings of the mind (Platek, Keenan, and Shackelford 2007). This evolutionary branch of neuroscience is hardly new, given the fact that neurobiology, long before the appearance of cognitive neuroscience, faced the problem of tracing the evolutionary history of sensory and nervous systems by means of the comparative method (Striedter 2006). Ever since anatomical and physiological techniques were in place, in the late 1800s, neurobiology has gone hand in hand with evolutionary biology, and many of the topics debated today in the light of discoveries in cognitive neuroscience could be traced back to debates among evolutionary neurobiologists. Interactions among the study of mind, behavior, and evolution benefited greatly from the advent of ethology, before the mid-1900s, in the wake of a genuinely Darwinian attitude toward behavior. This stance, affirmed in particular by European ethologists, promoted the understanding of behavior as an integral aspect of the species phenotype, largely innate but conceding windows of opportunity to experiential and environmental factors. In Konrad Lorenz's words in *The Foundations of Ethology* (1981, p. 100), "Under these circumstances a microsystematist on the lookout for comparable characters can hardly fail to notice that there are behavior patterns which represent just as reliable—and often particularly conservative—characteristics of species, genera, and even larger taxonomic groups, as do any morphological characteristics."

Evolutionary neurobiology increasingly found a necessary allied force in ethology, and the field of neuroethology (and the soon-to-be-born subfield of cognitive neuroethology; see Ewert 1982) is a good example of this alliance. If the coupling of neurobiology and ethology is a story of a relatively serene marriage, the same cannot be said about the relationship between genetics and the study of behavior. During the last century, population genetics and theoretical modeling helped to clarify many aspects of evolution, from the standpoint of genes, individuals, and groups. Probably most successful with respect to the specific issue of sexual selection—which already in the work of Darwin was deemed to be one of the key loci of selection—evolutionary explanations of behavior based on genetic data also brought us the controversial field of sociobiology (Wilson 1975). This much-criticized approach to behavior has not always been attacked for the best reasons, though it pushed an overly deterministic tie between behavior (at the individual or the group level, depending on one's preference for the locus of selection) and the genes responsible for behavior (Lewontin, Rose, and Kamin 1984). On the environmental side, the advent of behavioral ecology as a subfield of ethology strongly reinforced the principle that a driving force of behavior is the necessity of organisms to maximize access to available resources while minimizing risks associated with their pursuit—thus bringing economic principles of accounting for costs and benefits to the explanation of behavioral strategies (Krebs and Davies 1997).

A rather different story must be told about the adoption of evolutionary explanations in psychology. Once dominated by the behaviorist tradition, comparative psychology followed the cognitive revolution in pursuing a new approach to the study of the animal mind (Terrace 1984). The field of animal cognition rapidly progressed in studying the variability of species-specific mental abilities in the light of the different organismal constraints and ecological requirements that must have characterized species during their evolution. There has been much debate about whether and how the study of animal cognition can provide a framework for genuine evolutionary explanations of the mind (Bekoff et al. 2002) and this has become a particularly heated subject in discussions of the evolution of language and communication in human and nonhuman species (Hauser 1997).

However, animal cognition studies have taken advantage of an increasing interest in the comparative method for understanding the origins of mental abilities, and the rise of related disciplines such as cognitive ecology (a cross-breeding of animal cognition and behavioral ecology; Dukas 1998) and the previously noted field of cognitive neuroethology nicely represent the livelihood of the field in broader biological context. Another volume in the Vienna Series in Theoretical Biology (Heyes and Huber 2000) discussed the issue of evolution of cognitive abilities in animals with a special focus on nonhuman animals, and other important efforts have targeted the relationship between cognition and evolution (see, for instance, Shettleworth 1998).

Human psychology has been touched by the appeal of evolutionary explanations in a more dramatic (and often more dramatized) way. Though one can date quite precisely the birth of evolutionary psychology (Cosmides and Tooby 1987; Barkow et al. 1992), it is nonetheless hard to judge whether this discipline has safely emerged from its infancy. It has faced numerous difficulties, due to pressures stemming from a number of academic detractors in biology, psychology, and philosophy, although it is generally admitted that the basis of the approach of evolutionary psychology is more than respectable and should be pursued with the rigor of biological methodology (Richardson 2007; Buller 2005; de Waal 2002). The adoption of the evolutionary approach in the explanation of human cognition and behavior has focused mainly on the evolution of those neural and mental modules that qualify as optimal solutions of adaptive problems faced by our ancestors in their presumed environment and social milieu. The search for such adaptive specializations has ranged from nonselective learning modules that allow for the encoding of spatial and temporal contingencies (classical and operant conditioning) to modules sensitive to specific types of content, such as those sensitive to causes and effects in the physical environment (for example, folk physics), the features by means of which we recognize conspecifics (such as perception of faces and emotions), and the active understanding of the complex web of social relationships (theory of mind and aspects connected to mate choice, moral behavior, and the like). As already noted, evolutionary explanations of human cognition and behavior have provoked a number of criticisms. These have targeted principally the idea of adaptation, deemed to be too simplistic to explain the mechanics of human cognitive evolution as satisfactorily as it applies in the case of more classic subjects in organismal biology (Lewontin 1998). Despite the divergences, however, it is widely agreed that cognition should be considered not only an object of evolutionary explanation but also one agent whose action strongly impacts evolution, through the transmission of mental abilities and cultural innovations (Jablonka and Lamb 2005; Sperber 1996).

Last but not least, the dynamical dimension of evolution has largely increased its presence in the cognitive sciences via its relevance for both abstract and applied research carried out at the peculiar intersection of cognitive engineering and the life sciences, namely in the disciplines of artificial life and evolutionary computation. Although practitioners in these fields are not necessarily interested in modeling cognition per se, they have exploited notions of variation, reproduction, and selection in implementing software (genetic algorithms) and hardware (evolutionary robotics) whose main feature is that of changing through generations, showing fitter and fitter behavior in specific problem-solving contexts. As with the more traditional approaches of artificial intelligence, evolution-inspired cognitive engineering has made good use of well-known data to provide simulations and derive predictions about artificial systems, perhaps with the advantage of being a benchmark for otherwise impossible experimentation. In fact, given that the very large-scale temporal dimension can be made tractable when the availability of appropriate computational power is assumed, the field can contribute to an understanding of some aspects of the evolution of cognition in creative ways (see, for example, Cangelosi and Parisi 2001).

Development

The relevance of the developmental dimension to both biology and cognition is clear from the very moment one considers that development paves the way for organismal form and function, and that development represents the most plastic stage during an organism's life.

Studies of development, even of cognitive development, have been for a long time a district of psychology quite detached from the aims and objectives of the cognitive sciences. Piagetian theory, which was in itself a major pioneering contribution to cognitive theory, predating the birth of the cognitive sciences (Vauclair and Perret 2003), has been a particularly influential theory about cognition in infancy and childhood, positing that the acquisition of the fundamental elements of knowledge must pass through several stages in order to be fully mastered. Piagetian theory had many merits, chiefly that of devising clever ways to test what children can and cannot understand about a large number of knowledge categories, from the physics of containment to moral thought. Moreover, Piagetian theory, empirically targeting the mastering of numerous and diverse types of tasks, reinforced a vision of the developing mind as that of one system facing a number of separable problems, and established ad hoc experimental paradigms that allowed researchers to assess each of them. It is worth noting that many of those problems involve the types of representations that the contemporary cognitive sciences seek to understand, in that they are deemed to be the building blocks of cognition.

The interest of current developmental theory has recently zoomed in from the standard controversies over nativism or modularity writ large to selected types of content that largely cut across faculties and represent fundamental life aspects in an ecology of objects, events, and other organisms. It has been shown that there is much to learn about the nature of cognition from detailed analysis of the development of functions that allow children to encode and make use of specific forms of information in given contexts, disregarding any concern about the innateness or modularity of these functions: the empirical scenario is usually complex enough to satisfy a theorist's appetite, even (and especially) when starting from very specific aspects. Our ability to "understand" facial expressions, for instance, allows for a better coordination and regulation of a number of behaviors in the social structure that includes us, and this clearly involves the development of abilities that enable us to represent and manipulate facial information across perception, learning, memory, thought, and emotion.

The way these dedicated abilities develop over time is being better understood under the lens of neuroscience (see, for example, Nelson and Luciana 2001), with an increasing attention paid to aspects of neural development that might directly act as keys in the construction of cognition (see Mareschal et al. 2007).

We believe that recent fortunate changes in the fields of psychology and neuroscience have seen both comparative and developmental psychologists take a new direction that can help to delineate the future of the cognitive sciences. The core concepts of cognition and their levels of analysis (representations, computations and their function) are more likely to be uncovered through the adoption of a truly naturalistic perspective, one that merges cross-species research at various stages of development and at various levels of detail between brain and behavior—reflecting in a way the application of Tinbergen's four questions (Tinbergen 1963) on the levels of analysis set forth by David Marr (1982). This attitude has the added effect of forcing the careful consideration of many other aspects apart from evolution and development, such as ecology and genetics, that are clearly relevant in the definition of the biology of cognition.

Cognitive Biology

The reasons behind change in the history of science are not always clear. Sometimes change is produced by transformations from within, from the everyday activities and practices of scientists; at other times it reflects the action of political and cultural forces that define science as an aspect of society. If the study of evolution and development in the cognitive sciences is to be taken seriously, with attention to the proximate mechanisms and functions that underlie mind and behavior and their environmental and genetic constraints, it is clear that the enterprise is not logically separable from that of the life sciences. One of the central tenets of biology is that development, being a locus of variability, acts on evolution (Gilbert 2006). This is crucial because plasticity and developmental change become likely candidates for attaining one or another cognitive outcome, and many are the ways this can take place in ontogeny and phylogeny (Geary and Huffman 2002).

The idea that the cognitive sciences have inherited from biology more than the mere adoption of imaging techniques, constituting what we broadly refer to as "cognitive biology," is not new: the proposal that evolution and development are driving forces of a naturalistic approach to cognition is not new, nor is a sense that an evo-devo approach is important to the cognitive sciences (Hauser and Spelke 2004; Ellis and Bjorklund 2002; Langer 2000).[1] The editors of and contributors to this book hope to make the reader more familiar with the evo-devo approach, by presenting current research in a fashion that when seen from afar will convey the general picture of "cognitive biology"—but when seen from nearby will preserve the level of detail essential to the sciences of mind, brain, and behavior.

Note

1. Some time ago the expression "cognitive biology" was used very differently (Boden and Khin Zaw 1980), to refer to an approach to biology that made use of concepts usually associated with the language developed to speak about knowledge.

References

Barkow J, Cosmides L, Tooby J, eds (1992) The adapted mind: Evolutionary psychology and the generation of culture. New York: Oxford University Press.

Bechtel W, Abrahamsen A, Graham G (1998) The life of cognitive science. In: A companion to cognitive science (Bechtel W, Graham G, eds). Oxford: Basil Blackwell.

Bekoff M, Allen C, Burghardt GM, eds (2002) The cognitive animal: Empirical and theoretical perspectives on animal cognition. Cambridge, MA: MIT Press.

Boden M (2006) Mind as machine: A history of cognitive science. Oxford: Oxford University Press.

Boden M, Khin Zaw S (1980). The case for a cognitive biology. Proceedings of the Aristotelian Society, 54: 25–40.

Buller DJ (2005) Adapting minds: Evolutionary psychology and the persistent quest for human nature. Cambridge, MA: MIT Press.

Cacioppo JT, Berntson GG (2002) Social neuroscience. In: Foundations in social neuroscience (Cacioppo JT, Berntson GG, Adolphs RA, Carter CS, Davidson RJ, McClintock MK, McEwen BS, Meaney MJ, Schacter DL, Sternberg EM, Suomi SS, Taylor SE, eds), 3–10. Cambridge, MA: MIT Press.

Cangelosi A, Parisi D, eds (2001) Simulating the evolution of language. London: Springer-Verlag.

Christensen WD, Tommasi L (2006) Neuroscience in context: The new flagship of the cognitive sciences. Biol Theory 1: 78–83.

Cosmides L, Tooby J (1987) From evolution to behavior: Evolutionary psychology as the missing link. In: The latest on the best: Essays on evolution and optimality (Dupre J, ed), 277–306. Cambridge, MA: MIT Press.

de Waal FBM (2002) Evolutionary psychology: The wheat and the chaff. Curr Dir Psychol Sci 11: 187–191.

Dukas, R, ed (1998) Cognitive ecology: The evolutionary ecology of information processing and decision making. Chicago: University of Chicago Press.

Ellis BJ, Bjorklund DF, eds (2004) Origins of the social mind: Evolutionary psychology and child development. London: Guilford Press.

Ewert J-P (1982) Neuroethology: An introduction to the neurophysiological fundamentals of behaviour. New York: Springer-Verlag.

Gardner H (1985) The mind's new science: A history of the cognitive revolution. New York: Basic Books.

Geary DC, Huffman KJ (2002) Brain and cognitive evolution: Forms of modularity and functions of mind. Psych Bull 128: 667–698.

Gilbert S (2006) Developmental biology. 8th edition. Sunderland: Sinauer Associates.

Hauser MD (1997) The evolution of communication. Cambridge, MA: MIT Press.

Hauser MD, Spelke E (2004) Evolutionary and developmental foundations of human knowledge: A case study of mathematics. In: The cognitive neurosciences III (Gazzaniga MS, ed) 853–864. Cambridge, MA: MIT Press.

Heyes C, Huber L, eds (2000) The evolution of cognition. Cambridge, MA: MIT Press.

Jablonka E, Lamb MJ (2005) Evolution in four dimensions: Genetic, epigenetic, behavioral, and symbolic variation in the history of life. Cambridge, MA: MIT Press.

Krebs JR, Davies NB (1997) Behavioural ecology: An evolutionary approach. Oxford: Blackwell.

Langer J (2000) The descent of cognitive development. Dev Sci 3: 361–378.

Lewontin RC, Rose S, Kamin LH (1984) Not in our genes: Biology, ideology and human nature. New York: Pantheon Books.

Lewontin RC (1998) The evolution of cognition: Questions we will never answer. In: An Invitation to Cognitive Science. 2nd edition. Volume 4: Methods, models and conceptual issues (Scarborough D, Sternberg S, Osherson D, eds), 107–132. Cambridge, MA: MIT Press.

Lorenz KZ (1981) The foundations of ethology. New York: Springer-Verlag.

Mareschal D, Johnson MH, Sirois S, Spratling MW, Thomas MSC, Westermann G (2007) Neuroconstructivism I: How the brain constructs cognition. Oxford: Oxford University Press.

Marr D (1982) Vision. San Francisco: WH Freeman.

Nadel L, Piattelli Palmarini M (2003) What is cognitive science? In: Encyclopedia of cognitive science (Nadel L, ed), xiii–xli. London: Macmillan.

Nelson CA, Luciana M, eds (2001) Handbook of developmental cognitive neuroscience. Cambridge, MA: MIT Press.

Platek S, Keenan JP, Shackelford TK, eds (2007) Evolutionary cognitive neuroscience. Cambridge, MA: MIT Press.

Ramón y Cajal, S (1999; original 1899) Advice for a young investigator. Cambridge, MA: MIT Press.

Richardson RC (2007) Evolutionary psychology as maladapted psychology. Cambridge, MA: MIT Press.

Shettleworth SJ (1998) Cognition, evolution and behavior. New York: Oxford University Press.

Sperber D (1996) Explaining culture: A naturalistic approach. Oxford: Blackwell.

Striedter GF (2006) A history of ideas in evolutionary neuroscience. In: Evolution of nervous systems (Kaas JH, ed), 1–15. New York: Academic Press.

Terrace HS (1984) Animal cognition. In: Animal cognition: Proceedings of the Harry Frank Guggenheim Conference, June 2–4, 1982 (Roitblat HL, Bever TG, Terrace HS, eds), 7–28. Mahwah, NJ: Lawrence Erlbaum.

Tinbergen N (1963) On the aims and methods of ethology. Z Tierpsychol 20: 410–433.

Vauclair J, Perret P (2003) The cognitive revolution in Europe: Taking the developmental perspective seriously. Trends Cogn Sci 7: 284–285.

Weisberg DS, Keil FC, Goodstein J, Rawson E, Gray JR (2008) The seductive allure of neuroscience explanations. J Cogn Neurosci 20: 470–477.

Wilson EO (1975) Sociobiology: The new synthesis. Cambridge, MA: Belknap Press/Harvard University Press.

II SPACE

The first section of this volume deals with the domain of space, the study of which has in recent decades seen major advances in the spirit envisaged by the title of this book. Data from developmental, comparative, and cognitive psychology are being combined with data from computational and cognitive neuroscience as well as ecology and evolutionary neurobiology to explore questions that have long been fundamental to cognitive science: How is spatial knowledge represented in the mind/brain? How do these representations emerge in the course of an individual's development? What rules govern the processing of spatial knowledge, and are they the same as rules governing other knowledge domains? Much of the progress in this area dates from the discovery, thirty years ago, of cells in the hippocampus that govern an organism's perception of "place." This linkage between a complex cognitive function and a specific brain region that could be carefully studied in animal models has made it possible to relate details of anatomy and physiology to specific computational purposes, which themselves can be seen to fulfill certain adaptive functions.

In chapter 2, Lucia Jacobs discusses the evolution of the hippocampus, taking into consideration three major evolutionary forces that contributed to establishing the different degrees of hippocampal specialization observed in various species of vertebrates: natural selection, sexual selection, and social selection. These driving forces are exemplified by reviewing the evidence obtained in a number of behaviors in which space is an essential aspect of cognitive life, such as scatter hoarding, migration, and mating. Social selection, in particular, is invoked as a key to interpreting the variability of hippocampal size and specialization in the light of the competition among individuals involved by foraging and mate choice.

Alessandro Treves (chapter 3) focuses on a recent finding, the discovery of grid cells in the rat entorhinal cortex that has helped to clarify the microstructure of the neural bases of spatial cognition. This evidence, supported by the analysis of cortical lamination, suggests computational advantages not only for spatial cognition but extending also to the faculty of human language. Models such as this raise questions of modularity and the specificity of the rules by which different neurocognitive systems operate.

The three following chapters are linked by a common denominator, a focus on the biology of geometry. Neil Burgess, Christian Doeller, and Chris Bird (chapter 4) review human imaging and neuropsychological data obtained by means of spatial tasks originally inspired by rodent neurophysiology. They focus on the encoding of environmental geometry, and show how knowledge about the neural correlates of spatial cognition can illuminate theoretical controversies in the interpretation of purely behavioral evidence.

In chapter 5, Giorgio Vallortigara tackles the topic of geometry in the context of reorientation paradigms in human and nonhuman animals (particularly birds and fish). Successful encoding of geometry depends on the acquisition of basic building blocks such as sense (telling left from right) and distance (telling long from short). This kind of comparative work is particularly useful in examining hypotheses that give language a special role in spatial cognition—in this case the idea that combining landmark and geometric information in order to reorient depends on language. Since an ability to combine knowledge from multiple sources can be demonstrated in animals as well as humans, it is obvious that language is not critical, a point that Nora Newcombe and her colleagues make in the next chapter. Even though language can be disregarded, Vallortigara discusses aspects of hemispheric specialization in animals that will certainly be worth careful study in the future.

Finally, Nora Newcombe, Kristin Ratliff, Wendy Shallcross, and Alexandra Twyman (chapter 6) focus on the issues of modularity and experience in the acquisition and stabilization of geometric representations throughout human development, by making direct comparisons with data from research in other animal species. They challenge nativist positions based on hardwired modularity, emphasizing that multiple types of spatial information are recruited to recover environmental geometry after disorientation. Experiments on the effects of rearing and training on geometric encoding are also reviewed to further counter radically nativist positions.

2 The Role of Social Selection in the Evolution of Hippocampal Specialization

Lucia F. Jacobs

How Do Memory Specializations Evolve?

An important question facing both evolutionary biology and cognitive neuroscience is how the evolution of behavior might be constrained or, possibly, accelerated by innovations or limits to a species' memory capacity. Understanding how this memory capacity evolves may lead to a better understanding of how memory is (or is not) organized into specialized, dissociable memory systems (Sherry and Schacter 1987; Moscovitch et al. 2006). In the case of episodic memory, both its characteristics in humans and its scope and distribution in nonhumans remain a source of controversy (Hampton and Schwartz 2004). This remains the case even several decades after the term was first introduced by Tulving (1984) to characterize what appeared to be a unique ability of humans to recall an event from their personal past. Yet recalling events from the past is an attribute found widely in animals, both invertebrate and vertebrate. Even recalling information that is linked to a specific time and place has been described in insects, mammals, and birds (Gallistel 1990; Shettleworth 1998; Collett and Collett 2002). The knowledge of an event in the past also appears to be a common ability found in animals that store food. In species such as the common raven (*Corvus corax*) or the western scrub jay (*Aphelocoma californica*), individuals remember the association of a social event with a certain individual, such as being observed while caching (Bugnyar and Heinrich, 2006; Clayton et al. 2007). Individual scrub jays also use the time elapsed since caching to make economic decisions about cache retrieval, such as the decision to forgo a favorite but perishable food after long delays. The birds' ability to recall the location of each food type was a strong argument for the existence of an episodic-like memory in nonhumans (Clayton et al. 2001). Recent studies have demonstrated that nonhuman species peer not only into the past but also into the future. Two species of great ape, bonobos (*Pan paniscus*) and orangutans (*Pongo pygmaeus*), presciently took tools to bed that they needed not in the present but would need on the next day (Mulcahy and Call 2006). Western scrub jays, learning that their morning will be spent in a room without food, cache food in that room the day before (Raby et al. 2007).

None of the above examples supply proof of autonoesis, however, in light of Tulving's requirement that episodic memory also is a recollection of the self having had the experience. Self-awareness in nonhuman (and nonverbal) individuals has always been problematic (Griffin 1981), despite demonstrations of behaviors such as mirror-guided self-exploration (De Haan and van den Bos 1999) and, more recently, a demonstrated awareness of knowing (metacognition), both in the laboratory rhesus monkey (*Macaca mulatta*; see Hampton 2001) and the laboratory rat (*Rattus norvegicus*; see Foote and Crystal 2007). These results challenge our understanding of what self-awareness might look like in another species.

In the meantime, however, among us humans self-awareness is not only obvious but necessary for the whole concept of episodic memory. I give the following as an example of a typical episodic memory in humans, where the memory not only yields images of linked scenes located in time and space but also becomes incorporated into a sense of self as a "story with a moral," a causal explanation for an individual's later behavior (Campbell 1994).

Meeting Konrad Lorenz

On the afternoon of January 15, 1975, I stood in a room in an elegant villa in the village of Altenberg, Austria, not far from Vienna. Three decades later, in this very villa, we would hold the workshop that eventually resulted in the present book. In 1975 it was still Konrad Lorenz's study and I was a college freshman, home for Christmas. I had just returned from my first semester at Cornell, battered by the twin onslaughts of attending college in a foreign country and taking premed biology, after spending four years as a student at a tiny international school in Vienna. Perhaps this is why I had finally found the nerve to contact Lorenz, a Nobel laureate, as some kind of confirmation that I was on the right path—a path that his classic work, *King Solomon's Ring* (Lorenz 1952), had set me on when I was fourteen. I clutched my family's battered paperback copy of this book, which he had written to support his research after his return from a Soviet prisoner-of-war camp in 1948 (Lorenz 1996). I had telephoned the home of Professor Lorenz and his wife answered. I must have asked in German whether I could visit. She asked me whether a particular Thursday would be convenient for me. For a college freshman who had yet to meet a full professor at her own university, to be asked by the wife of a god if a Thursday was convenient made it already a memorable occasion. Even more remarkable was the atmosphere of collegiality and respect with which I was greeted upon my arrival at the Lorenz home—I was treated as a serious, if somewhat less experienced, colleague. I remember being taken to the greenhouse. Now the home for studies of cognition in captive marmosets at the Konrad Lorenz Institute for Evolution and Cognition Research, at that time it housed numerous aquaria filled with tropical fish. I remember feeling like a sparrow meeting a famous cobra, as I attempted to formulate intelligent sentences about animal behavior. I remember his fierceness, his enthusiasm, his dramatic white beard. I remember

a)

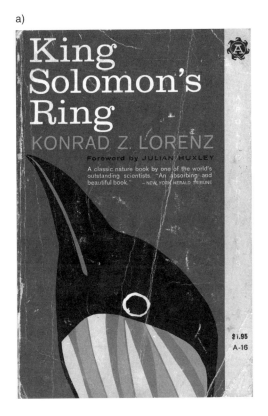

b)

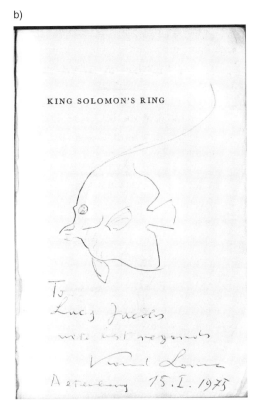

Figure 2.1
(a) Cover of *King Solomon's Ring* (Lorenz 1952) (b)Lorenz's autograph on the title page.

his speaking wistfully of the aquaria he had yet to build. Finally, I asked whether he would autograph the all-important beat-up paperback I had brought with me; he not only signed and dated it but added a brilliant illustration of an angelfish (see figures 2.1a and 2.1b). Later, I remember worrying that he had mistaken me for the daughter of a rich American who might be able to help his research, and not simply the humble fanatic that I was.

The next time I stood in his office, it was on the morning of June 16, 2006, and I was presenting my thoughts on the evolution of spatial and episodic memory.

The Birth of Ethology

How do we translate rich experiences, many of which may be tied up with human language, to the mind of another species? One answer, from Lorenz among others, was to understand, first, how minds evolve (Lorenz 1952). In the summer of 1937, at the Altenberg property, Konrad Lorenz and Niko Tinbergen dug ponds to study the development of behavior in the greylag goose (*Anser anser*). The two scientists had met a year earlier at a conference where they found themselves in enthusiastic agreement that behavior is constructed not just from malleable mortar—nurture—but also from the hard bricks of innate programs that they eventually would call releasers, fixed-action patterns, and innate releasing mechanisms. These species-specific bricks could be recognized, embedded in their mortar, not unlike fossilized bones embedded in geological layers. In the process Lorenz and Tinbergen also established the discipline of ethology, which they defined as the biological study of behavior (Lorenz and Tinbergen 1938). To dissect behavior they focused on behaviors with many such bricks: egg management by a brooding goose, conflict signals in the herring gull, courtship signals in the duck family Anatidae—all of these could be deconstructed into their sign stimuli and fixed-action patterns. The two pond-digging theorists also studied the mortar that held the bricks of such actions together—all the data that had to be learned for a greylag's survival, such as the recognition of nest or chick. Thus, Lorenz's studies of imprinting in the greylag geese that inhabited the ponds along with Tinbergen's study of spatial memory and orientation in the wasp known as the bee wolf (*Philanthus triangulum*; see Tinbergen 1972) together laid a foundation for the study of the ecology of animal cognition. This frame remained empty, however, not only for the duration of the war that engulfed and separated them but for many decades thereafter. Moreover, it was a mental outlook incompatible with radical behaviorism. Fortunately, scientific paradigms wax and wane, and the insights on animal cognition voiced by Lorenz, Tinbergen, von Frisch, Tolman, and others finally began to reemerge and gain traction in the late twentieth century (Zentall 1984; Wasserman 1997).

Cognitive Psychology—or Cognitive Biology?

Consequently it felt appropriate that the workshop where we struggled to come up with a new term for what we were discussing took place in the historic Lorenz villa. I call what I do "cognitive biology." The term subtly rearranges our assumptions as psychologists, effecting a quasi-Copernican reformulation. If cognitive biology is the goal, then the fundamental organizing principle is not cognition of the human species (as psychology is generally assumed to be) but cognition itself, regardless of species. The objects of study are not cognitive processes in humans but cognitive processes generally in the animal kingdom (the question of possible cognition in nonanimal kingdoms is one that perhaps can be raised in future conferences; see Trewavas 2005).

Let us return to episodic memory as an example of a phenomenon of cognition. It appears to be such an efficient way to organize recall that it would be puzzling if it were to be limited to our own species. Perhaps variants—without autonoesis, for example—are found in other species. An important structure in the mediation of episodic memory is the hippocampus (Burgess et al. 2002; see also chapter 4, this volume). Because this physiological structure has homologues in all vertebrates and is highly developed in birds and nonhuman mammals, it would be particularly intriguing to discover whether episodic-like memory occurs in such groups. At least one ancestral function of this structure, mapping allocentric space, appears to be highly conserved in vertebrates (Rodriguez et al. 2002; Jacobs and Schenk 2003).

So it is valid to ask how these two cognitive traits, spatial navigation and autonoetic memory for a location in space and time, are related. As with any biological trait, the evolution of a cognitive ability must proceed through stages that are each adapted to the current environment. It is reasonable to assume that vertebrates first learned to represent the world around them and only later used the hippocampus to compute abstract relations among objects. In this case the concrete functions of the hippocampus, such as allocentric navigation, preceded the evolution of abstract functions, such as episodic encoding. This is simply the more parsimonious explanation based on principles of brain evolution (Butler and Hodos 1996; Striedter 2005), although some argue that hippocampal abstract functions are ancestral to spatial functions (Eichenbaum et al. 2007). This question will no doubt be answered with future research, especially given the rapid pace of research in the field of comparative cognition (Bugnyar and Heinrich 2005; Csanyi 2005; Clayton et al. 2007; Tomasello and Carpenter 2007).

How shall we best study whether our nonhuman, nonverbal subjects manipulate representations of past and future time, such as in a recall of episodic memories? We could do worse than start with Tinbergen's exhortation to ethology. Building on the three fundamental levels of analysis proposed by Eric von Holst—phylogeny, function, and mechanism—Tinbergen demanded of himself and his fellow ethologists that they also understand the development of a behavior (Tinbergen 1963), a framework that has been described as the four "legs" of ethology.

In fact, though, a better metaphor might be the interacting gears of a clockwork mechanism, in which levels of analysis are geared together with feedback mechanisms (see figure 2.2). For example, phylogenetic constraints dictate the range of a physiological mechanism, the actions of other species dictate the size of a species's ecological niche, etc. In reality, therefore, any movement of one gear impedes or accelerates the movement of its neighbors—such is the dynamic interdependence of development, physiological mechanism, ecological function, and evolutionary history.

Take the question of human episodic memory as an example. If unique to humans, the answer could lie in phylogeny—there was a unique event—a novel mutation—in the hominin clade. This argument could be supported, as there is increasing evidence for novel alleles in our recent history (Pollard et al. 2006). Or the larger force could come from ontogeny: our peculiar, extended development and verbal language is necessary to support the development of this mental representation. There is also evidence for this point of view: the acceleration of episodic memory with language acquisition (de Haan et al. 2006). Or the best answer could be that it is simply the function, or adaptive value, in our species' cognitive niche that sustains and allows it. Other species have the potential for its development but they face less attractive cost/benefit ratios (being shorter-lived or working in less

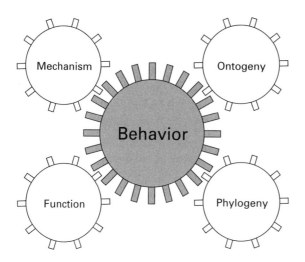

Figure 2.2
Schematic representation of Niko Tinbergen's four questions (Tinbergen 1963).

cooperative groups) for the use of such memory. Finally, the question might lie in mechanism: the computations require a certain circuitry of brain structures found only in the most recent hominin apes, i.e., our own species.

As the metaphor of interacting gears implies, the answer must always be all of the above. A hypothetical example would be the following: hominins, with their efficient cooperative hunting of high-protein food sources, were able to support the extended development required by this mental representation and subsequently required this mental representation to survive as an individual in our intensely competitive species. Thus, one gear, the ecological function of cooperative hunting, could have pushed another, brain size, which then pushed the length of development, allowing new ecological niches to be opened and exploited.

Another value of the geared-mechanism metaphor is that it identifies not only the all-important interdependence of levels but also sets up the important question: What first causes a certain gear to start to rotate more quickly than its fellows? The answer to this must ultimately come from understanding the interaction of development and evolution—how development is limited by evolutionary constraints and how developmental plasticity can be the engine for evolutionary acceleration (West-Eberhard 2003). The goal for the rest of this chapter is to answer the following question: Can we identify a gear whose acceleration could have led to episodic memory? And if so, can this help us analyze and predict its existence in other species? Because of the landmark work of Milner and colleagues (1998) and O'Keefe and Nadel (1978), we have a very good idea that the hippocampus plays a large role in spatial and episodic memory in humans (Burgess et al. 2002; see also chapter 4, this volume). What common function of the hippocampus can be found across vertebrates and what selective pressures might have led to the evolution of autonoetic memory for locations in space and time in our own species?

The Ecology of the Hippocampus

The phylogeny of the hippocampus, an ancient, conserved structure in vertebrates, is one of the best-documented cases of brain evolution (Striedter 2005). We can therefore proceed immediately to the current literature on functional patterns of spatial learning and its relation to the hippocampus or other medial pallium homologues. This literature now includes striking patterns of sex, season, species and/or population differences in birds, mammals, reptiles, and fish (see table 2.1), as well as strain differences within domesticated birds and mammals. Add to this the voluminous literature on the physiology of spatial cognition in laboratory-domesticated pigeons, rats, and mice, and we cognitive biologists should be grateful to have such a rich literature to ponder.

Instead of this pleasure, however, what we often feel is confusion. The studies and the field—whether you call it cognitive biology, neuroecology (Hampton et al. 2002), or evolutionary neuroscience (Striedter 2005)—is relatively new. Its adaptationist approach, with theory perhaps a nose ahead of the data, recently provoked fairly bitter attacks by skeptics (Macphail and Bolhuis 2001), engendering quick replies from those attacked (Hampton et al. 2002). This has had the healthy result of clarifying many issues, even the swapping of raw data for new analyses that have confirmed the original proposition that hippocampal size is related to spatial behavior (Lucas et al. 2004). For example, the greater variation of food-storing behaviors in Eurasian parids and corvids may be one reason for the stronger correlations between scatter hoarding and hippocampal size on that continent, compared to that of the more closely related birds studied so far in North America; however, there are also effects that cannot yet be explained by food hoarding (Garamszegi and Lucas 2005).

The patterns that have been documented are based on the assumption that the hippocampus "does" spatial learning. The results from studies summarized in table 2.1 imply that there are two ways to make your hippocampus bigger and better: storing food in scattered locations or searching for mates (Sherry et al. 1992). We cognitive biologists have long argued that the nature of selection on hippocampal size and function has therefore been one of two types: natural selection leading to differences among species or sexual selection leading to differences between the sexes within a species (Jacobs 1995, 1996a, 1996b, 2000). This is not inconsistent with what we know of brain evolution, for example, the models of concerted evolution of Finlay and Darlington (Finlay and Darlington 1995). In concerted evolution, developmental constraints strictly limit the degree to which an individual brain structure can be shaped by selection independent of other brain structures, as most changes in brain structures appear to occur in concert. In contrast, mosaic selection is the process by which an individual brain structure is independently selected for increased

Table 2.1
Studies of spatial cognition and correlations with hippocampus and medial pallium homologue structures among vertebrates

Taxonomic group	Spatial memory	Activity that brain structure is related to		
		Mating system	Foraging mode	Habitat use, including seasonal changes
Fish				
Cichlid: multiple-species study		Pollen et al. 2007		Pollen et al. 2007
Goldfish: single-species study	Rodriguez et al. 2002[b]			
Reptiles				
Lizards: multiple-species study	Day et al. 2001[b]		Day et al. 2001[b]	
Snake: single-species study	Holtzman et al. 1999			
Turtle: single-species study	Rodriguez et al. 2002[b]			
Mammals				Yaskin 1984[a]
Microchiropteran bats: multiple-species study			Safi and Dechmann 2005; Ratcliffe et al. 2006	Safi and Dechmann 2005; Ratcliffe et al. 2006
Bats: single-species study	Winter and Stich 2005	Ulanovsky and Moss 2007		
Voles and mice: multiple-species study	Gaulin and FitzGerald 1986; Galea et al. 1996	Jacobs et al. 1990[a]		Pleskacheva et al. 2000[a]
Voles and mice: single-species study	Galea et al. 1994[a]			Galea and McEwen 1999; Ormerod and Galea 2001
Sciuridae: multiple species			Barker et al. 2005[a]	
Sciuridae: single-species study	Jacobs and Liman 1991; Vander Wall 1991; Macdonald 1997; Jacobs and Shiflett 1999; Devenport et al. 2000; Vlasak 2006a, 2006b; Gibbs et al. 2007[a]			Lavenex et al. 2000a, 2000b[a]
Heteromyidae (kangaroo rats and pocket mice): multiple-species study	Daly et al. 1992; Leaver and Daly 2001; Preston and Jacobs 2005; Barkley and Jacobs 2007[a]	Jacobs and Spencer 1994[a]	Jacobs and Spencer 1994[a]	

Table 2.1 (continued)

| Taxonomic group | Spatial memory | Activity that brain structure is related to | | |
		Mating system	Foraging mode	Habitat use, including seasonal changes
Kangaroo rats: single-species study	Jacobs 1992b; Langley 1994; Barkley and Jacobs 1998; Preston and Jacobs 2001			
Birds			Healy and Hurly 2004	
Nonpasserines: single-species study	Bingman et al. 2003[b]			Volman et al. 1999; Abbott et al. 1999[a]
Passerines: multiple-species study	Brodbeck 1994		Hampton and Shettleworth 1996[b]; Lucas et al. 2004[a]	Lucas et al. 2004[a]
Cowbirds: single- and multiple-species studies		Sherry et al. 1993; Reboreda et al. 1996[a]		Clayton et al. 1997[a]
Corvids: multiple-species studies	Clayton and Krebs 1994; Balda and Kamil 1989			
Corvids: single-species studies	Bugnyar and Heinrich 2006; Clayton et al. 2007		de Kort and Clayton 2006	
Paridae: multiple-species studies	Biegler et al. 2001	Healy and Hurly 2004		
Paridae: single-species studies	Sherry et al. 1981; Sherry 1984; Herz et al. 1994	Petersen and Sherry 1996	Sherry et al. 1989; Smulders et al. 1995; Shiflett et al. 2002[a]	Pravosudov and Clayton 2002[a]

[a]Free-ranging subjects
[b]Lesion study

size or function (Striedter 2005). However, as Striedter has discussed, the scale of species differences in hippocampal size falls well under the ratios that concerted processes must be operating, namely, less than a factor of 2 or 3 (Striedter 2005, p. 149). Therefore, if we can assume that the patterns summarized in table 2.1 characterize typical species differences in vertebrates, then such medial pallium homologues could have arisen through mosaic selection, or at least through mosaic selection that is no doubt still influenced by concerted selection processes and could thus properly be called partial mosaic selection (Striedter 2005).

The next question is how this form of selection is driven by natural and sexual selection. I would like to introduce a third candidate into this discussion, one that has not been previously considered. This is social selection, an evolutionary process that is neither natural nor sexual selection but one that encompasses sexual selection and is distinct from natural selection (West-Eberhard 2003). In the next section I shall describe how adding social selection to the discussion of hippocampal evolution might help us understand its role not only in nonhuman cognition but also in human episodic memory.

Social Selection as an Evolutionary Force

In 1983, Mary Jane West-Eberhard formulated an important theory of evolutionary change: the concept of selection through social competition, or social selection (West-Eberhard 1983). Although Darwin had articulated the effects of social competition in the development of sexual selection, West-Eberhard expanded this to include all social competition, not just the intraspecific competition for reproductive partners, but all aspects of morphology and behavior driven by competition within a species. This landmark hypothesis continues to gain support as a model of the selective pressures unique to social interactions and has recently been reformulated in a book-length treatment (West-Eberhard 2003). West-Eberhard's theory should not be confused with Roughgarden's recent theory of social interaction, also called social selection (Roughgarden et al. 2006); the present discussion is in reference to the West-Eberhard concept.

Social selection is selection arising from competition within a species. An important implication of this definition is that sexual selection is part of social selection, and both are differentiated from natural selection. As West-Eberhard (1983) explains, "Seen in this broader perspective, sexual selection refers to the subset of social competition in which the resource at stake is mates. And social selection is differential reproductive success (ultimately, differential gene replication) due to differential success in social competition, whatever the resource at stake" (p. 158).

West-Eberhard identifies three critical characteristics of social selection: first, that social selection pressures differ from natural selection by having virtually no stasis. Competition within a species becomes a continual arms race, where the opponent can move competition into a new arena or to new levels, by introducing a new behavior or structure. The exaggeration of characters used in such competition is finally brought to a stop only by the cost of their production or use.

By contrast, change in ordinary or ecological characters—those responding to unchanging aspects of the physical environment, or organic aspects either not evolving or evolving very slowly in response to the adaptations in question—can approach a ceiling of perfection (optimum). Divergence in such characters in closely related species is therefore expected to be more limited than divergence in social traits (West-Eberhard 1983).

Second, social selection is constant. Because the trait exists in a species where there are always conspecifics attempting to solve the same problem in the same way, the pressure to improve in competition is unceasing. A response to a change in predation tactics or food distribution can be constructed and then an advantage can be enjoyed. But within a population, with genetic and cultural transmission, there is no such lag between competitors. As stated by West-Eberhard (1983), "Under intraspecific social competition every reproducing individual of every generation is involved in the same increasingly specialized unending contest" (p. 159). The implication of this is that greater evolutionary change is expected in species with greater social selection.

Third, there is the "accelerating effect of novelty" (West-Eberhard 1983). Successful competition within a species, to best one's conspecifics by means of overt or covert actions of song, deed, or wit often depends on the novelty of the production. For example, a new fighting maneuver, a new shortcut, or a new song—all of these behaviors depend on cognitive processes that will affect the outcome of social competition.

Social Selection and Social Intelligence

Despite the importance of these ideas for evolutionary biology, the connection has yet to be made between West-Eberhard's social selection and the rapidly emerging data sets and models for the evolution of social intelligence. Recent data and quantitative methods to test these ideas rigorously has led to an explosion of new results. Brain size has long been known to correlate with social factors, such as group size in primates (Harvey and Krebs 1990). More recently it has been shown that larger-brained bird species are more likely to use novel foraging techniques (Sol et al. 2005b), live longer (Sol et al. 2007), and be more successful at surviving in the new habitats that they occupy as invasive species (Sol et al. 2005a). Primate species with larger brains are more likely to show greater innovation, tool use, and, interestingly, social learning (Reader and Laland 2002). The dominant interpretation of these patterns has typically been that of Machiavellian intelligence, namely, it is necessary to have greater processing capacity (a larger brain) to keep track of and manipulate a quickly shifting social scene (Byrne and Whiten 1988). In their analysis, however, Reader and Laland offer an alternative view to the impact of social intelligence, asserting that the data suggest asocial innovation and social interaction cannot be distinguished as engines for change in brain size.

Social Selection and Hippocampal Evolution

In her original postulation, West-Eberhard used the example of signal evolution to illustrate the concept of social selection. Yet if we think of the hippocampus or spatial learning simply as a biological trait that has evolved, perhaps into quasi-independent modules

(Jacobs and Schenk 2003), then we can ask what the utility of this theory is to its evolution. In her 2003 book on development, plasticity, and evolution, West-Eberhard extends
this further, to the question of all interactions of plasticity and how these are shaped by
all evolutionary forces, including social selection, natural selection and even genetic drift.
She also addresses the question of learning, but as a biologist, not a cognitive biologist;
for example, she limited the 1983 discussion to "animals that can learn," even if it now
seems clear that all animals indeed can learn (Shettleworth 1998). In the 2003 book, learning is still discussed in circumscribed terms; there is no mention of spatial learning in this
(otherwise masterful!) book of 800-plus pages.

Yet there is an obvious relationship between sexually selected signals, such as birdsong,
and spatial learning in the context of mate competition. Both modes of competition can
be used to build predictive theories of sexual dimorphism in mammalian and other vertebrate brains (Jacobs 1996b).

What this leaves us with is a powerful theory of evolutionary change—social selection—that explicitly addresses the evolution of plastic behaviors (e.g., learning), yet is
currently unsophisticated about evolutionary neuroscience (Striedter 2005) or cognitive
biology. Yet the theory of social selection may be the key to the question of hippocampal
function and its evolution. Currently, there are at least three different patterns emerging
from the comparative literature on the hippocampus and its homologues (table 2.1). These
are: differences between females and males within a species; seasonal shifts in such sex
differences, and, finally, species differences, as a result of either the mating system, the
foraging mode, or habitat use. In the following sections, I shall discuss how these might
relate to West-Eberhard's framework of social selection.

Mating Systems and Social Competition

Social selection encompasses sexual selection as competition arising within a sex for
access to sexual partners and successful reproductive encounters with sexual partners.
Steve Gaulin first linked a century of documented sexual dimorphisms in spatial learning
in the lab rat with the mechanism and function of sexual selection and mate competition
(Gaulin and FitzGerald 1986). His work on voles was the first to predict the link between
mating system and spatial cognition, present in scramble polygynous species (where
roaming males physically contest each other for access to a female) and absent in monoga-
mous species, where the sexes defend a joint territory. We later made the link between
mating system and the relative volume of the hippocampus in voles (Jacobs et al. 1990);
this was inspired by David Sherry's discoveries of hippocampal size differences in
birds, with variations connected to both food-storing habits (Krebs et al. 1989; Sherry
et al. 1989) and to sex differences in eastern cowbirds (*Molothrus ater;* Sherry et al. 1993).
In both examples, the direction of the dimorphism could be predicted by sex-specific
behavior—the relatively larger hippocampus was found in the sex where successful competition required superior spatial orientation. In the polygamous meadow vole, it was the

males who had to relocate receptive females, while in the nest-parasitic cowbird, it was the females who had to relocate available host nests.

Even more convincing evidence of this functional link between hippocampal structure and social competition was the striking seasonal patterns of sex differences in both birds and mammals (Jacobs 1996b). Hippocampal and forebrain structures change with season in the eastern cowbird (Clayton et al. 1997), the meadow vole (*Microtus pennsylvanicus*) (Galea and McEwen 1999), the eastern gray squirrel (*Sciurus carolinensis*) (Lavenex et al. 2000a, 2000b), and many species of small mammals, such as shrews and voles (Yaskin 1984). Seasonal sex differences in spatial learning have also been demonstrated in deer mice and voles (Galea et al. 1996; Galea and McEwen 1999). Thus the social competition for mating opportunities, either the nests of a host bird species or a receptive female, can be seen to correlate directly with spatial ability and hippocampal structure.

Finally, some new results that are still being understood are interesting correlations between brain structures and mating systems in East African cichlid fish. The explosive speciation of these fish has been described as a natural laboratory of evolution (Pollen et al. 2007). The connection of changes in brain size to changes in mating systems in this highly complex and interesting group is clearly an area for future work.

The wealth of such patterns, however, could be the result of a sex-by-species predisposition for greater function or it could be the outcome of a life-long exercise of sex-specific spatial behaviors, in other words, the result and not the cause. Such sexual dimorphisms, however, have been documented in domesticated laboratory animals, with much less scope for sex-specific behaviors, long before these patterns were found in free-ranging animals. Second, if it were true that the hippocampus is monomorphic in females and males and it is only experience that induces sex differences, then it is still significant and important that social competition is capable of molding intraspecific variation. In this case, the capacity for such molding—the plasticity of the structure—is as much a trait under selection as the behavioral output. Indeed, the question of selection for "evolvability" has been an important new issue in the field of evolutionary developmental biology (West-Eberhard 2003). It could be the capacity for such molding and not what is learned that is under selection. The evolution of such plasticity has as much or more implications for cognitive evolution as a preprogrammed response to steroid hormones. Given the seasonal plasticity and the long evolutionary history of sex differences in vertebrates, it will probably turn out to be a combination of both. Referring once again to figure 2.2, the developmental and functional gears may be larger than those of the mechanism for plasticity or the phylogenetic constraints.

Scatter Hoarding as Social Competition

Of course the same argument applies equally to patterns of hippocampus development that vary with foraging mode, particularly with food storing. The idea that the hippocampus could vary in nature according to spatial behavior was first suggested in comparisons of scatter-hoarding bird species, described above. Here, too, the link between structure and function is one of interacting gears. Marsh tits (*Parus palustris*), a small scatter-hoarding passerine bird, have a relatively larger hippocampus than blue tits (*Parus caeruleus*), which scatter-hoard less. However, this is seen only when marsh tits are given access to the right combination of photoperiod and caching experience (Healy et al. 1994; Clayton 1995).

Sex differences clearly arise from social selection within a species. But food storing can also be seen as a competitive game (Andersson and Krebs 1978) and the social competition that arises with scatter hoarding could also be driving specializations in tracking items in space and time.

Any species that extracts food from a limited resource must negotiate with its fellows—a flock of sparrows jostling for crumbs is everyday evidence of this. Yet within food-storing strategies, scatter hoarding is an innately social competition. This relation of food storing to social competition may seem counterintuitive because at first glance, most scatter hoarders are either solitary or they store food in isolation. Yet no squirrel is an island: early experiments on the use of spatial memory in cache retrieval in mammals were specifically designed to simulate social competition. Mammalian scatter hoarders have a keen sense of smell and flexibly use odor or memory to retrieve caches, depending on environmental conditions (Vander Wall 2000).

In a typical experiment on scatter-hoarding mammals, gray squirrels cached nuts in a common arena. After a delay of several days the squirrel was faced with a social-competitive test: its ten caches were surrounded by ten other caches, nuts placed in sites chosen by seven competitors in the preceding week. A hungry squirrel responded by retrieving and eating more nuts from sites it had created then from the caches of its competitor (Jacobs and Liman 1991).

A study of Merriam's kangaroo rats (*Dipodomys*; Jacobs 1992b) also used social competition as an assay for the adaptive value of memory in cache retrieval. The cache distributions from a single individual were placed in the arena for solitary naïve competitors. Despite the small size of the arena (1 × 2 m) and plenty of time for the hungry pilferers to find the caches, their success rate was on average 30 percent less than that of the original owner (Jacobs 1992b).

Unlike birds, mammalian scatter hoarders can also identify the pilferer by the unique odor that the individual leaves behind in the form of scent marks, urine, and feces. Merriam's kangaroo rats, however, did not change their caching strategy or their behavior in the presence of this evidence that a conspecific had been present. But when these signs were accompanied by the sudden loss or redistribution of caches, kangaroo rats showed an increase in anxiety behaviors and a significant shift in foraging strategy (Preston and Jacobs 2001). A similar pattern was seen when the competitor was a heterospecific kangaroo rat species that co-occurs with the Merriam's, the Great Basin kangaroo rat (*Dipodomys microps*; see Preston and Jacobs 2005). These results nicely confirm Stephen Jenkin's prior work demonstrating population differences in cache distribution by kangaroo rats in the lab, with individuals from high-competition areas showing more distributed caches (Jenkins and Breck 1998). Such population differences in behavior have been found to predict patterns of caching behavior, memory, and hippocampal size in the black-capped chickadee (*Poecile atricapilla*) (Pravosudov and Clayton 2002).

It is important to try to disentangle the roles of natural and social selection in such guilds of competitive species, such as those of desert heteromyid rodents or passerine food-storing birds, where pilferage occurs both between and within species (Daly et al. 1992). The occurrence of pilferage and how caching can be maintained in the face of such pilferage is still not completely understood. Vander Wall and Jenkins have recently proposed a new model of scatter hoarding based on the idea of reciprocal pilfering (Vander Wall and Jenkins 2003). But social competition is present in all aspects of scatter-hoarding decisions, not simply cache maintenance but cache creation as well. After all, the goal of scatter hoarding is to compete with others over food items from a source that cannot be monopolized or defended (Jacobs 1995). All else being equal, it takes less time to hoard a large food item than to eat it. So when time—as at a rich but undefendable food source—is short, a scatter hoarder is able to "seclude" many more food items per unit time than it can consume, putting them in locations that it alone can relocate economically (Jacobs 1992a).

Scatter hoarding, then, is not simply about space—what was put where—but also reflects the difference between a foraging strategy that is socially mediated and one that is solitary. This could be the link between scatter hoarding and episodic memory. The ability of common ravens or western scrub jays to recall who was watching as they cached will not help them remember their cache locations—neither of these species encodes large numbers of caches. Obviously the importance of who was watching is a question of social competition: how to avoid the group member's later making off with the cache. Thus, among corvids, species that live in permanent competitive groups, such as piñon and Mexican jays (*Gymnorhinus cyanocephalus* and *Aphelocoma ultramarina*), can observe and remember where a conspecific is caching, but the solitary Clark's nutcracker apparently does not (Bednekoff and Balda 1996). Social competition in this case is not correlated with hippocampal size, since the Clark's nutcracker has a larger relative hippocampal size than the others (Basil et al. 1996). However, the question of phylogeny was not raised in these earlier studies; recent studies show a more complicated picture, indicating two lines of convergently evolving hippocampal specialization in corvids (de Kort and Clayton 2006).

In fact, the Clark's nutcracker is more closely related to Eurasian nutcrackers, all of whom have a group-specific larger hippocampus (Lucas et al. 2004). What this suggests is that hippocampus and brain structure in corvids might also show convergent evolution, with social selection for spatial memory to avoid cache pilferage in social jays, and natural selection for spatial memory to create and retrieve food distributions in nutcrackers. This social–natural selection hypothesis would lead to novel predictions not only for behavior but also for hippocampal function in these taxonomic groups.

Specialized Forms of Navigation: Migration and Echolocation

The example of convergent evolution in hippocampal size among corvids reminds us that such patterns must always be a product of more than one "gear" turning (see figure 2.2). If the hippocampus's role in spatial orientation evolved through natural selection, then specializations in navigational abilities that have no direct connections to social competition no doubt also arise via the same process. Two obvious examples are migratory patterns in songbirds and habitat-use patterns in microchiropteran bats (see table 2.1). Both of these behaviors—the continent-crossing migrations of songbirds and the ability of bats to navigate and forage using ultrasonic echolocation—are clearly remarkable feats of spatial orientation.

Nonetheless, it is worth considering whether the evolution of such specializations has been also affected by social selection. Migration is an old solution that decreases energy costs during the winter months and also reduces competition for food. But it is only one way to solve the problem of winter. There are two strategies, in terms of cognition, to survive this season: to stop thinking or to think harder (Jacobs 1996a). Nonstoring mammals use the first strategy—reduce activity by torpor or hibernation, often leading to a concomitant decrease in brain size. Scatter hoarders utilize the second strategy—though at a cost: the scatter-hoarding gray squirrel's brain is largest in October, when it is making thousands of scattered caches, but is significantly smaller in January and June (Lavenex et al. 2000a, 2000b).

Flying animals such as birds and insects instead use migration when temperatures drop and food is scarce. Although the act of migration itself is a remarkable act of spatial orientation, what the birds find on their arrival is an environment with warm temperatures and abundant food (the tropics in the winter for nonbreeding behavior; the Arctic in the summer for breeding behavior; Alerstam 1990). Exactly what one would expect from a specialized spatial orientation to a land of plenty has now been demonstrated: migrant species have smaller brains than resident species (Sol et al. 2005b), but those small brains have relative larger hippocampi (Healy et al. 1996). Given that we are comparing species, it is not clear whether the larger hippocampus is the result of a tradeoff, involving a loss of volume in another forebrain structure in birds. But it is clearly more parsimonious to conclude that such increases in hippocampal size are related to the actual migration, not to an increased difficulty of tracking food or social resources.

The pattern of structure and volume of the hippocampus in microchiropteran bats is another example that appears largely driven by natural selection. These patterns have been better documented in bats than in any other vertebrate group (Baron et al. 1996). In addition, there is now sophisticated research appearing on the spatial cognitive strategies of flower bats (Winter and Stich 2005; Toelch and Winter 2007). Yet attempts to correlate these patterns with behavior are still somewhat controversial. A first study reported that bat hippocampal size is related to habitat complexity and foraging style, specifically, a larger hippocampus is found in species that forage in cluttered environments than in open fields (Safi and Dechmann 2005). Yet a more recent study has reported no correlations of hippocampus size with foraging strategy but instead found an increase in isocortical volume in species that use both gleaning (picking prey from surfaces) and hawking (picking prey from midair) when compared to species that use only one of these strategies (Ratcliffe et al. 2006).

It is not clear what is driving the expression of this behavioral flexibility. It is possible that high levels of competition for prey force bats to search in many different habitats, which supports the notion of the role of social competition as a driver of hippocampal structure. Alternately, because the physiology of echolocation differs according to foraging substrate, with surface gleaners and aerial hawkers using different ultrasound frequencies, it may be that more complex input affects how the hippocampus computes locations. But recent work continues to underline similarities and differences between hippocampal function in terrestrial mammals and bats. As in laboratory rats and mice, single-unit recording from bat hippocampus confirmed the interplay between echolocation—whose function is to create a mental representation of space—and hippocampal activity (Ulanovsky and Moss 2007). In contrast to laboratory rodents, little to no adult neurogenesis was found in the hippocampus of nine species of microchiropteran bats (Amrein et al. 2007), however. Such results suggest that hippocampal function in flying mammals may be significantly different in form and function from that of rodents and primates. Understanding the bat hippocampus may thus allow us to understand the similarities and differences between bird and mammal hippocampus and to establish whether these are the results of homology or of convergent evolution, as Striedter (2005) has argued.

Conclusion

Let us return to the original question: How do memory specializations evolve? To answer this we must answer all of Tinbergen's questions. We need to understand not only memory's physiological mechanism but also its development, its adaptive value in light of the problems of living faced by a species, and, equally important, its evolutionary past. This means not only understanding the homologies in structure but also identifying the evolutionary processes that are at work. Although human episodic memory is clearly mediated by many brain structures, among them the hippocampus plays a major role. And because of hippocampal development in species, such as the western scrub jay, that appear to use episodic-like memory, asking what forces lead to this ability in nonhumans is a good place to start. West-Eberhard's theory of social selection has not been previously discussed as a force in hippocampal evolution. Viewing scatter hoarding, in particular, as a specialized foraging behavior that evolved in the forge of social competition from hoarding strategies that demand less cognitive capacity, such as larder hoarding, gives us a new perspective on hippocampal specialization. If the larger hippocampus seen in scatter-hoarding birds and mammals is related to tracking conspecific activity, then it is not significantly different in function from the larger hippocampus seen in polygynous male rodents or female nest-parasitic cowbirds (table 2.1). If these groups show a common ecological function, then understanding the selective forces underlying the evolution of the specialization in each group may lead to a better understanding of the physiological and anatomical homologies of the hippocampus in vertebrates.

These patterns of hippocampal increases in size and complexity suggest that episodic memory in humans may be derived from similar evolutionary forces as in the relevant animal species. Perhaps it was the need for social intelligence that led to the evolution of human episodic memory—the need for self-awareness and causal narrative to solve the great problems of within-species competition. Seen in this light, episodic memory, with or without its attendant specializations of autonoesis, might simply be one product of hippocampal evolution by social selection and one that we might already share with other species.

Acknowledgments

I would like to thank Luca Tommasi, Lynn Nadel, and Mary Peterson for organizing this remarkable conference and also the staff of the Konrad Lorenz Institute for providing an inspiring and gemütlich setting. For discussion of the ideas presented here, I would like to thank Tania Bettis, Becca Carter, Amy Cook, Nicole Vandersal, Anna Waisman and other members of Comparative Cognition Tea, John Campbell and other members of the Townsend Center for the Philosophy of Mind, and acknowledge my sabbatical support from the Santa Fe Institute.

References

Abbott ML, Walsh CJ, Storey AE, Stenhouse IJ, Harley CW (1999) Hippocampal volume is related to complexity of nesting habitat in Leach's storm-petrel, a nocturnal procellariiform seabird. Brain Behav Evol 53: 271–276.

Alerstam T (1990) Bird migration. Cambridge: Cambridge University Press.

Amrein I, Dechmann DK, Winter Y, Lipp HP (2007) Absent or low rate of adult neurogenesis in the hippocampus of bats (Chiroptera). PLoS ONE 2: e455.

Andersson M, Krebs JR (1978) On the evolution of hoarding behavior. Anim Behav 26: 707–711.

Balda RP, Kamil AC (1989) A comparative study of cache recovery by three corvid species. Anim Behav 38: 486–495.

Barker JM, Wojtowicz JM, Boonstra R (2005) Where's my dinner? Adult neurogenesis in free–living food-storing rodents. Genes Brain Behav 4: 89–98.

Barkley CL, Jacobs LF (1998) Visual environment and delay affect cache retrieval accuracy in a food-storing rodent. Anim Learn Behav 26: 439–447.

Barkley CL, Jacobs LF (2007) Sex and species differences in spatial memory in food-storing kangaroo rats. Anim Behav 73: 321–329.

Baron G, Stephan H, Frahm HD (1996) Comparative neurobiology in chiroptera: Brain characteristics in functional systems, ecoethological adaptation, adaptive radiation and evolution. Stuttgart: Birkhauser.

Basil JA, Kamil AC, Balda RP, Fite KV (1996) Differences in hippocampal volume among food storing corvids. Brain Behav Evol 47: 156–164.

Bednekoff PA, Balda, RP (1996) Observational spatial memory in Clark's nutcrackers and Mexican jays. Anim Behav 52: 833–839.

Biegler R, McGregor A, Krebs JR, Healy SD (2001) A larger hippocampus is associated with longer-lasting spatial memory. Proc Natl Acad Sci USA 98: 6941–6944.

Bingman VP, Hough GE, 2nd, Kahn MC, Siegel JJ (2003) The homing pigeon hippocampus and space: In search of adaptive specialization. Brain Behav Evol 62: 117–127.

Brodbeck DR (1994) Memory for spatial and local cues: A comparison of a storing and a nonstoring species. Anim Learn Behav 22: 119–133.

Bugnyar T, Heinrich B (2005) Ravens, Corvus corax, differentiate between knowledgeable and ignorant competitors. Proc Biol Sci 272: 1641–1646.

Bugnyar T, Heinrich B (2006) Pilfering ravens, Corvus corax, adjust their behaviour to social context and identity of competitors. Anim Cogn 9: 369–376.

Burgess N, Maguire EA, O'Keefe J (2002) The human hippocampus and spatial and episodic memory. Neuron 35: 625–641.

Butler AB, Hodos W (1996) Comparative vertebrate anatomy: Evolution and adaptation. New York: Wiley-Liss.

Byrne RW, Whiten A (1988) Machiavellian intelligence: Social expertise and the evolution of intellect in monkeys, apes and humans. Oxford: Clarendon Press.

Campbell J (1994) Past, space, and self. Oxford: Oxford University Press.

Clayton NS (1995) The neuroethological development of food-storing memory: A case of use it, or lose it. Behav Brain Res 70: 95–102.

Clayton NS, Dally JM, Emery NJ (2007) Social cognition by food-caching corvids. The western scrub-jay as a natural psychologist. Philos T Roy Soc Lond B 362: 507–522.

Clayton NS, Griffiths DP, Emery NJ, Dickinson A (2001) Elements of episodic-like memory in animals. Philos T Roy Soc Lond B 356: 1483–1491.

Clayton NS, Krebs JR (1994) One-trial associative memory: Comparison of food-storing and nonstoring species of birds. Anim Learn Behav 22: 366–372.

Clayton NS, Reboreda JC, Kacelnik A (1997) Seasonal changes of hippocampus volume in parasitic cowbirds. Behav Proc 41: 237–243.

Collett TS, Collett M (2002) Memory use in insect visual navigation. Nat Rev Neurosci 3: 542–552.

Csanyi V (2005) If dogs could talk: Exploring the canine mind. New York: North Point Press.

Daly M, Jacobs LF, Wilson MI, Behrends PR (1992) Scatter-hoarding by kangaroo rats (*Dipodomys merriami*) and pilferage from their caches. Behav Ecol 3: 102–111.

Day LB, Crews D, Wilczynski W (2001) Effects of medial and dorsal cortex lesions on spatial memory in lizards. Behav Brain Res 118: 27–42.

de Haan M, Mishkin M, Baldeweg T, Vargha-Khadem F (2006) Human memory development and its dysfunction after early hippocampal injury. Trends Neurosci 29: 374–381.

de Kort SR, Clayton NS (2006) An evolutionary perspective on caching by corvids. Proc Biol Sci 273: 417–423.

De Veer MW, van den Bos R (1999) A critical review of methodology and interpretation of mirror self-recognition research in nonhuman primates. Anim Behav 58: 459–468.

Devenport JA, Luna LD, Devenport LD (2000) Placement, retrieval and memory of caches by thirteen-lined ground squirrels. Ethology 106: 171–183.

Eichenbaum H, Yonelinas AP, Ranganath C (2007) The medial temporal lobe and recognition memory. Annu Rev Neurosci 30: 123–152.

Finlay BL, Darlington RB (1995) Linked regularities in the development and evolution of mammalian brains. Science, 268: 1578–1584.

Foote AL, Crystal JD (2007) Metacognition in the rat. Curr Biol 17: 551–555.

Galea LAM, Kavaliers M, Ossenkopp K-P (1996) Sexually dimorphic spatial learning in meadow voles *Microtus pennsylvanicus* and deer mice *Peromyscus maniculatus*. J Exp Biol 199: 195–200.

Galea LAM, Kavaliers M, Ossenkopp K-P, Innes D, Hargreaves EL (1994) Sexually dimorphic spatial learning varies seasonally in two populations of deer mice. Brain Res 635: 18–26.

Galea LA, McEwen BS (1999) Sex and seasonal differences in the rate of cell proliferation in the dentate gyrus of adult wild meadow voles. Neuroscience 89: 955–964.

Gallistel CR (1990) The organization of learning. Cambridge, MA: MIT Press.

Garamszegi LZ, Lucas JR (2005) Continental variation in relative hippocampal volume in birds: The phylogenetic extent of the effect and the potential role of winter temperatures. Biol Lett 1: 330–333.

Gaulin SJC, FitzGerald RW (1986) Sex differences in spatial ability: An evolutionary hypothesis and test. Amer Nat 127: 74–88.

Gibbs SEB, Lea SEG, Jacobs LF (2007) Flexible use of spatial cues in the southern flying squirrel (*Glaucomys volans*). Animal Cognition, 10: 203–209.

Griffin DR (1981) The question of animal awareness: Evolutionary continuity of mental experience. New York: Rockefeller University Press.

Hampton RR (2001) Rhesus monkeys know when they remember. Proc Natl Acad Sci USA 98: 5359–5362.

Hampton RR, Healy SD, Shettleworth SJ, Kamil AC (2002) "Neuroecologists" are not made of straw. Trends Cogn Sci 6: 6–7.

Hampton RR, Schwartz BL (2004) Episodic memory in nonhumans: What, and where, is when? Curr Opin Neurobiol 14: 192–127.

Hampton RR, Shettleworth SJ (1996) Hippocampus and memory in a food-storing and in a nonstoring bird species. Behav Neurosci 110: 946–964.

Harvey PH, Krebs JR (1990) Comparing brains. Science 249: 140–146.

Healy SD, Clayton NS, Krebs JR (1994) Development of hippocampal specialisation in two species of tit (*Parus* spp.). Behav Brain Res 61: 23–28.

Healy SD, Gwinner E, Krebs JR (1996) Hippocampal volume in migratory and non-migratory warblers: Effects of age and experience. Behav Brain Res 81: 61–68.

Healy SD, Hurly TA (2004) Spatial learning and memory in birds. Brain, Behavior and Evolution, 63: 211–220.

Herz RS, Zanette L, Sherry DF (1994) Spatial cues for cache retrieval by black-capped chickadees. Anim Behav 48: 343–351.

Holtzman DA, Harris TW, Aranguren G, Bostock E (1999) Spatial learning of an escape task by young corn snakes, *Elaphe guttata guttata*. Anim Behav 57: 51–60.

Jacobs LF (1992a) The effect of handling time on the decision to cache by grey squirrels. Anim Behav 43: 522–524.

Jacobs LF (1992b) Memory for cache locations in Merriam's kangaroo rats. Anim Behav 43: 585–593.

Jacobs LF (1995) The ecology of spatial cognition: Adaptive patterns of hippocampal size and space use in wild rodents. In: Studies of the brain in naturalistic settings (Alleva E, Fasolo A, Lipp H-P, Nadel L, eds), 301–322. Dordrecht: Kluwer Academic Publishers.

Jacobs LF (1996a) The economy of winter: Phenotypic plasticity in behavior and brain structure. Biol Bull 191: 92–100.

Jacobs LF (1996b) Sexual selection and the brain. Trends Ecol Evol 11: 82–86.

Jacobs LF (2000) Sexual differentiation and cognitive function. In: Gender and society (Blakemore C, Iversen S, eds), TK–TK. Oxford: Oxford University Press.

Jacobs LF, Gaulin SJC, Sherry DF, Hoffman GE (1990) Evolution of spatial cognition: Sex-specific patterns of spatial behavior predict hippocampal size. Proc Natl Acad Sci USA 87: 6349–6352.

Jacobs LF, Liman ER (1991) Grey squirrels remember the locations of buried nuts. Anim Behav 41: 103–110.

Jacobs LF, Schenk F (2003) Unpacking the cognitive map: The parallel map theory of hippocampal function. Psychol Rev 110: 285–315.

Jacobs LF, Shiflett MW (1999) Spatial orientation on a vertical maze in free-ranging fox squirrels (*Sciurus niger*). J Comp Psychol 113: 116–127.

Jacobs LF, Spencer WD (1994) Natural space-use patterns and hippocampal size in kangaroo rats. Brain Behav Evol 44: 125–132.

Jenkins SH, Breck, SW (1998) Differences in food hoarding among six species of heteromyid rodents. J Mammal 79: 1221–1233.

Krebs JR, Sherry DF, Healy SD, Perry VH, Vaccarino AL (1989) Hippocampal specialization of food-storing birds. Proc Natl Acad Sci USA, 86: 1388–1392.

Langley CM (1994) Spatial memory in the desert kangaroo rat (*Dipodomys deserti*). J Comp Psychol 108: 3–14.

Lavenex P, Steele MA, Jacobs LF (2000a) The seasonal pattern of cell proliferation and neuron number in the dentate gyrus of wild adult eastern grey squirrels. Eur J Neurosci 12: 643–648.

Lavenex P, Steele MA, Jacobs LF (2000b) Sex differences, but no seasonal variations in the hippocampus of food-caching squirrels: A stereological study. J Comp Neurol 425: 152–166.

Leaver LA, Daly M (2001) Food caching and differentail cache pilferage: A field study of coexistence of sympatric kangaroo rats and pocket mice. Oecologia, 128: 577–584.

Lorenz K (1952) King Solomon's ring. New York: Thomas Y. Crowell.

Lorenz K (1996) The natural science of the human species: An introduction to comparative behavioral research—"the Russian manuscript" (1944–1948). Cambridge, MA: MIT Press.

Lorenz K, Tinbergen N (1938) Taxis und Instinkthandlung in der Eirollbewegung der Graugans. Z Tierpsychol 2: 1–29.

Lucas JR, Brodin A, de Kort SR, Clayton NS (2004) Does hippocampal size correlate with the degree of caching specialization? Proc Biol Sci 271: 2423–2429.

Macdonald IMV (1997) Field experiments on duration and precision of grey and red squirrel spatial memory. Anim Behav 54: 879–891.

Macphail EM, Bolhuis JJ (2001) The evolution of intelligence: Adaptive specializations versus general process. Biol Rev 76: 341–364.

Milner B, Squire LR, Kandel ER (1998) Cognitive neuroscience and the study of memory. Neuron 20: 445–468.

Moscovitch M, Nadel L, Winocur G, Gilboa A, Rosenbaum RS (2006) The cognitive neuroscience of remote episodic, semantic and spatial memory. Curr Opin Neurobiol 16: 179–190.

Mulcahy NJ, Call J (2006) Apes save tools for future use. Science 312: 1038–1040.

O'Keefe J, Nadel L (1978) The hippocampus as a cognitive map. Oxford: Oxford University Press.

Ormerod BK, Galea LAM (2001) Reproductive status influences cell proliferation and cell survival in the dentate gyrus of adult female meadow voles: A possible regulatory role for estradiol. Neuroscience 102: 369–379.

Petersen K, Sherry DF (1996) No sex difference occurs in hippocampus, food-storing, or memory for food caches in black-capped chickadees. Behav Brain Res 79: 15–22.

Pleskacheva MG, Wolfer DP, Kupriyanova IF, Nikolenko DL, Scheffrahn H, Dell'Omo G, Lipp H-P (2000) Hippocampal mossy fibers and swimming navigation learning in two vole species occupying different habitats. Hippocampus 10: 17–30.

Pollard KS, Salama SR, Lambert N, Lambot MA, Coppens S, Pedersen JS, Katzman S, King B, Onodera C, Siepel A, Kern AD, Dehay C, Igel H, Ares M Jr, Vanderhaeghen P, Haussler D (2006) An RNA gene expressed during cortical development evolved rapidly in humans. Nature 443: 167–172.

Pollen AA, Dobberfuhl AP, Scace J, Igulu MM, Renn SCP, Shumway CA, Hofmann HA (2007) Environmental complexity and social organization sculpt the brain in Lake Tanganyikan cichlid fish. Brain Behav Evol 70: 21–39.

Pravosudov VV, Clayton NS (2002) A test of the adaptive specialization hypothesis: Population differences in caching, memory, and the hippocampus in black-capped chickadees (*Poecile atricapilla*). Behav Neurosci 116: 515–522.

Preston SD, Jacobs LF (2001) Conspecific pilferage but not presence affects Merriam's kangaroo rat cache strategy. Behav Ecol 12: 517–523.

Preston SD, Jacobs LF (2005) Cache decision making: the effects of competition on cache decisions in Merriam's kangaroo rat (*Dipodomys merriami*). J Comp Psychol 119: 187–196.

Raby CR, Alexis DM, Dickinson A, Clayton NS (2007) Planning for the future by western scrub-jays. Nature 445: 919–921.

Ratcliffe JM, Fenton MB, Shettleworth SJ (2006) Behavioral flexibility positively correlated with relative brain volume in predatory bats. Brain Behav Evol 67: 165–176.

Reader SM, Laland KN (2002) Social intelligence, innovation, and enhanced brain size in primates. Proc Natl Acad Sci USA 99: 4436–4441.

Reboreda JC, Clayton NS, Kacelnik A (1996) Species and sex differences in hippocampus size in parasitic and non-parasitic cowbirds. Neuroreport 7: 505–508.

Rodriguez F, Lopez JC, Vargas JP, Gomez Y, Broglio C, Salas C (2002) Conservation of spatial memory function in the pallial forebrain of reptiles and ray-finned fishes. J Neurosci 22: 2894–2903.

Roughgarden J, Meeko Oishi M, Akçay E (2006) Reproductive social behavior: Cooperative games to replace sexual selection. Science 311: 965–969.

Safi K, Dechmann DK (2005) Adaptation of brain regions to habitat complexity: A comparative analysis in bats (Chiroptera). Proceedings of the Royal Society B: Biological Sciences 272: 179–186.

Sherry DF (1984) Food storage by black-capped chickadees: Memory for the location and contents of caches. Anim Behav 32: 451–464.

Sherry DF, Forbes MRL, Kurghel M, Ivy GO (1993) Females have a larger hippocampus than males in the brood-parasitic brown-headed cowbird. Proc Natl Acad Sci USA 90: 7839–7843.

Sherry DF, Jacobs LF, Gaulin SJC (1992) Spatial memory and adaptive specialization of the hippocampus. Trends Neurosci 15: 298–303.

Sherry DF, Krebs JR, Cowie RJ (1981) Memory for the location of stored food in marsh tits. Anim Behav 29: 1260–1266.

Sherry DF, Schacter DL (1987) The evolution of multiple memory systems. Psychol Rev 94: 439–469.

Sherry DF, Vaccarino AL, Buckenham K, Herz RS (1989) The hippocampal complex of food-storing birds. Brain Behav Evolution 34: 308–317.

Shettleworth SJ (1998). Cognition, evolution, and behavior. Oxford: Oxford University Press.

Shiflett MW, Gould KL, Smulders TV, DeVoogd TJ (2002) Septum volume and food-storing behavior are related in parids. J Neurobiol 51: 215–222.

Smulders TV, Sasson AD, DeVoogd TJ (1995) Seasonal variation in hippocampal volume in a food-storing bird, the black-capped chickadee. J Neurobiol 27: 15–25.

Sol D, Duncan RP, Blackburn TM, Cassey P, Lefebvre L (2005a) Big brains, enhanced cognition, and response of birds to novel environments. Proc Natl Acad Sci USA 102: 5460–5465.

Sol D, Lefebvre L, Rodriguez-Teijeiro JD (2005b) Brain size, innovative propensity and migratory behaviour in temperate Palaearctic birds. Proc Biol Sci 272: 1433–1441.

Sol D, Szekely T, Liker A, Lefebvre L (2007) Big-brained birds survive better in nature. Proc Biol Sci 274: 763–769.

Striedter GF (2005) Principles of brain evolution. Sunderland, MA: Sinauer Associates.

Tinbergen N (1963) On the aims and methods of ethology. Z Tierpsychol 20: 410–433.

Tinbergen N (1972) On the orientation of the digger wasp *Philanthus triangulum* Fabr. I. In: The animal in its world (Tinbergen N, ed), 103–127. Cambridge, MA: Harvard University Press.

Toelch U, Winter Y (2007) Psychometric function for nectar volume perception of a flower-visiting bat. J Comp Physiol A 193: 265–269.

Tomasello M, Carpenter M (2007) Shared intentionality. Dev Sci 10: 121–125.

Trewavas A (2005) Plant intelligence. Naturwissenschaften 92: 401–413.

Tulving E (1984) Precis of Elements of Episodic Memory. Behav Brain Sci 7: 223–268.

Ulanovsky N, Moss CF (2007) Hippocampal cellular and network activity in freely moving echolocating bats. Nat Neurosci 10: 224–233.

Vander Wall SB (1991) Mechanisms of cache recovery by yellow pine chipmunks. Anim Behav 41: 851–864.

Vander Wall SB (2000) The influence of environmental conditions on cache recovery and cache pilferage by yellow pine chipmunks (Tamias amoenus) and deer mice (Peromyscus maniculatus). Behav Ecol 11: 544–549.

Vander Wall SB, Jenkins SH (2003) Reciprocal pilferage and the evolution of food-hoarding behavior. Behav Ecol 14: 656–667.

Vlasak AN (2006a) Global and local spatial landmarks: Their role during foraging by Columbian ground squirrels (Spermophilus columbianus). Anim Cogn 9: 71–80.

Vlasak AN (2006b) The relative importance of global and local landmarks in navigation by Columbian ground squirrels (Spermophilus columbianus). J Comp Psychol 120: 131–138.

Volman SF, Grubb TC, Schuett KC (1997) Relative hippocampal volume in relation to food-storing behavior in four species of woodpeckers. Brain Behav Evol 49: 110–120.

Wasserman EA (1997) The science of animal cognition: Past, present, and future. J Exp Psychol Anim B 23: 123–136.

West-Eberhard MJ (1983) Sexual selection, social competition, and speciation. Quart Rev Biol 58: 155–183.

West-Eberhard MJ (2003) Developmental plasticity and evolution. Oxford: Oxford University Press.

Winter Y, Stich KP (2005) Foraging in a complex naturalistic environment: Capacity of spatial working memory in flower bats. J Exp Biol 208: 539–548.

Yaskin VA (1984) Seasonal changes in brain morphology in small mammals. Carnegie Mus Nat Hist Spec Publ 10: 183–193.

Zentall TR, ed (1984) Animal cognition: A tribute to Donald A. Riley. Hillsdale, NJ: Lawrence Erlbaum.

3 Spatial Cognition, Memory Capacity, and the Evolution of Mammalian Hippocampal Networks

Alessandro Treves

Beyond the Grid, There Is Not Much Space

The discovery of grid cells in the medial entorhinal cortex (MEC) of the rat (Fyhn et al. 2004) and of the precise triangular pattern of their firing fields (Hafting et al. 2005) requires a substantial reformulation of the questions relating to spatial cognition. It now appears, more clearly than before, that spatial computations per se are largely performed by the rat brain before the hippocampus is ever accessed, and culminate in a sort of universal map of allocentric space, in MEC layer II. Only a portion of the EC participates in such a map, which is applied and used irrespective of context, but in combination with context-specific signals that determine the activity of other parts of entorhinal cortex. The hippocampus operates on the universal map and on context-specific signals to create context-specific metric representations of space, which are stored in memory. The capacity of the hippocampus to rapidly switch between the representations of different contexts is illustrated by hippocampal global "remapping," i.e., the transition to new, unrelated arrangements of place fields by the same population of recorded cells, after suitable behavioral manipulations, and without concurrent MEC remapping (Fyhn et al. 2007). Consequently, understanding the circuitry of the hippocampus crucially involves understanding this capacity for decorrelating spatial representations, at least in rodents. It could well be that in other species complex memories of a less spatial nature take a more prominent role, in which case it would be even more appropriate to approach hippocampal decorrelation and memory processes at an abstract level, and independent of the possibly species-specific spatial processes so finely investigated with the rat model (see also chapter 2 of this volume, by Lucia F. Jacobs).

Which approaches can take us beyond a mere functional description of the role of different networks in the brain, and lead us to understand, in evolutionary terms, their design principles? In recent years I have studied three apparently disparate topics from a computational viewpoint: the lamination of the sensory cortex, the differentiation into subfields of the mammalian hippocampus, and the neuronal dynamics that might underlie the faculty for language in the human frontal lobes. These studies share a common perspective: they all discuss the evolution of cortical networks in terms of their computations, quantified by simulating simplified formal models. They all dwell on the interrelationship between qualitative and quantitative change. Finally, they all include, as a necessary ingredient of the relevant computational mechanisms, a simple feature of pyramidal cell biophysics: firing-rate adaptation. In this chapter I formulate this general viewpoint, which does not usually find space in individual papers, and then I focus on the computational approach to hippocampal network design, seen in the context of the other two problems.

Looking at the Past Through a Spin Glass

To approach each of the three problems, I have used the simulation of drastically simplified network models as the primary tool for analysis. Although the details of the models used were specific and were adapted to the problem being considered, the underlying approach has been similar across studies, and this is what I want to briefly discuss first.

An assumption motivating my approach is that the most important steps in the evolution of the nervous system are those that address *computational* demands, demands that are part of the "job specification" of the brain as an information-processing system, rather than steps that address, say, physiological or anatomical constraints. Among genuine information-processing problems, one that has been quantified through the use of formal models is the limit on the storage of memories that is imposed by the connectivity of a system of neuron-like units. Considering this limit is partly motivated by the observation that most gray-matter volume appears to be devoted to synaptic contacts (Braitenberg and Schüz 1991), as if the cortex had evolved to maximize connectivity and ultimately memory storage. The mathematical procedures that have been used to obtain a proper quantification of the relation between connectivity and memory were originally developed to analyze the physics of a class of materials known as spin glasses (see, e.g., Amit 1989). Spin glasses are endowed with interactions that can be characterized as disordered and hence as interfering with each other, somewhat as, in a neural network, distinct memory representations interfere with each other at retrieval. Although spin glasses have nothing deeper in common with memory systems than this analogy and the mathematical procedures useful in analyzing them, the effectiveness and generality of these procedures have led some of us to approach many information- processing problems by relying on the analysis of spin glasses as a basic paradigm. Unwrapped from its technicalities, the spin-glass approach reduces essentially to the idea that cortical systems face a crucial connectivity constraint on extensive memory storage, that the constraint results from interference among memories, and that to analyze such interference we can borrow techniques from statistical physics.

The three problems I have considered are all, to some extent, spin-glass problems in disguise.

The Phase Transition That Made Us Mammals

Mammals originate from the therapsids, one order among the first amniotes, or early reptiles, as they are commonly referred to. They are estimated to have radiated away from other early reptilian lineages, including the anapsids (the progenitors of modern turtles) and diapsids (out of which other modern reptilians, as well as birds, derive) some 300 million years ago (Carroll 1988). Perhaps mammals emerged as a fully differentiated but still rather homogeneous class out of the third-to-last of the great extinctions, in the Triassic period, with their explosive diversification occurring much later (Bininda-Emonds et al. 2007). The changes in the organization of the nervous system that mark the transition from proto-reptilian ancestors to early mammals can be reconstructed only indirectly. Along with supporting arguments from the examination of endocasts (the inside of fossil skulls; Jerison 1990) and of presumed behavioral patterns (Wilson 1975), the main line of evidence is the comparative anatomy of present-day species (Diamond and Hall 1969). Among a variety of quantitative changes in the relative development of different structures—changes that, by tuning the expression of specific genes (Mallamaci and Stoykova 2006) have been extended, accelerated, and diversified during the entire course of mammalian evolution (Finlay and Darlington 1995; Barton 2007)—two major qualitative changes in the forebrain stand out: two new features that, once established, characterize the cortex of mammals as distinct from that of reptilians and birds. Both these changes involve the introduction of a new "input" layer of granule cells.

In the first change, it is the medial pallium (the medial part of the upper surface of each cerebral hemisphere, as it bulges out of the forebrain) that reorganizes into the modern-day mammalian hippocampus. The crucial step is the detachment of the most medial portion, which loses both its continuity with the rest of the cortex at the hippocampal sulcus and its projections to the dorsolateral cortex (Ulinski 1990). The rest of the medial cortex becomes Ammon's horn and retains the distinctly cortical pyramidal cells, while the detached cortex becomes the dentate gyrus, with its population of granule cells, which now project, as a sort of preprocessing stage, to the pyramidal cells of field CA3 (Amaral, Ishizuka, and Claiborne 1990). In the second change it is the dorsal pallium (the central part of the upper surface) that reorganizes internally, in areas that process topographic modalities, to become the cerebral neocortex. Aside from special cases, most mammalian neocortices display the characteristic isocortical pattern of lamination, or organization into distinct layers of cells (traditionally classified as 6, in some cases with specialized sublayers; see Yamamori and Rockland 2006). A prominent step in lamination is granulation, whereby the formerly unique principal layer of pyramidal cells is split by the insertion of a new layer of excitatory, but intrinsic, granule cells, in between the pyramidal cells of the infragranular and supragranular layers. This is layer IV, where the main ascending inputs to cortex terminate (Diamond et al. 1985).

Lamination May Reconcile Memory with Topography

I have formulated a hypothesis (Treves 2003) that accounts for granulation, and for the differentiation between supra- and infragranular pyramidal layers, as advantageous to support fine topography in the sensory maps that mammals have evolved, over and beyond the gross topography that limits the usefulness of sensory maps in reptiles. Fine topography implies a generic distinction between "where" information, explicitly mapped on the cortical sheet, and "what" information, represented in a distributed fashion as a distinct firing pattern across neurons. Memory patterns can be stored on recurrent collaterals in the cortex, and such memory can help substantially in the analysis of current sensory input. The effective use of recurrent collaterals, because of the "spin-glass" limit on memory storage load, requires afferent projections to the cortex that are spread over a large patch; whereas the precise localization of a stimulus on the sensory map requires narrowly focused afferents (see Treves 2003 for the complete argument; Roudi and Treves 2006 for the analytical treatment of a single-layer model). The simulation of a simplified network model demonstrates that a nonlaminated patch of cortex with a single characteristic spread of afferent connections must compromise between transmitting "where" information or retrieving "what" information. The differentiation of a granular layer affords a quantitative advantage by allowing focused afferents to the granular units together with widespread afferents to pyramidal units. For this purely anatomical differentiation to be effective, however, it must be accompanied by a physiological differentiation: pyramidal units must adapt their firing—that is, decrease their response to steady inputs—much more than granular units. With this further difference, the pyramidal layers can select the correct attractor for memory retrieval before the granular layer, which adapts less, partially takes over the dynamics, and focuses activity on the cortical spot that most accurately reflects the position of the sensory input.

Adaptation thus effectively separates out in time, albeit only partially, two information-processing operations that occur in different spaces: the retrieval of memories in the abstract space of attractors and the accurate relay of stimulus position in the physical space of the cortical surface. The advantage of the differentiation is quantitatively minor (see figure 3.1). My hypothesis is that a major qualitative step, the transition from a simpler paleocortex to a more elaborate isocortex, came about just in order to gain a few percent more bits in the average combined value of "what" and "where" information.

The Phase Transition That Made Us Human

Our lineage is estimated to have radiated away genetically from those of other great apes perhaps 5 million to 6 million years ago. Functionally, a number of lines of evidence point at a stage of accelerated change and complexification in human behavior, a so-called cognitive revolution, taking place much later, perhaps 50,000 years ago. In terms of the organization of the nervous system, no salient qualitative trait distinguishes us from our

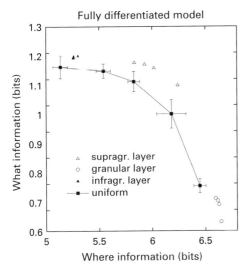

Figure 3.1
Combination of what and where information that can be extracted from neural activity in model cortical patches of different architectures. The "uniform" model is made up of three statistically identical layers of units, each of which produces the same what-where mix at some location on the solid line, depending on the spread of afferent inputs. The "differentiated" model includes three layers with distinct connectivity and adaptation properties, each of which affords a different what-where mix, but always beyond the limit reached by the uniform model. Simulation details in Treves (2003).

closest cognates, such as chimps or gorillas. The only clear structural pattern is one of quantitative change: with respect to other primates—but not necessarily with respect to all other mammals (Goffinet 2006)—an increase is observed in some key parameters of cortical extension, arealization (Krubitzer and Huffman 2000), and connectivity (Elston 2000). It seems unlikely, therefore, that a new gene may have triggered the development of uniquely human capacities without apparently inducing any detectable change of design in the brain. Yet the scientific community has been reluctant to abandon the expectation, naively raised by popular media, of a quick and ready-to-use solution to the question of what makes us human. Many respectable scientists have continued to harbor the hope that—if not a gene, if not a magic molecule—at least a dedicated piece of neural circuitry may be found that could explain, for example, the human faculty of language.

Understanding the neural basis of higher cognitive functions such as those involved in language requires in fact a shift from a localization approach to an analysis of network operation. Localization approaches have run their course, and they have highlighted a substantial continuity between the cortical areas most directly implicated in language functions in the human brain and homologue areas in other primates. Finding out where language "is" has not provided a shred of a clue as to how it came about. Hauser and colleagues, in a recent proposal (2002), point instead to *infinite recursion* as the core process involved in several higher functions, including language, forcefully arguing for the hypothesis that the roots of language may be in a new process rather than in a new structure. The proposal offers a way out of the reductionist cul-de-sac and it challenges cortical-network theorists to describe network behavior that could subserve infinite recursion.

Building on a variant of the notion that language may have evolved out of the semantic and procedural memory systems (Ullman 2001) I have been exploring the hypothesis that a capacity for infinite recursion may be associated with the natural adaptive dynamics of large semantic associative networks (Treves 2005). I have used a network of Potts (multistate) units to simulate a semantic memory system distributed over many cortical modules, and I have tested its joint ability to both retrieve a semantic memory based on a partial cue and, subsequently, when deprived of further inputs, also to follow a latching dynamics in attractor space, jumping from one memory to the next with structured transition probabilities. While the retrieval ability is limited by an appropriate variant of the spin-glass constraint (first considered by Kanter 1988), the latching ability requires a sufficient density of attractors. Since the spin-glass constraint limits the number of attractors proportionally to the connectivity (Kropff and Treves 2005), the joint ability for retrieval and latching can be realized only once the connectivity of the modular system becomes, in evolution, sufficiently extensive. At that point, after a kind of percolation-phase transition, the system is both able to retrieve and to support structured transition probabilities between global network states. The crucial development endowing a semantic system with a non-random dynamics would thus be an increase in connectivity, perhaps to be identified with the dramatic increase in spine numbers recently observed in the basal dendrites of pyramidal cells in human and Old World monkey frontal cortex (Elston 2000). Once again the crucial step in the argument is a quantitative analysis based on network simulations, which spin-glass mathematical methods promise to consolidate, to describe a phase transition that could not be accessed with mere qualitative reasoning.

The Differentiation of the Hippocampus

Focusing now on the hippocampus, one may ask, what is the evolutionary advantage, for mammals, brought about by the changes mentioned above, in its internal organization? Since the seminal paper by David Marr (1971), and well before awareness developed among modelers of the evolutionary specificity of hippocampal organization (Treves et al. 2008), attempts to account for its remarkable differentiation into three main subfields have been mostly based on the computational analysis of the role of the hippocampus in memory. With the simultaneous discovery of place cells (O'Keefe and Dostrovsky 1971), the rodent model seemed to point at a special hippocampal role for spatial representation and spatial memory. Although an accumulating body of evidence has suggested that hippocampal activity may not be exclusively related to space (Eichenbaum 2000), the prevalence of spatial correlates in the rat has encouraged speculations on the evolution of the hippocampus based on spatial function. The hippocampus, however, is important for spatial memory also in birds (Bingman and Jones 1994; Clayton and Krebs 1995; Clayton et al. 2003; Bingman and Sharp 2006). The avian and mammalian hippocampi are structurally very different, with birds perhaps having stayed close to their reptilian progenitors in this respect, and mammals having detached the dentate gyrus from Ammon's Horn, as mentioned above and further discussed by Treves and colleagues (2008). A reasonable hypothesis may then be that the new mammalian design somehow enhances the capability of the hippocampus to serve as a memory store, perhaps with the nuance of a prevailingly spatial memory store.

It is plausible that the primitive cortical tissue in early reptile-like ancestors of both mammals and birds was rich in recurrent collaterals, much like region CA3 in the modern mammalian hippocampus. Simplified models show how a recurrent network can naturally retrieve distributions of activity from partial cues as an autoassociative memory (Hopfield 1982), provided the synapses on the recurrent connections among its pyramidal cells are endowed, as likely was the case for primitive cortex, with associative, "Hebbian," plasticity, such as that based on NMDA receptors (Collingridge and Bliss 1995). That cortex can then be conceptualized as having operated, at least, as a content-addressable memory for distributed activity patterns—provided it had an effective way of distinguishing its operating modes. A generic problem with associative memories based on recurrent connections is to distinguish a storage mode from a retrieval mode. To be effective, recurrent connections should dominate the dynamics of the system when it is operating in retrieval mode. While storing new information, instead, the dynamics should be primarily determined by afferent inputs, with limited interference from the memories already stored in the recurrent connections, which should, however, modify their weights to store the new information (Treves and Rolls 1992).

Distinguishing Storage from Retrieval

The most phylogenetically primitive solution to effect the dual operating mode is to use a modulator that acts differentially on the afferent inputs (originally, those arriving at the apical dendrites) and on the recurrent connections (predominantly lower on the dendritic tree). Acetylcholine (ACh) can achieve this effect, exploiting the orderly arrangement of pyramidal cell dendrites in the cortex (Hasselmo and Schnell 1994). Acetylcholine is one of several very ancient neuromodulating systems, well conserved across vertebrates, and it is likely that it operated in this way already in the early reptilian cortex, throughout its subdivisions. Mike Hasselmo has emphasized this role of ACh in memory with a combination of slice work and neural network modeling (Hasselmo et al. 1995, 1996). This work has been focused on the hippocampus, originally the medial wall, and on piriform cortex, originally the lateral wall. The proposed mechanism, however, has no reason to be circumscribed to these regions, and it could well operate across cortical systems involved in memory storage.

One flaw of an ACh-based mechanism is that it requires an active process that distinguishes storage from retrieval periods, and regulates Ach release accordingly. In the hippocampus, however, it appears that mammals have devised a more refined expedient to separate storage from retrieval, which can efficiently perform both functions also in a passive mode: inserting a preprocessor before the CA3 memory network. The preprocessor should instruct which units in CA3 should fire in a new distribution of activity to be stored as the memory trace of a new item to be remembered. As a simplest model, one can think of a preprocessing network without recurrent connections, which simply forms new arbitrarily determined representations on the fly, and through a system of one-to-one connections ("detonator" synapses) imposes these new representations onto CA3 (McNaughton and Morris 1987). In fact, the one-to-one correspondence is not needed: what enriches the representation to be stored of meaningful content, against the interference of recurrent connections, is just a system of sparse and strong connections from a sparsely coded feedforward network. Developing the preprocessor notion, we have proposed a quantitative estimate of the amount of new information that could be encoded in CA3 representations with different input systems (Treves and Rolls 1992; see figure 3.2).

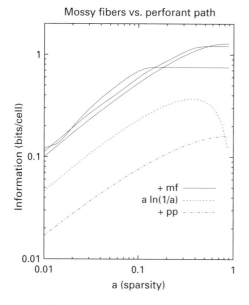

Figure 3.2
Information per unit in a model CA representation, as a function of its sparsity. The dashed line is the amount that can be associatively retrieved; the dash-dotted line is what can be stored by inputs with the characteristics of the perforant path to CA3, and the three solid lines are three estimates of what can be stored through mossy fiber inputs (the estimates differ in the sparsity of the dentate). Analytical derivation in Treves and Rolls (1992).

The argument is based on the "quasi-theorem," which has never been satisfactorily proved but empirically holds true, that an associative memory can hold up to $I/(NC) \approx$ 0.2 0.3 bits of information per synapse, where N is the number of units and C the average number of connections, or synapses, per unit. Since the storage capacity, or maximum number of discrete patterns of activity that can be individually retrieved, is estimated as $p_c \approx 0.2$–0.3 $C/[a \ln(1/a)]$, where a is the sparsity of the stored representation (see Treves and Rolls 1991), information-theoretical efficiency requires that each such representation should contain at least roughly $i \approx N$ a $\ln(1/a)$ bits of new information. Per unit, this is the amount of information of a noiseless binary variable (in the sparse $a \ll 1$ regime and apart from the $\ln(2)$ factor). Thus, efficient storage requires that CA3 pyramidal units be as informative about new contents as, roughly, binary units can be. The challenge for afferent inputs is to prevail over the recurrent connections, which do not impart new contents to a pattern of activity to be stored. Figure 3.2 shows that this challenge can be met by afferent inputs with the characteristics of the mossy fibers, but not by those with the characteristics of the perforant path to CA3 (Treves and Rolls 1992).

Mapping Continuous Attractors onto Discrete Memories

The argument above has been worked out for the case of discrete memory items, which can be taken as a model of episodic memory. Initially, in fact, the neural network approach, aiming at quantifying the capacity of associative memories, has been formulated in terms of fully connected recurrent architectures and discrete memory states, conceived—in the limit of no fluctuations—as points in the multidimensional space in which each component corresponds to the firing rate or in general to the activity of one unit (Hopfield 1982). This formulation, which was the starting point for physicists interested in applying powerful mathematical analysis techniques, had been preceded by the more rudimentary analysis of David Marr. Marr also thought in terms of discrete memory states, and had guessed the importance of recurrent collaterals, a prominent feature of the CA3 subfield (Amaral et al. 1990), even though his own model was not really affected by the presence of such collaterals, as shown later (Willshaw and Buckingham 1990). Although the paper by Marr was nearly simultaneous with two of the most exciting experimental discoveries related to the hippocampus, that of place cells (O'Keefe and Dostrowski 1971) and that of long-term synaptic potentiation (Bliss and Lømo 1973), for a long time it did not seem to inspire further theoretical analyses, with the exception of an interesting discussion of the collateral effect in a neural network model (Gardner-Medwin 1976). One factor was probably the mathematical "technology" available to Marr, inadequate to really investigate his models quantitatively. Marr himself become disillusioned with his youthful enthusiasm for unraveling brain circuits, and in his mature years took a much more sedate, and less neural, interest in vision. From the 1987 paper by McNaughton and Morris, however, an increasing number of other investigators rediscovered the young Marr, and tried to elaborate those ideas in order to understand the operation of hippocampal circuits. Edmund Rolls (1989) and others again emphasized the crucial role probably played by the CA3 recurrent collaterals and made explicit the relation to the auto-associative memory networks studied quantitatively by the physicists (Amit et al. 1987). In establishing the relation, the salient spatial character of hippocampal memory correlates was provisionally neglected, to take advantage of the formal models based on discrete attractor states.

As a matter of fact, an autoassociator may subserve both the storage of discrete memories as point-like attractor states or of more complex memories—for example, synfire chains (Abeles 1991), which can be individually distinct and discrete or organized in arbitrary branching patterns—or continuous attractors, when network dynamics converges to fixed points that are continuously arranged on some manifold in the high–dimensional activity space. Simple examples of continuous attractors are present in models of orientation selectivity by horizontal interaction in visual cortex (Sompolinsky and Shapley 1987) or of the head direction system (Skaggs et al. 1995). These models do not store information in long-term memory, and in the continuum limit their fixed points comprise a single (in these particular cases, 1D) manifold. Samsonovich and McNaughton's multiple-chart model (1997) demonstrated instead, in the context of a model for path integration, how one could conceive of fixed points organized in multiple 2D continuous manifolds, each of which maps the animal position in a distinct environment. Exploration of a new environment leads to the formation of a new chart (*ab initio,* or using some prewired connectivity; it may be difficult to distinguish the two possibilities). The question then arises of how many charts a given recurrent network can hold in long-term memory.

The storage capacity of a multichart recurrent autoassociator was analyzed by Battaglia and Treves (1998), who extracted a simple rule of thumb for assessing the memory load of a chart. A chart that maps a finite environment onto the activity of place-cell-like units is equivalent, capacitywise, to as many discrete attractor states as there are locations, in the environment, for which the activity vectors are pairwise decorrelated. If the 2D environment is represented by place-cell-like units, which are quiescent outside their place field, the decorrelation radius is roughly the radius of the typical place field, which is itself proportional to the linear size of the environment times the square root of the sparsity of the neural representation. Thus, if, say, some dozen typical CA3 fields "fit", once properly juxtaposed, in a typical rat recording box, the memory load of the chart corresponding to that box is roughly equivalent to a dozen discrete memories of equal sparsity. The number of such charts, or distinct environments that can be held simultaneously in the network, is limited by the critical value $p_{charts} \approx 0.1\ C\ /\ \ln(1/a)$ (see figures 1 and 2 in Battaglia and Treves 1998). The apparent paradox that fewer charts can be stored if they are sparser (a lower a parameter makes the denominator larger) can be understood by considering that sparser activity, in a large net, leads to better spatial resolution, and hence requires more discrete fixed-point attractors to cover, as effectively smaller tiles, the whole environment. This chart capacity again respects the unproven associative memory theorem mentioned earlier, in that the maximum amount of information that can be retrieved per synapse is about 0.15 bits, as shown in figure 5 of Battaglia and Treves (1998).

The Dentate Gyrus as a Chart Preprocessor

This mapping quantifies the retrieval capacity for charts and opens the way for once more investigating the issue of whether enough new information can be stored in each representation to fully exploit the network capacity for information retrieval. In other words, a quantitative analysis of information storage in a model CA3 network, operating with and without dentate gyrus, would be needed to assess again any information-theoretical advantage in forming new representations. Unfortunately, the very 2D nature of charts makes a simplified mathematical analysis of information storage like the one in Treves and Rolls (1992) not applicable, because neighboring locations on one new chart generate correlated activity that cannot be easily dissected from the interfering correlations with other, unrelated, charts. Mathematical tools based on the newly revealed spatial representation in the dentate are being developed (Treves, Cerasti, and Papp 2008); meanwhile I have reported simplified simulations (Treves 2004). Within their limits, the simulations confirm the essential role of the inputs from the dentate gyrus to CA3 in guiding the learning of a new chart (see figure 3.3).

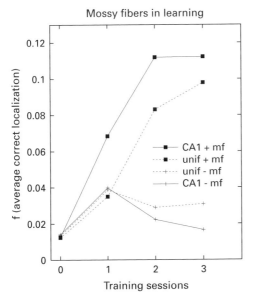

Figure 3.3
Localization accuracy as a function of training session in hippocampal network models with and without the differentiation between CA3 and CA1, and with and without mossy fiber inputs. In the differentiated model, the position of the virtual rat is decoded from the CA1 representation. With reference to figure 3.4, cue size is $Q = 0.2$. Other details in Treves (2004).

It is worth noting that the beneficial forcing effect of mossy fiber inputs to CA3 is even more salient when assessed indirectly in the information content or localization accuracy afforded by representations in CA1, whose units are only indirectly influenced by dentate gyrus activity.

These simple simulations, while supportive of a specific role of the dentate gyrus in information storage, did not take into consideration two major recent findings. One concerns the differences emerging between CA3 and CA1 in the representation of similar, correlated environments; these will be discussed further. The other is the novel observation that the activity of dentate units, previously deemed to be very sparse, seems to be concentrated on a relatively small fraction of newly generated granule cells (Ramirez-Amaya et al. 2006), which are biophysically indistinguishable from older neurons (Laplagne et al. 2006) but appear to "take care" of representing new information more than older, and perhaps already committed, neurons. New recording experiments (Leutgeb et al. 2007) may help clarify how space is coded by dentate granule cells.

At any rate, the crucial prediction of the argument based on the analysis of discrete memories, if applied to charts, is that the inactivation of the mossy fiber synapses should impair the formation of new charts, but not the retrieval of previously stored ones. This prediction has recently been supported at the behavioral level (Lassalle et al. 2000): mice with a temporary inactivation supposedly selective for the mossy synapses were impaired in finding the hidden platform in a Morris water maze, but not if they had learned its location the previous week. A consistent result was more recently obtained in rats with a different, irreversible procedure of selective lesions, and using indicators that only very approximately dissociate storage from retrieval (Lee and Kesner 2004): the strong double dissociation found between perforant path and dentate lesions is remarkable, given the overlapping nature of the behavioral measures. While waiting for neurophysiological experiments to test the prediction at the neural level, the tentative conclusion from behavioral tests in rodents is that indeed the dentate gyrus may have evolved in order to facilitate the storage of new information in the recurrent CA3 network. If validated, this hypothesis suggests that a quantitative information-theoretical advantage may have favored a qualitative change, such as the insertion of the dentate gyrus in the hippocampal circuitry.

CA1 as a Cleanup Device?

The DG argument does not itself address the CA3-CA1 differentiation, which is equally prominent in the mammalian hippocampus. If DG can be understood as a CA3 preprocessor, perhaps CA1 should be understood as a CA3 postprocessor. In reptiles, CA3 and CA1 are structurally homogeneous contiguous portions of the dorsomedial cortex. As this is reorganized into the mammalian hippocampus, CA3 and CA1 differentiate in two important ways. First, only CA3 receives the projections from the dentate gyrus, the mossy fibers. Second, only CA3 is dominated by recurrent collaterals, whereas most of the inputs to CA1 cells are the projections from CA3, the Schaffer collaterals (Amaral et al. 1990).

The simplest version of the postprocessor notion is that it may be useful to add a further feedforward associative network, to clean up memory representations already retrieved, but in incomplete form, by the CA3 network. The extra stage of recoding, if based on more neurons (there are more pyramidal cells in CA1 than in CA3 across all species where numbers have been estimated) could also add robustness to the retrieved representation. Yet a mathematical network analysis of the cleanup notion—in the framework of discrete "episodic memory" fixed-point attractors and neglecting the separate entorhinal cortex inputs directly to CA1—failed to illustrate impressive advantages to adding such a post-processing stage (Treves 1995). Information content grows from CA3 to CA1, but by a minor amount.

A more interesting suggestion comes from a review of neuropsychological studies in rats (Kesner et al. 2002) that indicate a more salient role for CA1 along the temporal dimension. CA3 may specialize in associating information that was experienced strictly at the same time, whereas CA1 may more than CA3 link together information across adjacent times. This may lead to the storage of sequences of instantaneous events, that together build up an episode, or, if the events are not parsed, to effectively continuous attractors along the temporal dimension. A way to formulate a qualitative implication of such a putative functional differentiation is to state that CA1 is important for prediction, i.e., for producing an output representation of what happened just after whatever is represented by the pattern of activity retrieved at the CA3 stage. Note, however, that reading the review by Kesner and colleagues (2002) in full indicates that the table at the end is a well-meaning simplification. Their figure 31.2 suggests that CA3 may be involved in temporal pattern separation just as much as CA1. Moreover, the role of either DG or CA3 in temporal pattern association has not been satisfactorily assessed. Further, available studies on the role of CA1 fail to make a clear distinction between tasks in which massive hippocampal outputs to the cortex are crucial and tasks in which a more limited hippo-campal influence on the cortex may be sufficient. In the first case, lesioning CA1 should have an effect independent of what CA1 specifically contributes to information processing, simply because one is severing the main hippocampo-cortical output pathway. In the second, CA3 outputs through the fimbria/fornix could enable hippocampus-mediated influences to be felt, even if the specific CA1 contribution is absent.

Testing the Prediction of Predictive Coding

I have explored the hypothesis that the differentiation between CA3 and CA1 may help solve precisely the computational conflict between pattern completion, or integrating current sensory information on the basis of memory, and prediction, or moving from one pattern to the next in a stored continuous sequence. To obtain results comparable with typical rat experiments, I have used the same neural network simulations of a virtual rat exploring a small toroidal environment as the ones analyzing the role of dentate inputs to CA3 (Treves 2004). The network model was thus trained to acquire a chart representation of the explored environment as a spatially continuous attractor. Temporal continuity along each trajectory was used to assess the extent to which CA3 would take care of (spatial) pattern completion, while CA1 would concentrate on prediction (i.e., temporal pattern completion). With the simulations one can, at the price of some necessary simplification, compare the performance of the differentiated circuit with a "uniform," nondifferentiated circuit of equal number and type of components (one in which CA3 and CA1 have identical properties, e.g., both receive mossy fibers and are interconnected with recurrent collaterals). Lesion studies, by contrast, can only compare the normal circuit with others with missing components, making it difficult to assess the significance of a differentiation.

The functional differentiation hypothesis was not really convincingly supported by neural network simulations. The conflict between spatial pattern completion, as quantified by localization accuracy, and temporal prediction indeed exists, but two mechanisms that would more directly relate to a functional CA3-CA1 differentiation were found unable to produce genuine prediction. Instead, a simple mechanism based on firing-frequency adaptation in pyramidal cells was found to be sufficient for prediction, with the degree of adaptation as the crucial parameter balancing retrieval with prediction. This is evident from the simulations of the nondifferentiated model. The differentiation between the connectivity of CA3 and CA1 does not really influence the predictiveness, or degree of anticipation, of hippocampal activity. The differentiation has a significant positive effect, however, and, in particular for a given anticipatory interval, it significantly increases, in the model, the information content of hippocampal outputs, making the CA1 representation more informative than the CA3 one (or the nondifferentiated one) when used to decode the position of the virtual rat. Different degrees of adaptation in CA3 and CA1 cells were not, however, found to lead to better performance, further undermining the notion of a full qualitative functional dissociation. There may, therefore, be just a plain quantitative advantage in differentiating the connectivity of the two fields, just as the hypothesis about isocortical lamination holds that there may be just a plain quantitative advantage in differentiating connectivity across layers. In a sense, the outcome of the simulations supports a revised version of the postprocessing cleanup notion. As figure 3.4 shows, the information content in CA1 in the differentiated model is higher than in CA3, with the nondifferentiated model midway between the two.

Correlated Environments Stimulate Orthogonal Ideas

As for the lamination study, the analysis of this hypothesis about the differentiation of hippocampal subfields was based on the simulation of two simplified models, uniform and differentiated, tested on the same task, in this case acquiring a memory chart for a single spatial environment. The accuracy of spatial memory retrieval is subject to the general "spin-glass" limit, and it is further modulated by connectivity details. Recent results obtained recording the activity of multiple hippocampal cells in the labs of Edvard and May-Britt Moser (Leutgeb et al. 2004) and of James Knierim (Lee et al. 2004) indicate a

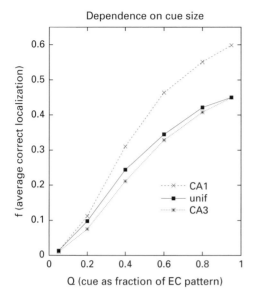

Figure 3.4
Localization accuracy as a function of cue size, after extensive training, in hippocampal network models with and without the differentiation between CA3 and CA1 (and with mossy fiber inputs). In the differentiated model, the position of the virtual rat is better decoded from the CA1 than from the CA3 representation. Simulation details in Treves (2004).

potentially much more dramatic differentiation between CA3 and CA1 units, which has to do with their ability to distinguish among several spatial environments. Activity in CA3 and CA1 was found to differ remarkably when rats were asked to explore environments that some cues suggested were the same, and others, that they were different. CA3 appears to take an all-or-none decision, usually allocating nearly orthogonal neural representations to even very similar environments and switching to essentially identical representations only above a high threshold of physical similarity. Activity in CA1, on the other hand, varies smoothly to reflect the degree of similarity. This functional differentiation and the finding that new representations in CA3 emerge slowly, presumably through iterative processing, are entirely consistent with the recurrent character of the CA3 network and the prevailing feedforward character of the CA1 network. Further surprises have come from applying a "morphing" paradigm, to test spatial representations in environments quasi-continuously changed between two well-learned extremes (Willis et al. 2005; Leutgeb et al. 2005).

In their original form (Treves 2004), the connectivity differentiation models addressed the mechanism linking firing-rate adaptation to the prediction of spatial position within a single environment but could not capture any advantage brought about by the connectivity differentiation having to do with multiple maps. The experimental results have stimulated the development of more elaborate computational models, which however still have to satisfactorily find their way around the spin-glass limit on memory retrieval (see Papp et al. 2007). In fact, training virtual rats on several virtual environments, correlated or not, requires them to be endowed with large virtual brains. Simulations with networks of a thousand units or so, which were adequate for the single-environment case, have to be extended to networks larger by one or two orders of magnitude, which have become time-consuming to simulate extensively. Even then, because of the heavy memory load for multiple environments (Battaglia and Treves 1998), the representations tend to collapse on each other, making the comparison with real rat data more problematic (Papp and Treves 2008). One observation that emerges from this study, already at this stage, is that CA3 representations tend to be more fragmented, in the sense that neural activity in pairs of separate locations can be identical, or quite different, in violation of the metric nature of the environment. CA1 representations tend to be relatively smoother, with a higher match between the distance among locations and the difference among their neural activity vectors. This smoothing function for CA1 strongly resembles the cleanup notion originally investigated for discrete memories, which was relevant also to the notion of prediction, that implies continuity in time but which now finds a more interesting role in reproducing the continuity of physical space. Thanks to the experimental findings with correlated environments, we may be beginning to finally "understand" CA1 and to make some (spatial) sense of the events that drastically altered the structure of our medial pallium hundreds of millions of years ago.

Quality vs. Quantity and the Need to Adapt

All three studies reviewed here require firing-rate adaptation as a crucial ingredient in producing, respectively, a separation between the processing of "what" and "where" information, transitions to different semantic attractor states, and the prediction of future locations in a spatial environment. In all three, memory retrieval is limited by the "spin-glass" constraint. A fundamental dissimilarity is in the relation between qualitative and quantitative changes. In the two "mammalian" studies, the hypothesis is that a major *qualitative* structural change may have served to produce a solely *quantitative* functional advantage. Although the first such hypothesis seems a posteriori more convincing than the second, both are methodologically valid a priori, and in fact it has been noted (Carroll 1988) that often in evolution major steps may subserve only "small" improvements in survival ability. In the "human" study, the hypothesis considered has the opposite flavor: a quantitative change in connectivity (admittedly, a *major* change) would be enough to produce a phase transition to an entirely novel computational faculty—namely, infinite recursion—with its collateral effects including the emergence of language in humans. Although all these hypotheses require much further testing, they serve to underscore the often subtle relations between structure and function that can apply to cortical networks, mediated by the collective emergent dynamics of large populations of neurons.

Acknowledgments

I am grateful to colleagues in the lab of Edvard and May-Britt Moser for letting me participate in their investigations.

References

Abeles M (1991) Corticonics: Neural Circuits of the Cerebral Cortex. Cambridge: Cambridge University Press.

Amaral DG, Ishizuka N, Claiborne B (1990) Neurons, numbers and the hippocampal network. Prog Brain Res 83: 1–11.

Amit DJ (1989) Modeling Brain Function. Cambridge: Cambridge University Press.

Amit DJ, Gutfreund H, Sompolinsky H (1987) Statistical mechanics of neural networks near saturation. Ann Phys (N.Y.) 173: 30–67.

Barton RA (2007) Evolutionary specialization in mammalian cortical structure. J Evolution Biol 20: 1504–1511.

Battaglia FP, Treves A (1998) Attractor neural networks storing multiple space representations: A model for hippocampal place fields. Phys Rev E 58: 7738–7753.

Bingman VP, Jones T-J (1994) Sun-compass based spatial learning impaired in homing pigeons with hippocampal lesions. J Neurosci 14: 6687–6694.

Bingman VP, Sharp PE (2006) Neuronal implementation of hippocampal-mediated spatial behavior: A comparative evolutionary perspective. Behav Cogn Neurosci Rev 5: 80–90.

Bininda-Emonds ORP, Cardillo M, Jones KE, MacPhee RDE, Beck RMD, Greyner R, Price SA, Vos RA, Gittelman JL, Purvis A (2007) The delayed rise of present-day mammals. Nature 446: 507–512.

Bliss TV, Lømo T (1973) Long-lasting potentiation of synaptic transmission in the dentate area of the anaesthetized rabbit following stimulation of the perforant path. J Physiol 232: 331–356.

Braitenberg V, Schüz A (1991) Anatomy of the cortex. Berlin: Springer-Verlag.

Carroll RL (1988) Vertebrate paleontology and evolution. New York: WH Freeman.

Clayton NS, Bussey TJ, Dickinson A (2003) Can animals recall the past and plan for the future? Nat Rev Neurosci 4: 685–691.

Clayton NS, Krebs JR (1995) Memory in food-storing birds: From behaviour to brain. Curr Opin Neurobiol 5: 149–154.

Collingridge GL, Bliss TV (1995) Memories of NMDA receptors and LTP. Trends Neurosci 18: 54–56.

Diamond IT, Conley M, Itoh K, Fitzpatrick D (1985) Laminar organization of geniculocortical projections in *Galago senegalensis* and *Aotus trivirgatus*. J Comp Neurol 242: 584–610.

Diamond IT, Hall WC (1969) Evolution of neocortex. Science 164: 251–262.

Eichenbaum H (2000) A cortical-hippocampal system for declarative memory. Nat Rev Neurosci 1: 41–50.

Elston GN (2000) Pyramidal cells of the frontal lobe: All the more spinous to think with. J Neurosci 20: RC95(1–4).

Finlay BL, Darlington RB (1995) Linked regularities in the development and evolution of mammalian brains. Science 1268: 1578–1584.

Fyhn M, Hafting T, Treves A, Moser EI, Moser M-B (2007) Hippocampal remapping and grid realignment in entorhinal cortex. Nature 446: 190–194.

Fyhn M, Molden S, Witter MP, Moser EI, Moser M-B (2004) Spatial representation in the entorhinal cortex. Science 305: 1258.

Gardner-Medwin AR (1976) The recall of events through the learning of associations between their parts. P Roy Soc Lond B Bio 194: 375–402.

Goffinet AM (2006) What makes us human? A biased view from the perspective of comparative embryology and mouse genetics. J Biomed Discov Collab 1: 16.

Hafting T, Fyhn M, Molden S, Moser M-B, Moser EI (2005) Microstructure of a universal spatial map in the entorhinal cortex. Nature 436: 801–805.

Hasselmo ME, Schnell E (1994) Laminar selectivity of the cholinergic suppression of synaptic transmission in rat hippocampal region CA1: Computational modeling and brain slice physiology. J Neurosci 14: 3898–3914.

Hasselmo ME, Schnell E, Barkai E (1995) Dynamics of learning and recall at excitatory recurrent synapses and cholinergic modulation in rat hippocampal region CA3. J Neurosci 15: 5249–5262.

Hasselmo ME, Wyble B, Wallenstein G (1996) Encoding and retrieval of episodic memories: Role of cholinergic and GABAergic modulation in hippocampus. Hippocampus 6: 693–708.

Hauser MD, Chomsky N, Fitch WT (2002) The faculty of language: What is it, who has it, and how did it evolve? Science 298: 1569–1579.

Hopfield JJ (1982) Neural networks and physical systems with emergent collective computational abilities. Proc Natl Acad Sci USA 79: 2554–2558.

Jerison HJ (1990) Fossil evidence of the evolution of the brain. In: Comparative structure and evolution of cerebral cortex, vol. 8A (Jones EG, Peters A, eds) 285–309. New York: Plenum Press.

Kanter I (1988) Potts-glass models of neural networks. Phys Rev A 37: 2739–2742.

Kesner RP, Gilbert PE, Lee I (2002) Subregional analysis of hippocampal function in the rat. In: Neuropsychology of memory (Squire LR, Schacter DL, eds), 395–411. New York: Guilford Press.

Kropff E, Treves A (2005) The storage capacity of Potts models for semantic memory retrieval. J Stat Mech 2: P08010.

Krubitzer L, Huffman KJ (2000) Arealization of the neocortex in mammals: Genetic and epigenetic contributions to the phenotype. Brain Behav Evol 55: 322–335.

Laplagne DA, Esposito MS, Piatti VC, Morgenstern NA, Zhao C, van Praag H, Gage FH, Schinder AF (2006) Functional convergence of neurons generated in the developing and adult hippocampus. PLoS Biol 4: e409.

Lassalle J-M, Bataille T, Halley H (2000) Reversible inactivation of the hippocampal mossy fiber synapses in mice impairs spatial learning, but neither consolidation nor memory retrieval, in the Morris navigation task. Neurobiol Learn Mem 73: 243–257.

Lee I, Kesner RP (2004) Encoding versus retrieval of spatial memory: Double dissociation between the dentate gyrus and the perforant path inputs into CA3 in the dorsal hippocampus. Hippocampus 14: 66–76.

Lee I, Yoganarasimha D, Rao G, Knierim JJ (2004) Comparison of population coherence of place cells in hippocampal subfields CA1 and CA3. Nature 430: 456–459.

Leutgeb JK, Leutgeb S, Moser M-B, Moser EI (2007) Pattern separation in the dentate gyrus and CA3 of the hippocampus. Science 315: 961–966.

Leutgeb S, Leutgeb JK, Treves A, Moser M-B, Moser EI (2004) Distinct ensemble codes in hippocampal areas CA3 and CA1. Science 305: 1295–1298.

Leutgeb JK, Leutgeb S, Treves A, Meyer R, Barnes CA, McNaughton BL, Moser M-B, Moser EI (2005) Progressive transformation of hippocampal neuronal representations in "morphed" environments. Neuron 48: 345–358.

Mallamaci A, Stoykova A (2006) Gene networks controlling early cerebral cortex arealization. Eur J Neurosci 23: 847–856.

Marr D (1971) Simple memory: A theory for archicortex. Philos T Roy Soc Lond B 262: 24–81.

McNaughton BL, Morris RGM (1987) Hippocampal synaptic enhancement and information storage. Trends Neurosci 10: 408–415.

O'Keefe J, Dostrovsky J (1971) The hippocampus as a spatial map: Preliminary evidence from unit activity in the freely moving rat. Brain Res 34: 171–175.

Papp G, Treves A (2008) Network analysis of the significance of hippocampal subfields. In: Hippocampal place-fields: Relevance to learning and memory (Mizumori S, ed), 328–342. New York: Oxford University Press.

Papp G, Witter MP, Treves A (2007) The CA3 network as a memory store for spatial representations. Learn Memory 14: 732–744.

Ramirez-Amaya V, Marrone DF, Gage FH, Worley PF, Barnes CA (2006) Integration of new neurons into functional neural networks. J Neurosci 26: 12237–12241.

Rolls ET (1989) Functions of neuronal networks in the hippocampus and cerebral cortex in memory. In: Models of brain function (Cotterill R, ed), 15–33. New York: Cambridge University Press.

Roudi Y, Treves A (2006) Localized activity profiles and storage capacity of rate-based autoassociative networks. Phys Rev E 73: 061904.

Samsonovich A, McNaughton BL (1997) Path integration and cognitive mapping in a continuous attractor neural network model. J Neurosci 17: 5900–5920.

Skaggs WE, Knierim JJ, Kudrimoti HS, McNaughton BL (1995) A model of the neural basis of the rat's sense of direction. In: Advances in neural information processing systems (Tesauro G, Touretzky D and Leen T, eds), 173–180. Cambridge, MA: MIT Press.

Sompolinsky H, Shapley R (1997) New perspectives on the mechanisms for orientation selectivity. Curr Opin Neurobiol 7: 514–522.

Treves A (1995) Quantitative estimate of the information relayed by the Schaffer collaterals. J Comput Neurosci 2: 259–272.

Treves A (2003) Computational constraints that may have favoured the lamination of sensory cortex. J Comput Neurosci 14: 271–282.

Treves A (2004) Computational constraints between retrieving the past and predicting the future, and the CA3-CA1 differentiation. Hippocampus 14: 539.

Treves A (2005) Frontal latching networks: A possible neural basis for infinite recursion. Cognitive Neuropsych 21: 276–291.

Treves A, Cerasti E, Papp G (2008) The dentate gyrus and the formation of new spatial representations in CA3. 6th FENS Forum abstract 225.25.

Treves A, Rolls ET (1991) What determines the capacity of autoassociative memories in the brain? Network 2: 371–397.

Treves A, Rolls ET (1992) Computational constraints suggest the need for two distinct input systems to the hippocampal CA3 network. Hippocampus 4: 374–391.

Treves A, Tashiro A, Witter ME, Moser EI (2008) What is the mammalian dentate gyrus good for? Neuroscience 154: 1155–1172.

Ulinski PS (1990) The cerebral cortex of reptiles. In: Cerebral cortex, volume 8A: Comparative structure and evolution of cerebral cortex (Jones EG, Peters A, eds), 139–215. New York: Plenum Press.

Ullman MT (2001) A neurocognitive perspective on language: The declarative/procedural model. Nat Rev Neurosci 2: 717–726.

Willis TJ, Lever C, Cacucci F, Burgess N, O'Keefe J (2005) Attractor dynamics in the hippocampal representation of the local environment. Science 308: 873–876.

Willshaw D, Buckingham J (1990) An assessment of Marr's theory of the hippocampus as a temporary memory store. Philos T Roy Soc Lond B 329: 205–215.

Wilson EO (1975) Sociobiology. The new synthesis. Cambridge, MA: Harvard University Press.

Wilson MA, McNaughton BL (1993) Dynamics of the hippocampal ensemble code for space. Science 261: 1055–1058.

Yamamori T, Rockland KS (2006) Neocortical areas, layers, connections, and gene expression. Neurosci Res 55: 11–27.

4 Space for the Brain in Cognitive Science

Neil Burgess, Christian F. Doeller, and Chris M. Bird

The focus of cognitive science is to understand behavior at the algorithmic level, aiming to understand how the amazing competences of humans and animals in their daily tasks could be achieved. A substantial proportion of cognitive scientists have argued that the brain could safely be ignored in this endeavor, since neuroscience research simply did not provide data at the appropriate level. And for many decades they were largely correct in this view and in good company with many researchers in artificial intelligence and the traditional wing of psychology in which the emphasis was strictly on the "psyche". Despite the pioneering advances in electrophysiology in the 1960s and 70s, inspiration was predominantly sought from the concurrent explosion in digital computing (both advances driven by the breakthrough in semiconductor devices).

Here we provide two examples from spatial cognition of why, in our view, cognitive neuroscience is now becoming a serious source of inspiration to cognitive science, in the same way that artificial computers, production systems, and the like were previously. In some ways this chapter parallels other chapters in this volume which describe how cognitive science is waking up to the inspiration available from other aspects of biology, as exemplified by the developmental and evolutionary approaches to cognition. And, in common with these chapters, we apologize to the increasingly many readers who will say "but of course, cognitive science has always been open to such sources of inspiration." To those readers we merely point out the, hopefully decreasingly few, cognitive scientists resolutely refusing to be contaminated by impure thoughts about the brain, or being dragged reluctantly, kicking and screaming, in that direction.

We argue that recent and not-so-recent advances in cognitive neuroscience, particularly single-unit recording, in combination with neuropsychology and fMRI (functional magnetic resonance imaging), provides valuable insights into the organization of spatial cognition. In some cases these insights provide clear added value to the inferences that can be made from behavioral studies alone. Here we focus on memory for locations in large-scale space, a paradigm that benefits from being applicable to humans and other animals in rather similar forms. We argue that the representations and processes underlying this type of spatial memory can be understood in terms of the brain systems in medial temporal lobe, neostriatum, and parietal cortex, which support them. In this endeavor, computational modeling provides an important bridge between the various levels of analysis (neuronal or synaptic, systems neuroscience, behavior).

To illustrate these points we focus on a number of current controversies in spatial cognition. First, we examine the proposal that object locations are solely represented in an egocentric fashion by well-oriented participants (e.g., Wang and Spelke 2002). That is, object locations are represented relative to the participant, and are not represented relative to the locations of other objects or landmarks within the environment. Having argued for the existence of allocentric as well as egocentric representations, we go on to explore whether multiple types of allocentric representations exist. Specifically, we explore the proposal that the surface geometry of the environment is processed in an independent manner from environmental features (also known as a "geometric module" within spatial cognition; see, e.g., Gallistel 1990). Evidence for a geometric processing system exists, but there is little support for the proposal that these representations are "encapsulated" and thus unavailable to other parallel spatial representations. Last, we present evidence that the processing of the surface geometry of the surrounding environment obeys different learning rules than the processing of local environmental features. In all these cases, we argue that evidence from neuroscience inspired the novel behavioral tests that have shed light upon these controversies.

Egocentric vs. Allocentric Representations

It has often been argued that the presence of "allocentric," or "geocentric" (world-centered), representations of location cannot be inferred from behavioral results alone, as alternative explanations requiring solely "egocentric" (body-centered) representation can often be found (e.g., Bennett 1996). A refinement of this position was recently provided by Wang and Spelke (2002), which provides an interesting model of spatial cognition in its own right. This model holds that the basic cognitive functions supporting spatial behavior depend solely upon egocentric representations, plus the use of a separate "geometric module" (e.g., Cheng 1986; Gallistel 1990). The egocentric processes include viewpoint-dependent scene recognition and spatial updating of egocentric locations by self-motion information, whereas the geometric module is solely used for reorientation of disoriented subjects.

Evidence from Neuroscience

Egocentric representations of the location of a stimulus or the end-point of an action abound in the sensory and motor cortices (e.g., neurons responding to visual stimulation in a specific retinal location in visual cortical areas; or neurons responding to an action in a particular reaching direction in motor cortical areas). Nonetheless, it is important to be aware of the diversity of the multiple, often redundant, parallel representations available in the brain. Thus, allocentric representation of one's own location relative to the surrounding environment can be seen in the mammalian hippocampus of rats (O'Keefe 1976) and primates (Ono et al. 1991). This representation is supported by representations of orientation (Taube 1998) and a gridlike representation suitable for path integration (Hafting et al. 2005) in nearby regions, both also environment-centered (see next section for details). These representations appear to be available to guide behavior, and do so in spatial memory paradigms in which simple egocentric representations do not suffice to guide behavior (reviewed in detail in a later section). In these more complex situations, behavioral responses match the firing of the cells (Lenck-Santini et al. 2001; Lenck-Santini et al. 2005; O'Keefe and Speakman 1987), and hippocampal lesions or inactivation impair performance (e.g., Morris et al. 1982; Packard and McGaugh 1996).

These results were found in nonhuman animals, but there are reasons to believe that they may generalize to humans. Thus, making use of virtual environments, responses resembling those of place cells have been found in the human brain, clustered in the hippocampus (Ekstrom et al. 2003), while functional neuroimaging (Maguire et al. 1998; Hartley et al. 2003; Iaria et al. 2003) and neuropsychological (Abrahams et al. 1997; Spiers et al. 2001a, 2001b; King et al. 2002; King et al. 2004) data confirm the involvement of the human hippocampus in spatial memory in similar memory paradigms to those in which the hippocampus has been implicated in other animals. Hartley and colleagues (2004) reported purely behavioral data that are consistent with similar spatial representations being present in humans as in other animals. The authors trained participants to learn the positions of objects in a rectangular arena surrounded by distant landmarks, and subsequently replace these objects in their correct locations. On some trials, the dimensions of the arena were varied between presentation and test. These spatial manipulations modulated the participants' responses, in line with a model of spatial memory based on storing hippocampal place cell representations (the boundary vector cell model; discussed in a later section).

One of the three experiments in which Wang and Spelke developed their 2002 hypothesis was performed by Wang and Simons (1999). In this experiment (see figure 4.1), participants view a spatial array of objects on a circular table, and their memory is tested after a short delay by asking them which object in the array had been moved. By cleverly varying the participant's viewpoint and the orientation of the array, it was possible to probe for the presence of two types of representations of the locations of objects in the array. The first type of representation, "visual snapshots," are viewpoint-dependent representations of the appearance of the array, and these would aid behavior if the participant's view of the array was the same at presentation and test. The second type of representation, egocentric representations of location which are automatically updated by the participant's movement, would aid behavior if the object locations remained stationary while the subject

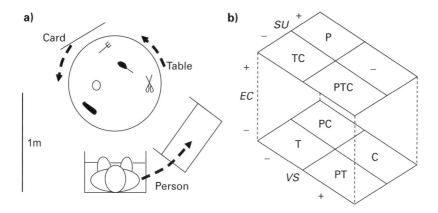

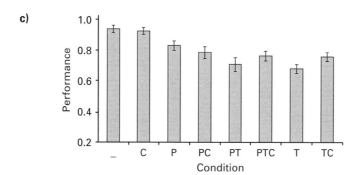

Figure 4.1

Spatial-memory performance is consistent with the presence of (at least) three representations of location: *visual snapshots* (VS); egocentric representations that are *spatially updated* by self-motion (SU); allocentric representations of location relative to an *external cue* (EC). (a) Participants view an array of five phosphorescent objects on a round table and a phosphorescent card (the EC) in the dark. After a brief delay, they are asked to indicate which of the objects has been moved. (b) Between viewing and test, any combination of the person (P), table (T) or card (C) may move so that the test configuration is consistent (+) or inconsistent (−) with VS, SU, or EC representations in a 2 × 2 × 2 factorial design. (c) Performance (proportion of trials correct) shows beneficial effects of consistency with all three types of representation. Conditions corresponding to no change (_), and movement of P, PT, and T replicate the effects of consistency with SU (helping when the table does not rotate compared to when it does) and VS (helping when the table stays or rotates in synch with the person) found by Wang and Simons (1999); the additional effect of the EC can be seen in the other four conditions (helping when it moves with the table: PTC versus PT, TC versus T; hindering when it moves without the table, C versus _, PC versus P). Error bars show the standard error of the mean. Adapted from Burgess et al. (2004).

moved. The experiment found evidence for both kinds of egocentric representation, with the greatest effect for spatially updated representations.

However, baseline performance, when the array is rotated alone (and so is incompatible with both kinds of representation) is quite good, allowing for the possibility that other types of representation are present in parallel that aid performance. In addition, no direct experimental manipulation was made that would affect any allocentric representations that might be present. Indeed, the test conditions compatible with egocentric spatial updating are also compatible with allocentric representations: in these conditions the array remained fixed relative to the testing room, which was fully visible. To attempt to control for this, Simons and Wang (1998) performed a separate experiment in the dark in which they used phosphorescent objects; again they found an effect of consistency with spatial updating. However, no direct comparison between the experiments was performed, and an apparent reduction in performance in the dark may indeed reflect the use of allocentric representations in the light.

To test for the presence of allocentric representations we performed a third variation: explicitly manipulating a single large visual cue, external to the array (see figure 4.1). Thus, by employing a fully factorial design, we were able to separately examine three types of representations: visual snapshots; egocentric representations updated by self-motion; and representations relative to the external cue (Burgess et al. 2004). Improved performance was seen whenever the test array was oriented consistently with any of these stored representations. Therefore, there is evidence that all three representations are available to participants and independently contribute to performance (see Burgess 2006 for further discussion).

Another interesting phenomenon that has been used to investigate the nature of spatial representations is the "disorientation effect" (Wang and Spelke 2000). In these experiments, participants learn the locations of several objects in a room. They are then asked to point to the remembered locations of the objects both before and after a disorientation procedure (which is ostensibly to remove path integration). The variability in the pointing errors increased significantly after disorientation, which was interpreted by Wang and Spelke as evidence that relatively precise egocentric representations of space underpin spatial memory, and these representations are degraded after disorientation. They concluded that the relatively inaccurate performance following disorientation cast doubt on the existence of enduring allocentric representations. Nevertheless, there is evidence that whilst allocentric representations may be less precise than egocentric representations, they are more enduring and are favored in certain circumstances. For example, Waller and Hodgson (2006) replicated Wang and Spelke's disorientation effect, but further showed that equivalent levels of performance decrement were observed after a rotation of 135 degrees, even though the participants were not disoriented. Furthermore, disorientation had no effect on pointing errors to objects made on the basis of long-term memory (objects in the participants' bedrooms) and it actually facilitated judgments of relative directions between newly learned object locations. In another series of experiments investigating the disorientation effect, Mou and colleagues (2006) demonstrated that allocentric representations of object arrays are favored when a large number of objects are to be learned, particularly when they are viewed from outside of the array and when the layout of the objects has salient intrinsic axes. Evidence for multiple spatial representations was also reported by Schmidt and Lee (2006) on the basis of both reaction time and pointing errors on two immersive spatial learning tasks. One task investigated the effect of object-centered representations (learning the location of surrounding objects configured in a triangular arrangement) or salient environmental representations (learning the location of surrounding objects in a neutral configuration surrounded by a triangular room). In addition to strong egocentric effects, retrieval accuracy was improved when imagined heading direction was consistent with both object- and environment-centered representations.

In summary: By looking at the neural representations of location in animals, we were inspired to search for behavioral evidence of allocentric spatial representations that had been previously overlooked (Wang and Spelke 2002). It is now apparent that multiple, parallel forms of spatial representations (including allocentric) exist, all of which can influence behavior, with specific representations favored in certain circumstances, contingent upon task demands. In the next section we discuss the characteristics of these different putative spatial representations in more detail.

Distinct Neural Systems for Specific Types of Spatial Information: Reinterpretation of the "Geometric Module"

Animals can navigate to an unmarked location using a variety of strategies. For example, assuming that animals are capable of judging directions, the relative angles to three or more identifiable landmarks can unambiguously define a location in (two-dimensional) space. In an enclosed area, assuming animals are capable of judging distance, one or more sufficiently distant landmarks can specify orientation so that a location can then be defined in terms of distance and direction to a local landmark or to the boundary of the arena. Last, a single local landmark that includes an unambiguous heading direction and distance (such as a signpost) can also specify a location. In this section we discuss the middle example, where distal landmark information determines the subject's orientation, and this must be integrated with information about the location of a boundary, or a local landmark (with no intrinsic axis), referred to here as boundary and landmark learning, respectively. We will argue that all three types of information processing (orientation relative to distal landmarks and bearings to boundaries or to local landmarks) have distinct neuroanatomical substrates.

As noted, neurons in different parts of the brain appear to represent different types of spatial information. Here we consider how evidence from neuroscience relates to proposals based on analyses of behavior, that distinct processing modules support different aspects of behavior by performing different types of computation. First we briefly review the neuroscientific evidence that three specific types of information are represented by different neuronal systems: orientation relative to the environment; locations defined relative to environmental surface geometry; locations defined relative to local landmarks. We then consider how these systems for defining locations combine in human spatial memory, and whether they operate under the same or different learning rules. Finally, we consider how our neuroscience-inspired categorization of function compares to a closely related proposal from cognitive science: that of a "geometric module" for reorientation that processes surface geometry as opposed to local landmarks or featural information (Cheng 1986; Cheng and Newcombe 2005; Gallistel 1990).

Head-Direction Cells and Orientation

In 1990, Taube and colleagues identified a class of neurons that appear to provide a metric for orientation (Taube et al. 1990a, 1990b). The cells were tuned to discharge whenever an animal's head faces a particular direction, irrespective of its location within an environment. These units have become known as "head-direction cells." Head-direction-cell firing is largely independent of the animal's ongoing behavior (whether the animal is moving or stationary) and these cells maintain their directional preferences in the dark, demonstrating that they can be driven by purely idiothetic information, such as proprioceptive inflow and motor outflow (also known as "efference copy"). In the light, however, head-direction cells can be controlled by visual landmarks, and rotation of the landmark leads to a corresponding shift in the directional preferences of the cells (Taube et al. 1990b). Furthermore, head-direction cells are driven by distal, background cues rather than local foreground cues (Zugaro et al. 2001). When head-direction cells are recorded simultaneously with place cells, it is possible to investigate whether the spatial representations in these two systems are consistent with each other. It was shown that both head-direction cells and place cells may be driven by idiothetic or distal visual cues, and when the directional firing of head-direction cells rotates following a manipulation of one of these sources of input, the place cell ensemble also rotates in the same direction by the same amount (Hargreaves et al. 2007). Head-direction cells are found throughout Papez's circuit, including the postsubiculum, anterior thalamus, and retrosplenial cortex.

Is there any direct evidence that head-direction-cell firing encodes the animal's sense of direction? Dudchenko and Taube (1997) used a radial arm maze task to demonstrate that not only were head-direction cells usually controlled by a distal orienting cue but also that behavioral responses in the task were consistent with head-direction-cell firing. Critically, on the few occasions when a rat's behavioral responses did not shift following a cue rotation, the head-direction cells also did not shift their firing patterns. Lesions of the head-direction system, caused by cytotoxic injections in the anterior thalamic nuclei, cause profound spatial impairments in rats (Aggleton et al. 1996). Using a variant of the well-known Morris Water Maze, it was shown that lesioned rats were impaired in their ability to navigate to a hidden platform on the basis of distal landmarks. Interestingly, the same rats were also unable to navigate to the hidden platform on the basis of a local landmark—they could not derive the correct directional heading from the landmark from the distal cue (Wilton et al. 2001). In contrast, anterior thalamic lesions do not impair rats' ability to navigate to a visible landmark (Sutherland and Rodriguez 1989).

Hippocampus and Location Relative to Environmental Geometry

Over the past thirty years there has been a wealth of studies investigating the spatial firing properties of hippocampal "place cells" in rats. For example, the receptive fields of place cells in open field environments are independent of the animal's orientation (Muller and Kubie 1989). In enclosed environments, place cell firing is strongly driven by the presence of continuous boundaries. O'Keefe and Burgess (1996) recorded from the same cells in similar (rectangular) environments that differed in their dimensions. They observed that the location of peak firing typically remained in a constant position relative to the nearest walls and additionally, several of the fields were stretched along the axes of the environment. On the basis of these and related findings, it was proposed that place cells received inputs that are tuned to respond to the presence of a barrier at a given distance along a given allocentric direction—the so-called boundary vector cell (BVC) model (Barry et al. 2006; Hartley et al. 2000; see figure 4.2). The allocentric direction is likely to be set by head-direction cells since the place cell ensemble rotates so as to be consistent with them (see earlier discussion). The BVC model has been used to successfully predict the pattern of place cell firing in novel environments (Hartley et al. 2000; O'Keefe and Burgess 1996). Studies have also shown that place cell firing corresponds to behavioral choices in spatial memory tasks (O'Keefe and Speakman, 1987; Lenck-Santini et al. 2001). Moreover, the BVC model also predicted the behavior in humans performing a spatial memory task, suggesting that similar environmental cues are used to remember unmarked locations across species (Hartley et al. 2004, reviewed in the previous section; see Ekstrom et al. 2003, for evidence of place cells in humans). In contrast to the robust effect of environmental boundaries on place cell firing, discrete landmarks within an environment have very little effect on place cell firing (Cressant et al. 1997).

The single-unit data, summarized briefly earlier, seems to indicate preferential processing of the surface geometry of the environment by a specific brain region, the hippocampus, a region identified as providing a "cognitive map" (see O'Keefe and Nadel 1978). There is considerable evidence that the hippocampus plays a critical role in aspects of spatial memory functions. Hippocampal lesions dramatically impair performance on the

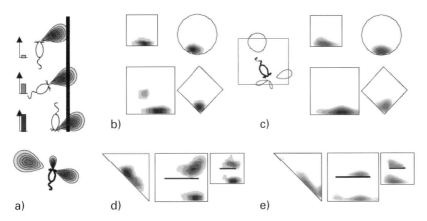

Figure 4.2
Model of the influence on place cell firing of the surface geometry of the environment, given that a stable directional reference frame is provided by distal cues. Place cell firing fields ("place fields") are a thresholded linear sum of the firing of "boundary vector cells" (BVCs). (a) Above: Each BVC has a Gaussian tuned response to the presence of a boundary at a given distance and bearing from the rat (independent of the rat's orientation). Below: The sharpness of tuning of a BVC decreases as the distance to which it is tuned increases. The only free parameters of a BVC are the distance and direction of peak response. (b): Place fields recorded from the same cell in four environments of different shape or orientation relative to distal cues. (c): Simulation of the place fields in (b) by the best-fitting set of four BVCs constrained to be in orthogonal directions (BVCs shown on the left, simulated fields on the right). The simulated cell can now be used to predict firing in novel situations. Real and predicted data from three novel environments are shown in (d) and (e), respectively, showing good qualitative agreement. Adapted from Hartley et al. (2000).

classic version of the water maze, where rats must use distal landmark information as well as distance to the maze boundary to locate a hidden platform (Morris et al. 1982). Interestingly, the maze wall is a powerful cue used to locate the platform, even when it is transparent, illustrating the importance of continuous boundaries for navigation (Maurer and Derivaz 2000). Similar to rats with lesions to the anterior thalamus (with presumed disruption of the head-direction system), hippocampal lesions do not disrupt the ability to navigate toward a visible landmark. It is, however, important that unlike anterior thalamic lesions, hippocampal damage does not impair the ability of rats to locate a hidden platform when its position is indicated by the combination of a local cue and distal landmarks (Pearce et al. 1998). Thus, the hippocampus may not be necessary to derive a heading direction from distant landmarks.

Another paradigm used to assess spatial memory is the plus maze, which consists of four arms arranged in a cross. In the plus maze task rats are trained in an initial learning phase to retrieve food from the end of one arm (e.g., West), starting from another arm (e.g., South). This paradigm can be used to elegantly study whether rats learn to navigate to the food through learning a stereotyped response (turn left), or through learning the place within the test room (presumably defined by distal cues in the environment). The use of a response or a place strategy can be assessed during a probe trial in which rats start from a novel arm (e.g., North). The rat could either follow the learned response—turning left and thus search for food in the East arm (response strategy)—or follow a place strategy and searching in the original food arm (West). In probe trials after eight and sixteen days of training, healthy rats shifted from approaching the "place" associated with food after eight days to making the turn "response" associated with food after sixteen days. However, injections of lidocaine to inactivate the hippocampus abolished place learning (Packard and McGaugh 1996).

Striatum and Location Relative to Local Landmarks

Although the hippocampus has been implicated in spatial processing of distal landmarks and environmental boundaries, other systems are involved in learning sequences of behavioral responses to visual cues. This system involves a part of the basal ganglia, the dorsal striatum, and has been conceptualized as "habit learning" (see Yin and Knowlton 2006). Lesion studies in rodents have provided evidence for the independence of this system from the other systems just described. Packard and McGaugh demonstrated that injection of lidocaine into the dorsal striatum of rats left place learning in the plus maze intact, but impaired the ability of rats to learn to use a response strategy. In the water maze, basal ganglia lesions impair rats' ability to learn to swim to a safe platform identified by a distinctive pattern. In contrast, the same rats are capable of learning to swim to a safe platform that remains in a constant location relative to external landmarks (Packard and McGaugh 1992; McDonald and White 1994).

To summarize, these double dissociations between information-processing systems illustrate that different types of representations are available to animals when they are solving spatial tasks. As described, the head-direction system found throughout Papez's circuit may provide a metric for orientation, whereas the hippocampus has been identified with environment-centered representations of locations and the dorsal striatum has been associated with approach responses to a single landmark. It is reasonable to assume that the striatal system would be necessary to locate unmarked locations by using a visible local landmark in conjunction with external orienting cues. Taking these studies as inspiration, we investigated whether there was evidence for similar dissociable neural substrates of spatial learning systems in the human brain.

Neural Systems for Processing Boundaries vs. Landmarks in Humans: How They Learn and How They Combine

We recently investigated spatial memory in a paradigm designed to dissociate memory for locations relative to either an environmental boundary or to a local landmark, and to investigate the learning rules used within each type of memory. Using desktop virtual reality we created an object-location memory task in which some objects, without being distinguished by any explicit instructions, maintained a fixed relation to the environmental boundary while others maintained a fixed relation to a single intramaze landmark. Functional MRI was used to examine the neural bases of learning and remembering the locations of the objects (Doeller et al. 2008), while a series of behavioral experiments tested the associative properties of the learning to either type of environmental cue (Doeller and Burgess 2008).

Participants explored a virtual-reality arena bounded by a circular wall, containing a single landmark, and surrounded by distant orientation cues. Within this arena they encountered four objects in four different locations (see figure 4.3). On each subsequent trial they saw a picture of one of the objects (the "cue phase") and indicated its location within the arena by navigating to it from a random start location and making a button-press response (the "replace" phase). Following this, the object then appeared in its correct location and was collected (the "feedback" phase). Each set of sixteen trials (four per object) made up a block, with four blocks in the entire experiment. Critically, the landmark and boundary were moved relative to each other between blocks, with two objects maintaining their location relative to the boundary and two relative to the landmark. Within each block, participants gradually learned the relationship between object locations and landmark or boundary, using the feedback provided. "Memory performance" was measured in terms of the proximity of response location to the correct location, and "learning" during the feedback phase, as the improvement in performance on the next trial with the same object. The relative influence of landmark or boundary on responding was reflected implicitly by the distance of the indicated location from the locations predicted by either cue. Both cues played functionally equivalent roles in the task and were not distinguished in the participants' instructions, and their relation to the distant orientation cues remained unchanged, as these were projected at infinity.

On a behavioral level, participants learned both types of cue associations in a similar manner. A performance increase could be observed within and across blocks (figure 4.4). Interestingly, participants' responses were influenced by both cues when both types of object were replaced. As well as quantifying the influence of each cue on responses, we also quantified the extent to which responses reflected use of the incorrect cue. Our results indicate that inaccurate responses largely reflected use of the incorrect cue early in each block.

These analyses established that participants were able to learn the positions of the objects relative to both landmarks and boundaries. Behaviorally they did not appear to favor one type of cue over the other. However, according to our hypothesis, learning to the landmark should engage components of the basal ganglia while learning to the boundary should engage the hippocampal system. This hypothesis was supported by the imaging data. At the neural level, activity in the right caudate nucleus, which is part of the dorsal

a) Virtual reality environment

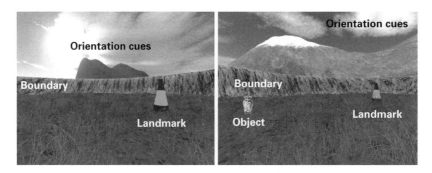

b) Trial structure

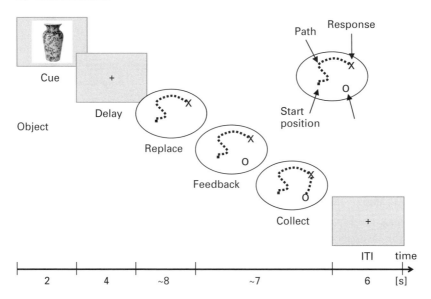

Figure 4.3
A virtual-reality paradigm for separating the contributions of an environmental boundary and an intramaze landmark on memory for object locations. (a): The virtual arena from the participant's perspective (different viewpoints) showing the intramaze landmark (traffic cone), the boundary (circular wall), the distal orientation cues (mountains, which were projected at infinity) and one object (vase). (b): Trial structure. Participants are cued with an object followed by the replace phase after a short delay. Here participants have to indicate the location of the cued object by navigating to the object's expected location and pressing a button. This phase was followed by presentation of the object at the correct position, which the participants then had to collect (feedback phase). The replace phase is assumed to reflect spatial memory, whereas spatial learning is assumed to occur during the feedback phase. Trials occur in blocks, between which the intramaze landmark and boundary can be moved relative to each other: the correct location for "landmark-related" objects maintains its position relative to the landmark; the correct location for "boundary-related" objects maintains its position relative to the boundary. Adapted from Doeller et al. (2008).

a) Behavioral results

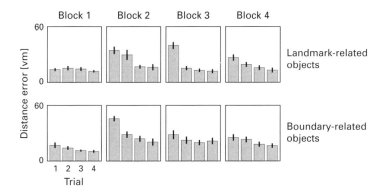

b) fMRI results

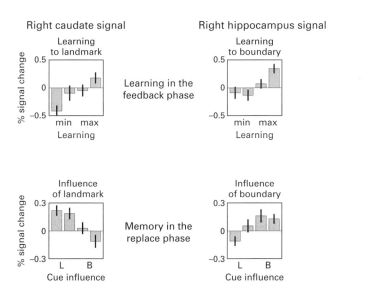

Figure 4.4
fMRI study of the neural bases of landmark and boundary processing in spatial memory. (a) Mean performance (distance to the correct object location) is depicted separately for landmark-related objects (top row) and boundary-related objects (bottom row), separately for each block and trial (±SEM). The performance measures are collapsed across both objects per object type and averaged across all participants. As apparent from the figure, performance is roughly equivalent for each object type and increases at similar rates within and across blocks. (b) Bar plots show mean fMRI signal in the right caudate and right posterior hippocampus in the feedback phase (above) and replace phase (below). Above: Activation in the feedback phase was analyzed as a function of the amount learned from the feedback received. For each object type, amount learned was parameterized as the improvement in performance from the current trial to the next trial for that object. Landmark-related learning corresponded to significant activation of the right caudate nucleus. Boundary-related learning corresponded to activation of the right posterior hippocampus. Below: Activation in the replace phase was analyzed as a function of the relative influence of each cue on replacement. This was parameterized by the relative proximity of the replacement location to the two locations predicted by the relationship to the landmark and boundary in the previous block. The influence of the landmark corresponded to the activation of the right caudate. The influence of the boundary corresponded to the activation of the right hippocampus. Adapted from Doeller et al. (2008).

striatum correlated with the amount of learning relative to the landmark, whereas learning of boundary-related objects corresponded to right posterior hippocampal activity during the feedback phase. This dissociation between both systems was also observed during the replace phase, with landmark-based trials associated with increased caudate activity and with right posterior hippocampus involvement in boundary-based trials (see figure 4.4). Thus, differential activity seen in the caudate and hippocampus corresponded to the acquisition and expression of information about locations derived from environmental landmarks or boundaries, respectively.

Our results suggest that human spatial memory recruits two distinct systems (hippocampus and striatum) to process information about different aspects of the environment during navigation (boundaries vs. landmarks). These data are entirely consistent with studies of the neural substrates of spatial behavior in rats and primates (see earlier discussion). Given that these systems appear to be neurally dissociable, we further investigated whether they obeyed different learning rules.

Associative learning theory has been proposed as a general model for animal learning (Pavlov 1927; Rescorla and Wagner 1972; Mackintosh 1975; Dickinson 1980; Pearce and Hall 1980). This type of (incremental) associative learning on the basis of a single common error signal, and its more recent incarnation as "reinforcement learning" (Sutton and Barto 1988), in which error is signaled by dopamine (Waelti et al. 2001; Schultz et al. 1997), makes explicit predictions about patterns of learning to multiple cues. In these models of learning, environmental cues are associated with expected reinforcement, and a global error signal (the difference between the actual and the expected reinforcement) is used to modify these associations. The extent to which one cue already accurately predicts feedback will reduce the learning of associations from other cues, because it reduces the global error. Thus, when prior learning to one cue allows accurate prediction of reinforcement, it is said to "block" subsequent learning to other cues. Similarly, if learning to two cues occurs concurrently, the presence of one or other cue may "overshadow" learning to the other.

In the spatial domain, previous studies in humans and rats found evidence that the key predictions of reinforcement learning on the basis of a single error term appear to hold in spatial tasks, e.g., blocking (Hamilton and Sutherland 1999) or overshadowing (Chamizo et al. 2003) between distal cues, or blocking and overshadowing between distal cues and asymmetrical boundary geometry (Pearce et al. 2006). However, a qualitatively different form of learning, depending only on co-occurrence (Hebb 1949), has long been proposed for some aspects of spatial learning, in which "incidental" and "latent" learning occurs in the absence of reinforcement or behavioral outcome (Tolman 1948; Gallistel 1990), and is associated with the hippocampus (O'Keefe and Nadel 1978). Given the results of the fMRI analysis, we hypothesized that learning to the landmark, associated with the dorsal striatum, would conform to the predictions of "associative" or "reinforcement" learning, whereas learning to the boundary, associated with the hippocampus, would be incidental, and not show these predictions.

In several behavioral studies we examined the nature of learning in both systems in more detail (figure 4.5). We predicted that learning relative to the landmark would show overshadowing and blocking whereas learning relative to the boundary would continue, irrespective of learning to the other cues.

In the first experiment we examined overshadowing between landmark and boundary as cues to object location (in all cases the distal orientation cues were present, as we wanted to avoid disorientation as a potentially confounding variable). Four groups of subjects were tested while they were performing the equivalent of block 1 in the fMRI task described earlier. In a first learning phase, feedback regarding the object's correct location was provided after each response. Groups 1 and 3 learned four object locations with both cues (landmark and boundary) present. Group 2 learned object locations with only the boundary present, and group 4 learned object locations with only the landmark present.

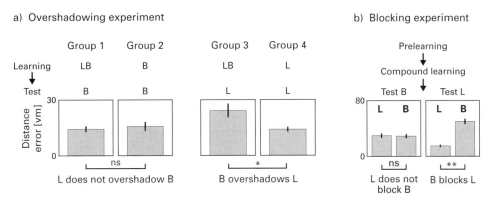

Figure 4.5
Landmark-related learning obeys associative error correction but boundary-related learning does not. Reinforcement learning with a single error term (including "associative learning theory" based on the Rescorla-Wagner rule) predicts that learning to behave on the basis of one cue will reduce the error term and thus reduce learning to behave on the basis of a second cue. Learning to the second cue is said to be "overshadowed" if learning to both cues occurs concurrently, or "blocked" if learning to the first cue precedes learning to the second. (a) Overshadowing experiment. Four different groups (columns) learned four object locations with either or both landmark (L) and boundary (B) present and were tested with either landmark or boundary alone. When both cues are present, learning to the boundary overshadows learning to the landmark (see replacement error for groups 3 and 4), but learning to the landmark does not overshadow learning to the boundary (see groups 1 and 2). (b) Blocking experiment. Participants performed "prelearning" of eight object locations (eight blocks with different configurations of landmark versus boundary; four object locations paired with the landmark, four with the boundary) followed by "compound learning" (with both cues fixed). Performance was tested with either cue alone (left: test with boundary; right: test with landmark). Right: When participants were tested with the landmark, their performance on objects associated with the boundary during prelearning (bar B) was worse than on objects associated with the landmark during prelearning (bar L). The prior learning to the boundary blocked learning to the landmark during the compound learning phase. Left: When tested with the boundary, performance was equally good on objects associated with either landmark or boundary during prelearning (bars L and B). Prior learning to the landmark did not block learning to the boundary during the compound learning phase. Adapted from Doeller and Burgess (2008).

Memory performance was then tested in the presence of either the boundary (group 1 and 2) or the landmark (group 3 and 4) alone (without feedback). No performance difference was observed between both groups tested with the boundary (group 1 and 2), indicating that participants had learned the relationship to the boundary equally well, irrespective of whether the landmark was also available. By contrast, during the landmark test, performance was impaired in group 3 relative to group 4. These data indicate that the presence of the boundary for group 3 had overshadowed learning to the landmark, which had occurred much more strongly in the absence of the boundary for group 4. Thus, learning to the landmark was overshadowed by the boundary, but learning to the boundary had not been overshadowed by the landmark. Furthermore, in two control experiments we ruled out that the overshadowing effect was due to the salience of the boundary or a generalization decrement after removing the boundary in group 3.

In a second experiment, we examined blocking. In a first phase, participants underwent a prelearning session, with landmark and boundary moving relative to each other at the beginning of each block. During prelearning the locations of four objects were associated with the landmark (maintaining a constant position relative to the landmark), and four other object locations were associated with the boundary (maintaining a constant position relative to the boundary). During a second phase, both the landmark and the boundary were fixed and could thus be associated to the positions of all eight objects (the "compound learning" phase). During two final test phases (without feedback), memory performance was tested in the presence of the landmark or the boundary alone. When tested with the boundary, performance did not differ between objects associated with landmark or boundary during prelearning: their locations relative to the boundary were learned equally well during the compound learning phase—prior association to the landmark did not block subsequent learning to the boundary. However, when tested with the landmark, performance was much worse for the objects associated with the boundary during prelearning. Their prior association to the boundary blocked learning to the landmark during the compound phase. Thus the boundary blocked the landmark but not vice versa.

In summary, two qualitatively different types of allocentric spatial representations supported by two distinct neural systems in the hippocampus and striatum respectively appear to exist. The former system may well support a geometric module, in the sense that it is tuned to environmental geometry. Interestingly, these two distinct representations are subserved by learning mechanisms that obey different learning rules. Spatial learning relative to environmental boundaries is supported preferentially by the hippocampus and is incidental and invulnerable to competition with other spatial cues available. By contrast, spatial learning relative to discrete environmental landmarks is supported by the striatum and follows the rules of "associative" or "reinforcement" learning with a single error term: being blocked and overshadowed by boundaries.

Reinterpretation of the Geometric Module

The animal literature and the human study reported here demonstrate that a variety of spatial representations are available to animals for the purposes of behavior. One of these, which is hippocampal dependent, is specialized for processing location on the basis of environment-centered coordinates. Although the link with the literature on place cell firing in rats was not made at the time, the related idea of a "geometric module" (Cheng 1986; Gallistel, 1990) was proposed sometime later on purely behavioral grounds. A "module" only operates on certain inputs, and the information it processes is "encapsulated," in other words, it comprises only a subset of all the information available to the animal (Fodor 1983). Thus, the hypothesized geometric module processes metric information such as the lengths and angles of walls, as well as distinguishing right and left. However, featural information such as the color of walls or distinguishing landmarks would be neither processed nor accessible to it. In this section we briefly review some of the evidence for this proposal so that we can then compare it with the neuroscientific information reviewed above.

So-called *reorientation* paradigms have been a popular source of data in the debate about whether a geometric module exists (see Cheng and Newcombe 2005). In such paradigms, an animal learns a goal location in one corner of a rectangular arena. Following disorientation by being rotated in the absence of stable sensory cues, the animal reenters the arena and searches for the goal location. In the absence of any featural information, the animal could theoretically choose the correct location 50 percent of the time, with the other 50 percent spent searching the diagonally opposite corner, since these are geometrically indistinguishable. The addition of some form of featural information predicts the goal location with 100 percent accuracy. Most vertebrates are able to use geometry for orientation purposes, but seem to differ in their ability to use featural information (see Cheng and Newcombe 2005). For example, disoriented rats are poor at using featural information, as are prelinguistic human children and adult humans, if required to perform a concurrent verbal shadowing task (repeating verbal material as it was being spoken). These observations provided some support for the proposal that geometric information was indeed encapsulated, although in humans featural and geometric information could be integrated via verbal mediation (Hermer-Vazquez et al. 1999).

Subsequent research has demonstrated that several species are capable of integrating featural and geometric information to solve reorientation tasks. Thus, many nonlinguistic species, including fish (Sovrano et al. 2003) and monkeys (Gouteux et al. 2001), use both types of information on at least some versions of the task. Importantly, prelinguistic humans are only impaired at using featural information in a *small* room (Learmonth et al. 2002). Furthermore, the finding that verbal mediation is required to integrate featural and geometric information has been challenged. Ratliff and Newcombe (2005) demonstrated that adults' performance on the task improves if the instructions are made more explicit, and additionally, they showed that a concurrent nonverbal task interfered with integration of featural and geometric information, provided that the interference task had a spatial component. In addition, Hupbach et al. (2006) found that reorientation by featural information in a large square room is impaired by a concurrent spatial task, but not by a verbal shadowing (see also chapters 5 and 6 in this volume).

The BVC model, which is based upon the spatial firing properties of hippocampal neurons, posits a role for the hippocampus in processing environmental geometry, particularly the directions and distances of boundaries (i.e., a neural substrate for the "geometric module"). However, several cross-species findings using reorientation paradigms have demonstrated not only that is geometric processing of the environment possible in many vertebrates but that local featural information can also be utilized for navigation (that is, the geometric information is not encapsulated). Interestingly, we learned from the single-unit studies that disorientation paradigms are not the best way to isolate the hippocampal contribution to spatial memory. This is because many types of cue interact to determine orientation, including local cues, distal cues, and environmental geometry, and do so within the head-direction system (see, e.g., Taube 1998) rather than the hippocampus. Despite the intriguing paradigm of Cheng (1986), in which geometry dominates, in general, which cues dominate orientation depends on many factors, including each cue's apparent stability (Jeffery et al. 1997; Jeffery and O'Keefe 1999), its distal or proximal location (Cressant et al. 1997), whether the rat is systematically disoriented (Knierim et al. 1995), environmental size (see chapter 5 and 6, this volume), as well as cue abstractness, subject gender, and task instructions.

In summary, there may well be something resembling a geometric module in the brain. That is, there is a (hippocampal) system specifically tuned to surface geometry and operating under different learning rules to (striatal) processing of discrete featural information. However, the reorientation paradigms traditionally associated with this proposition actually tap into a different but closely related system, the head-direction system, in which distinctions between which cues are used and in which circumstances are much less clear.

Conclusions

Using examples from research into spatial memory, we have argued that knowledge of the neural underpinnings of cognitive processes can inform our understanding of these processes at an algorithmic level. The first lesson from the brain is the existence of multiple parallel (and often redundant) spatial representations that operate in both egocentric and allocentric reference frames. Thus, electrophysiological studies of hippocampal place cells in rats implied that allocentric representations of the environment do exist, even if they may not have been apparent from previous behavioral studies. When suitable behavioral tasks have been designed to specifically probe these representations (by manipulating allocentric orientation cues, in our example), they have been shown to be present.

With regard to the geometric module, proposed by Cheng and Gallistel (Cheng 1986; Gallistel 1990) on the basis of behavioral findings (see also Hermer and Spelke 1994), the presence of a system specialized for processing the surface geometry of an environment is supported by a wealth of neuroscientific evidence concerning the hippocampus. By considering the neural representations found in the hippocampi of freely moving rats, we were able to find a task to cleanly dissociate the hippocampal contribution to location judged relative to environmental geometry from location judged relative to discrete landmarks. In addition, we were able to show that associations to the two types of cue were formed using distinct incidental and associative learning rules. However, the hypothesis that there is an "encapsulated" geometric module can be rejected: objects can be located using (hippocampally mediated) environmental geometry alone, or in combination with (striatally mediated) landmark information.

Interestingly, the behavioral basis for the initial proposal of a geometric module rested on "reorientation" paradigms, which do not directly depend on hippocampal functioning, but rather on a closely related system for representing head direction. Although this system does respond to environmental geometry, it also responds to many other types of cues, including distal featural information. One critical aspect of our behavioral paradigm was to control orientation via salient distal cues and use of a circular boundary so that the distinct representations of location relative to the boundary or the landmark could then be revealed. When orientation is not carefully controlled, the complex interplay between multiple factors used to determine heading direction can result in a confusing pattern of data, such as that recently reported in the various implementations of reorientation paradigms.

More generally, it seems likely that direct examination of the neural representations actually being used in the brain will help to resolve further controversies in the cognitive literature. Of course, the complexities of both brain and behavior, and of the link between the two, will require that a careful path be tread, and misinterpretations are likely to occur. However, the increasing opportunities for carefully controlled investigations using multiple convergent technologies points toward rejection of cognitive science's traditional council of despair that the brain should be ignored.

Acknowledgments

This work was supported by the Medical Research Council and Biotechnology and Biological Sciences Research Council of the United Kingdom.

References

Abrahams S, Pickering A, Polkey CE, Morris RG (1997) Spatial memory deficits in patients with unilateral damage to the right hippocampal formation. Neuropsychologia 35: 11–24.

Aggleton JP, Hunt PR, Nagle S, Neave N (1996) The effects of selective lesions within the anterior thalamic nuclei on spatial memory in the rat. Behav Brain Res 81: 189–198.

Barry C, Lever C, Hayman R, Hartley T, Burton S, O'Keefe J, Jeffery KJ, Burgess N (2006) The boundary vector cell model of place cell firing and spatial memory. Rev Neurosci 17: 71–97.

Bennett AT (1996) Do animals have cognitive maps? J Exp Biol 199: 219–224.

Burgess N (2006) Spatial memory: How egocentric and allocentric combine. Trends Cogn Sci 10: 551–557.

Burgess N, Spiers HJ, Paleologou E (2004) Orientational manoeuvres in the dark: Dissociating allocentric and egocentric influences on spatial memory. Cognition 94: 149–166.

Chamizo VD, Aznar-Casanova JA, Artigas AA (2003) Human overshadowing in a virtual pool: Simple guidance is a good competitor against locale learning. Learn Motiv 34: 262–281.

Cheng K (1986) A purely geometric module in the rat's spatial representation. Cognition 23: 149–178.

Cheng K, Newcombe NS (2005) Is there a geometric module for spatial orientation? Squaring theory and evidence. Psychon B Rev 12: 1–23.

Cressant A, Muller RU, Poucet B (1997) Failure of centrally placed objects to control the firing fields of hippocampal place cells. J Neurosci 17: 2531–2542.

Dickinson A (1980) Contemporary Animal Learning Theory. Cambridge: Cambridge University Press.

Doeller CF, Burgess N (2008) Distinct error-correcting and incidental learning of location relative to landmarks and boundaries. Proc Natl Acad Sci USA 105: 5909–5914.

Doeller CF, King JA, Burgess N (2008) Parallel striatal and hippocampal systems for landmarks and boundaries in spatial memory. Proc Natl Acad Sci USA 105: 5915–5920.

Dudchenko PA, Taube JS (1997) Correlation between head direction cell activity and spatial behavior on a radial arm maze. Behav Neurosci 111: 3–19.

Ekstrom AD, Kahana MJ, Caplan JB, Fields TA, Isham EA, Newman EL, Fried I (2003) Cellular networks underlying human spatial navigation. Nature 425: 184–188.

Fodor J (1983) The Modularity of mind. Cambridge, MA: MIT Press.

Gallistel CR (1990) The organization of learning. Cambridge, MA: MIT Press.

Gouteux S, Thinus-Blanc C, Vauclair J (2001) Rhesus monkeys use geometric and nongeometric information during a reorientation task. J Exp Psychol Gen 130: 505–519.

Hafting T, Fyhn M, Molden S, Moser MB, Moser EI (2005) Microstructure of a spatial map in the entorhinal cortex. Nature 436: 801–806.

Hamilton DA, Sutherland RJ (1999) Blocking in human place learning: evidence from virtual navigation. Psychobiology 27: 453–461.

Hargreaves EL, Yoganarasimha D, Knierim, JJ (2007) Cohesiveness of spatial and directional representations recorded from neural ensembles in the anterior thalamus, parasubiculum, medial entorhinal cortex, and hippocampus. Hippocampus 17: 826–841.

Hartley T, Trinkler I, Burgess N (2004) Geometric determinants of human spatial memory. Cognition 94: 39–75.

Hartley T, Burgess N, Lever C, Cacucci F, O'Keefe J (2000) Modeling place fields in terms of the cortical inputs to the hippocampus. Hippocampus 10: 369–379.

Hartley T, Maguire EA, Spiers HJ, Burgess N (2003) The well-worn route and the path less traveled: Distinct neural bases of route following and wayfinding in humans. Neuron 37: 877–888.

Hebb DO (1949) The Organization of behavior. New York: Wiley.

Hermer L, Spelke ES (1994) A geometric process for spatial reorientation in young children. Nature 370: 57–59.

Hermer-Vazquez L, Spelke ES, Katsnelson AS (1999) Sources of flexibility in human cognition: Dual-task studies of space and language. Cognitive Psychol 39: 3–36.

Hupbach A, Hardt O, Nadel L, Bohbot V (2006) Spatial reorientation: Effects of verbal and spatial shadowing. Spatial Cognit Comput 7: 213–226.

Iaria G, Petrides M, Dagher A, Pike B, Bohbot VD (2003) Cognitive strategies dependent on the hippocampus and caudate nucleus in human navigation: Variability and change with practice. J Neurosci 23: 5945–5952.

Jeffery KJ, Donnett JG, Burgess N, O'Keefe JM (1997) Directional control of hippocampal place fields. Exp Brain Res 117: 131–142.

Jeffery KJ, O'Keefe JM (1999) Learned interaction of visual and idiothetic cues in the control of place field orientation. Exp Brain Res 127: 151–161.

King JA, Burgess N, Hartley T, Vargha-Khadem F, O'Keefe J (2002) Human hippocampus and viewpoint dependence in spatial memory. Hippocampus 12: 811–820.

King JA, Trinkler I, Hartley T, Vargha-Khadem F, Burgess N (2004) The hippocampal role in spatial memory and the familiarity-recollection distinction: A single case study. Neuropsychology 18: 405–417.

Knierim JJ, Kudrimoti HS, McNaughton BL (1995) Place cells, head direction cells, and the learning of landmark stability. J Neurosci 15: 1648–1659.

Learmonth AE, Nadel L, Newcombe NS (2002) Children's use of landmarks: Implications for modularity theory. Psychol Sci 13: 337–341.

Lenck-Santini PP, Rivard B, Muller RU, Poucet B (2005) Study of CA1 place cell activity and exploratory behavior following spatial and nonspatial changes in the environment. Hippocampus 15: 356–369.

Lenck-Santini PP, Save E, Poucet B (2001) Evidence for a relationship between place–cell spatial firing and spatial memory performance. Hippocampus 11: 377–390.

Mackintosh NJ (1975) A theory of attention: Variations in the associability of stimuli with reinforcement. Psychol Rev 82: 276–298.

Maguire EA, Burgess N, Donnett JG, Frackowiak RS, Frith CD, O'Keefe J (1998) Knowing where and getting there: A human navigation network. Science 280: 921–924.

Maurer R, Derivaz V (2000) Rats in a transparent Morris water maze use elemental and configural geometry of landmarks as well as distance to the pool wall. Spatial Cognit Comput 2: 135–156.

McDonald RJ, White NM (1994) Parallel information processing in the water maze: Evidence for independent memory systems involving dorsal striatum and hippocampus. Behav Neural Biol 61: 260–270.

Morris RGM, Garrud P, Rawlins JN, O'Keefe J (1982) Place navigation impaired in rats with hippocampal lesions. Nature 297: 681–683.

Mou W, McNamara TP, Rump B, Xiao C (2006) Roles of egocentric and allocentric spatial representations in locomotion and reorientation. J Exp Psychol Learn Mem Cogn 32: 1274–1290.

Muller RU, Kubie JL (1989) The firing of hippocampal place cells predicts the future position of freely moving rats. J Neurosci 9: 4101–4110.

O'Keefe J (1976) Place units in the hippocampus of the freely moving rat. Exp Neurol 51: 78–109.

O'Keefe J, Burgess N (1996) Geometric determinants of the place fields of hippocampal neurons. Nature 381: 425–428.

O'Keefe J, Nadel L (1978) The hippocampus as a cognitive map. Oxford: Oxford University Press.

O'Keefe J, Speakman A (1987) Single unit activity in the rat hippocampus during a spatial memory task. Exp Brain Res 68: 1–27.

Ono T, Nakamura K, Fukuda M, Tamura R (1991) Place recognition responses of neurons in monkey hippocampus. Neurosci Lett 121: 194–198.

Packard MG, McGaugh JL (1992) Double dissociation of fornix and caudate nucleus lesions on acquisition of two water maze tasks: Further evidence for multiple memory systems. Behav Neurosci 106: 439–446.

Packard MG, McGaugh JL (1996) Inactivation of hippocampus or caudate nucleus with lidocaine differentially affects expression of place and response learning. Neurobiol Learn Mem 65: 65–72.

Pavlov IP (1927) Conditioned reflexes. Oxford: Oxford University Press.

Pearce JM, Graham M, Good MA, Jones PM, McGregor A (2006) Potentiation, overshadowing, and blocking of spatial learning based on the shape of the environment. J Exp Psychol Anim Behav Process 32: 201–214.

Pearce JM, Hall G (1980) A model for Pavlovian learning: Variations in the effectiveness of conditioned but not of unconditioned stimuli. Psychol Rev 87: 532–552.

Pearce JM, Roberts AD, Good M (1998) Hippocampal lesions disrupt navigation based on cognitive maps but not heading vectors. Nature 396: 75–77.

Ratliff KR, Newcombe NS (2005) Human spatial reorientation using dual task paradigms. Proceedings of the Annual Cognitive Science Society 27: 1809–1814.

Rescorla RA, Wagner AR (1972) A theory of Pavlovian conditioning: Variations in the effectiveness of reinforcement and non-reinforcement. In: Classical Conditioning II. Current Research and Theory. (Black AH, Prokasy WF, eds), 64–99. New York: Appleton-Century-Crofts.

Schmidt T, Lee EY (2006) Spatial memory organized by environmental geometry. Spatial Cognition and Computation 6: 345–368.

Schultz W, Dayan P, Montague PR (1997) A neural substrate of prediction and reward. Science 275: 1593–1599.

Simons DJ, Wang RF (1998) Perceiving real-world viewpoint changes. Psychol Sci 9: 315–320.

Sovrano VA, Bisazza A, Vallortigara G (2003) Modularity as a fish (*Xenotoca eiseni*) views it: Conjoining geometric and nongeometric information for spatial reorientation. J Exp Psychol Anim B 29: 199–210.

Spiers HJ, Burgess N, Hartley T, Vargha-Khadem F, O'Keefe J (2001a) Bilateral hippocampal pathology impairs topographical and episodic memory but not visual pattern matching. Hippocampus 11: 715–725.

Spiers HJ, Burgess N, Maguire EA, Baxendale SA, Hartley T, Thompson P, O'Keefe J (2001b) Unilateral temporal lobectomy patients show lateralised topographical and episodic memory deficits in a virtual town. Brain 124: 2476–2489.

Sutherland RJ, Rodriguez AJ (1989) The role of the fornix/fimbria and some related subcortical structures in place learning and memory. Behav Brain Res 32: 265–277.

Sutton RS, Barto AG (1988) Reinforcement Learning: An Introduction. Cambridge, MA: MIT Press.

Taube JS (1998) Head direction cells and the neuropsychological basis for a sense of direction. Prog Neurobiol 55: 225–256.

Taube JS, Muller RU, Ranck JB, Jr (1990a) Head-direction cells recorded from the postsubiculum in freely moving rats. I. Description and quantitative analysis. J Neurosci 10: 420–435.

Taube JS, Muller RU, Ranck JB, Jr (1990b) Head-direction cells recorded from the postsubiculum in freely moving rats. II. Effects of environmental manipulations. J Neurosci 10: 436–447.

Tolman EC (1948) Cognitive maps in rats and men. Psychol Rev 55: 189–208.

Waelti P, Dickinson A, Schultz W (2001) Dopamine responses comply with basic assumptions of formal learning theory. Nature 412: 43–48.

Waller D, Hodgson E (2006) Transient and enduring spatial representations under disorientation and self-rotation. J Exp Psychol Learn 32: 867–882.

Wang RF, Simons DJ (1999) Active and passive scene recognition across views. Cognition 70: 191–210.

Wang RF, Spelke E (2000) Updating egocentric representations in human navigation. Cognition 77: 215–250.

Wang RF, Spelke ES (2002) Human spatial representation: Insights from animals. Trends Cogn Sci 6: 376–382.

Wilton LA, Baird AL, Muir JL, Honey RC, Aggleton JP (2001) Loss of the thalamic nuclei for "head direction" impairs performance on spatial memory tasks in rats. Behav Neurosci 115: 861–869.

Yin HH, Knowlton BJ (2006) The role of the basal ganglia in habit formation. Nat Rev Neurosci 7: 464–476.

Zugaro MB, Berthoz A, Wiener SI (2001) Background, but not foreground, spatial cues are taken as references for head direction responses by rat anterodorsal thalamus neurons. J Neurosci 21: RC154.

5 Animals as Natural Geometers

Giorgio Vallortigara

A substantial amount of contemporary research has focused on the possibility of elucidating the evolutionary, cognitive, and neurobiological bases of natural geometrical cognition (see, e.g., Dehaene et al. 2006; Biegler et al. 1999; Kamil and Jones 1997; Burgess 2006). Under some conditions, animals can use geometry to determine their orientation, to identify landmarks, or to find a place; that is, they can identify spatial locations not by their appearance but by their spatial relationships to other locations; for example, they can use information equivalent to "in the center of such an enclosed space" or "to the left to this blue wall" (Cheng 1986; Vallortigara et al. 1990; Hermer and Spelke 1994; review by Cheng and Spetch 1998). It is important to stress that this use of geometry does not necessarily imply use of allocentric representations based on aspects of the external environment (see Burgess 2006). Wang and Spelke (2002), for instance, suggested a model of spatial cognition that relies upon two types of egocentric processes and a "geometric module." According to this view, egocentric processes provide viewpoint-dependent scene recognition and spatial updating of egocentric locations by self-motion information. The geometric module represents the surface geometry of the surrounding environment, and is used by organisms to reorient themselves, but plays no direct role in representing object locations. Explicit allocentric representations of location are absent in this model. However, Wang and Spelke (2002) argue that, unique among living organisms, humans can go beyond these basic processes by using natural language to combine each with the other, as well as by using cognitive prostheses such as symbolic spatial maps.

Here I will concentrate on some particular aspects of the animals' ability to deal with natural geometry, focusing in particular on spatial reorientation mechanisms.

Spatial Reorientation: Encoding Geometric and Landmark Information

When an animal is disoriented (say, when it is subjected to several rotations in the absence of stable sensory cues) it must reorient itself with respect to the surrounding environment before it can navigate to a remembered location. Such a reorientation ability has been extensively investigated in recent years, from both a comparative and a developmental perspective.

In 1994 Hermer and Spelke compared human adults and young children in a task modeled on tasks previously developed by comparative psychologists—most notably by Cheng (1986). Subjects were shown a goal-object hidden in one corner of a rectangular enclosure one of whose walls was colored blue and the others were all white. Then the subjects were removed from the enclosure and disoriented. When reintroduced into the enclosure adults searched mainly in the correct location, whereas children searched equally at the target corner and at the corner located at a 180° rotation from the target, i.e., a location that had the same geometric relationship to the shape of the environment as the target location itself. To understand the significance of these findings let us consider the task in more detail.

Imagine you are located in a rectangular room with identically colored walls and no intra- or extra-room cues. In a corner there is something very interesting to you (figure 5.1a). Then you are displaced from the room and with your eyes closed you are turned passively a few times. Finally you are reintroduced into the room. The goal object is no

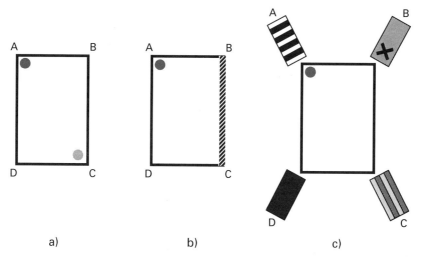

a)   b)   c)

Figure 5.1
Schematic representation of the geometrical information available in a rectangular environment. The target (darker circle) stands in the same geometric relation to the shape of the environment as its rotational equivalent (lighter circle). Metric information (the distinction between a short and a long wall) together with sense (the distinction between left and right) suffices to distinguish between locations AC and locations BD, but not to distinguish between A and C (or between B and D). When some featural information is available (such as a blue wall, figure 5.1b), the combination of geometric and featural information provides a complete disambiguation of the task, and the correct A corner can be easily distinguished from its geometrical equivalent C corner. When panels are added at the corners (figure 5.1c), featural information alone can provide a way to uniquely identify the location of each corner.

longer visible. Your task is to find the corner where the goal object was previously located. Apparently, there is no solution to the problem and perhaps you would predict random choices: 25 percent of the search would be associated with each corner.

However, if you ponder the problem a little bit, you realize that a partial (not a complete) disambiguation of the problem is possible. This is because you are located in an environment with a certain shape: a rectangular, not a square, environment. In a rectangular environment you can use metric properties of the surfaces (short vs. long walls) and what is called in geometry "sense" (left vs. right) in order to (partially) disambiguate the task. Let's suppose you are facing corner A, the correct corner during initial training. On the right you have a short wall and on the left, a long wall (figure 5.1a). There is only one other location that stands in the same geometric relationships with respect to the shape of the environment: this is corner C, its rotational (geometric) equivalent. In fact, when you are facing corner C once again you have on the right a short wall and on the left a long wall. Thus, corners A and C cannot be distinguished from each other—they are geometrically equivalent—but they can be distinguished from corners B and D, so, using the shape of the environment to reorient yourself, you now actually have a 50 percent (not 25 percent) probability of being correct.

This white-walls version of the task has been used with a variety of species, including fish (Sovrano et al. 2002; Vargas et al. 2004), birds (Vallortigara et al. 1990; Kelly et al. 1998), and mammals (Cheng 1986; Gouteux et al. 2001). All these species proved to be capable of encoding purely geometric information to partially disambiguate the task.

Now imagine you are located again in a rectangular room but, this time, there is a nongeometrical feature (i.e., a salient visual cue) like a blue wall as shown in figure 5.1b. In this condition the reinforced corner A can be easily distinguished from its geometric equivalent (corner C) because it lacks any blue wall. Thus, you have 100 percent probability of being correct in your choice. However, results with the blue-wall version of the task varied somewhat depending on species and developmental level.

In the original study by Cheng (1986), rats (*Rattus norvegicus*) were shown the location of a food reward in a corner of a rectangular room (120 × 60 cm) with several visual and olfactory cues; the rats were then removed from the room, passively disoriented, and finally returned to the room and allowed to search for food. Results showed that rats searched equally at the target corner and at the corner located at a 180-degree rotation from the target. Surprisingly, rats did not make any use of the nongeometric cues (visual and olfactory) to distinguish between the two geometrically equivalent locations. As mentioned, a subsequent series of studies in the laboratory of Elizabeth Spelke demonstrated that children (eighteen-to-twenty-four-month-olds), like adult rats, reorient using the geometric features of the environment and ignore obvious nongeometric features (Hermer and Spelke, 1994, 1996). Children and adults were tested in a rectangular room (4 × 6 ft) with either all-white walls or with three white walls and one blue wall. In the all-white-walls condition, in which only geometric cues were available, both children and adults searched for an out-of-sight toy equally in the correct and in the geometrically equivalent corners. In the blue-wall condition, however, adults readily used the presence of the blue wall to search only in the correct corner, whereas children performed like rats, systematically confusing the two geometrically equivalent corners.

Spelke and coworkers suggested that these results indicate that children must possess some sort of innate "geometric module" and that with the development of spatial language the module may be overridden to allow for the conjoining of geometric and nongeometric information (Spelke 2003; Wang and Spelke 2002). This hypothesis is sustained by data showing that once children acquire spatial language abilities (Hermer-Vazquez et al. 2001) they can conjoin geometric and nongeometric information in the blue-wall task. Indeed, the ability to correctly orient in the blue-wall task (Hermer and Spelke 1994) correlated with the ability of children to produce and use phrases involving "left" and "right" when describing the locations of hidden objects (MacWhinney 1991). The developmental time course of the ability to conjoin geometric and nongeometric information thus suggests that language acquired by children, starting at two to three years of age, would soon allow them, at five to seven years of age, to perform as well as adults (see Hermer-Vazquez et al. 2001).

Recently, however, it has been shown that many nonlinguistic animals can, unlike rats, integrate the two sources of information (fish: redtail splitfins (*Xenotoca eiseni*), Sovrano et al. 2002, 2003; goldfish (*Carassius auratus*), Vargas et al. 2004; birds: domestic chicks (*Gallus gallus*), Vallortigara et al. 1990; pigeons (*Columba livia*), Kelly et al. 1998; mammals: rhesus monkeys (*Macaca mulatta*), Gouteux et al. 2001; tamarins (*Saguinus oedipus*), Deipolyi et al. 2001). Moreover, it has become apparent that even rats can, in some circumstances, integrate geometric and nongeometric (landmark) cues—in reference-memory tasks but not in working-memory tasks; see the original Cheng (1986) paper.

It should be noted, however, that it remains perfectly possible (and maybe also likely) that humans do prefer using language to integrate geometric and nongeometric information, even though such integration can in principle be obtained in other ways (as shown by nonlinguistic animals). In fact, Carruthers (2002) provided a way to face the potential challenge offered by comparative data with nonhuman species to the hypothesis that integration of information from different modules would not be possible without language. The idea would be that even though other species are able to solve the spatial disorientation problem, this does not prove that they are able to integrate geometric with landmark information into a single belief or thought, for it could be that they are making use of the information *sequentially*. According to this view, the difference between species such as chicks, pigeons, rhesus monkeys, and fish, on the one hand, and rats and (prelinguistic) children, on the other hand, would simply be that the former use nongeometric information first, before using geometry, whereas the latter use geometry exclusively. But this hypothesis meets with some difficulties as recent evidence shows that under certain conditions, both rats (when tested in escape tasks; see Golob and Taube 2002) and prelinguistic children (when tested in large rooms; see Learmonth et al. 2001; Learmonth et al. 2002; see also Hupbach and Nadel 2005) can combine geometric and nongeometric information. Moreover, it is difficult to imagine how the distinction between a "sequential" and a simultaneous use of geometric and nongeometric information can be tested empirically. Let us consider some recent results obtained in our laboratory to explain the nature of the difficulty (see also Vallortigara and Sovrano 2002 for a more extensive discussion).

We trained redtail splitfins fish in a rectangular tank with four distinctive panels located at the corners (see figure 5.1c). In this case no integration of geometric and nongeometric information is needed to solve the reorientation task: each corner can be identified without any ambiguity on the sole basis of the featural information provided by the panels. We found that the fish managed the task (Sovrano et al. 2003). According to Carruthers's hypothesis, they (like chickens and monkeys) should possess an innate predisposition to seek landmark information first, only using geometric information to navigate in relation to a known landmark. However, given that in this case geometric information was not necessary for reorientation, we should probably have expected that no encoding of such information would occur at all. Surprisingly, however, when tested after removal of all the panels, fish did not choose locations randomly, but searched systematically in the two locations specified by purely geometric information (Sovrano et al. 2003). Similar results have been obtained with chicks (Vallortigara et al. 1990) and pigeons (Kelly et al. 1998). This clearly provides evidence that fish encode geometric information even when not required, that is, even when featural information suffices to solve the task. But does this provide evidence that fish had encoded geometric and nongeometric information in a single belief? Probably not, for it can be claimed that encoding of geometric and nongeometric information by two separate modules occurs anyway, even when this is not required by the task, but that information from these modules can then be *used* only sequentially. Thus, the data cast doubt on the account provided by Carruthers, because it seems that there is a "primacy" of geometric information even in those species such as fish and chickens that solve the spatial reorientation task. Nonetheless, the data do not disrupt Carruthers's central tenet, for the crucial hypothesis is that information is used sequentially, but the order in which information is used can well vary in different species. Carruthers's hypothesis thus does not seem to be easily subjected to empirical control: whatever behavioral performance we could document in animals, it would be always possible to explain it as a result of a sequential, rather than a simultaneous, use of information from different modules.

Integrating Landmark and Geometric Information in Environments of Different Spatial Scale

As alluded to previously, an interesting finding on spatial reorientation in the blue-wall task has recently been reported, namely, that the spatial scale of the environment in which the children are tested can play a crucial role in their ability to conjoin geometric and landmark information. Learmonth and colleagues (2001, 2002) replicated the original finding of Hermer and Spelke (1994), and concluded that children failed to conjoin geo-metric and landmark information in a small room (4 × 6 ft), but demonstrated that the same children succeeded in a large room (8 × 12 ft).

We also conducted a series of comparative studies on the effects of the spatial scale on reorientation. Besides providing comparison with developmental data, we were also inter-ested in verifying that animals can generalize spatial reorientation to environments of dif-ferent size. After learning to reorient in an enclosure of a certain size, would animals be able to reorient immediately when located in a larger or smaller enclosure? The issue is relevant to the problem of whether animals (as well as humans) encode absolute or relative metric properties of an environment (see Tommasi and Vallortigara 2000, 2001). Evidence for use of absolute metrics has come from several studies in which a goal was hidden at a fixed location relative to an array of landmarks. On array expansion-contraction tests, several species (gerbils: Collett et al. 1986; pigeons: Spetch et al. 1997) have been proved to search at locations that maintained the approximate training vector (distance and direction) from individual landmarks. However, when trained with continuous surfaces instead of discrete landmarks, animals seem to show relational rather than absolute encoding during expansion-contraction tests (chicks: Tommasi et al. 1997; Tommasi and Vallortigara 2000; pigeons: Gray et al. 2004). Perhaps orienting on the basis of distances from surfaces or the geometric arrangements of walls may promote different encoding strategies than orienting based on discrete local landmarks (for a review see Vallortigara 2006). Alternatively, the crucial difference could be in the availability of external visual cues (see Gray and Spetch 2006). However, little research has been done on this issue using the rectangular-cage task. The problem can be addressed through size transformation tests, which preserve shape but alter absolute metrics. Work carried out with pigeons (Kelly and Spetch 2001) showed that these animals encoded the relative geometry of the enclosure. However, pigeons were tested in a rectangular enclosure without any nongeo-metric cues available. It would thus be interesting to know whether, when geometric and nongeometric information must be conjoined for spatial reorientation, any change in the absolute size of the experimental enclosure would affect encoding of metric properties of the environment.

We tested redtail splitfins fish and failed to reveal any difference in conjoining geometric and featural information in a large (31 × 14 × 16 cm) tank and in a small (15 × 7 × 16 cm) tank (Sovrano et al. 2005). Interestingly, however, we found that when tested for transfer from a large to a small experimental space or vice versa, redtail splitfins tended to make relatively more errors based on geometric information when transfer occurred from a small to a large space, and to make relatively more errors based on landmark information when transfer occurred from a large to a small space.

Domestic chicks also appeared to be able to conjoin geometric and nongeometric (landmark) information to reorient themselves in both a large and a small enclosure (Vallortigara et al. 2005). Moreover, chicks reoriented immediately when displaced from a large to a small experimental space and vice versa, without showing any difference in the amount of geometric and nongeometric errors. Thus, chicks seemed to differ from fish in this regard. However, some interesting results were obtained when chicks were tested with a transformation (affine transformation) that alters the geometric relations between the target and the shape of the environment. In the affine transformation, each of the four panels is moved to the adjacent corner in the same direction, say, clockwise, in such a way that the panel in corner A moves to B, the one in B moves to C and so on; the result of such a geometric transformation is that the previously correct, reinforced, panel is located in a novel, and geometrically incorrect, location at test (figure 5.2). Results with the affine transformation showed that chicks tended to make more errors on the basis of geometric information when tested in the small than in the large space (figure 5.2; see Vallortigara et al. 2005). Thus, there seems to be a general similarity in the overall pattern of results obtained with these three very different species (humans, redtail splitfins, and chicks), in that in all cases geometric information seems to be more prominent in a small than in a large environment.

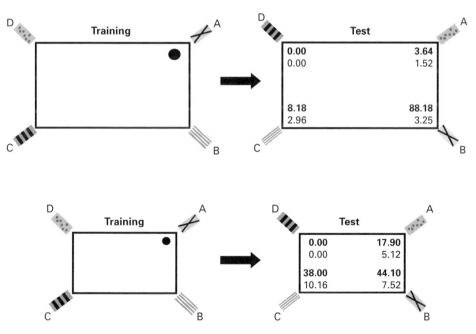

Figure 5.2
Results of an experiment in which chicks were trained in either a large (top) or a small (bottom) rectangular enclosure with panels at the corners, and then tested in the same-size enclosure after an affine transformation of the spatial arrangements of panels (rightmost figures), so that contradictory geometric and nongeometric information were provided. Note that after the affine transformation, the correct panel is located in a geometrically incorrect corner. Mean percentages of choices for each corner are shown in bold (with SEM below). Adapted from Vallortigara et al. (2005).

Further work confirmed this view. In some experiments we tried to disentangle the relative contribution of geometry and landmark cues as a function of the size of the experimental space (see Chiandetti et al. 2007). Domestic chicks were trained to find food in a corner of either a small or a large rectangular enclosure. A distinctive panel was located at each of the four corners of the enclosures. After removal of the panels, chicks tested in the small enclosure showed better retention of geometrical information than chicks tested in the large enclosure. In contrast, after changing the enclosure from a rectangular to a square one, chicks tested in the large enclosure showed better retention of landmark (panels) information than chicks tested in the small enclosure.

Overall, these findings suggest that the reliance on the use of geometric information regarding the spatial scale of the environment is not restricted to the human species. It remains unclear, however, why geometric information should be more important in small environments. One possibility suggested by various authors is that organisms are "prepared" to use only distant featural information as landmarks (Wang and Spelke 2002; Spelke 2003; Nadel and Hupbach 2006). However, one problem with this view is that, given the evidence for a primacy of geometric information over nongeometric information, the basic issue is not to explain why organisms do not use featural information in small spaces (they could do that simply because of the primacy of geometric information), but rather to explain why they do not continue to use geometric information even when tested in large spaces. This is particularly intriguing, because it has been frequently argued that geometric information may provide more stable and reliable information than local environmental features such as landmarks (Cheng and Newcombe 2005). Indeed, using geometric information for spatial reorientation makes sense ecologically. The large-scale shape of the landscape does not change across seasons, whereas there are important seasonal changes in the nongeometric properties of the landscape, such as the appearance of grass and vegetation, snow cover and snow melting, and so on. But of course this is true both in a small and in a large environment.

We thus tried to explore a different avenue. The solution of the blue-wall task encompasses the combined use of two sources of information, geometric information provided by the shape of the room (the arrangements of surfaces as surfaces) and nongeometric, landmark information provided by the blue wall. However, geometric information actually has two aspects, which have not been considered separately in previous work, namely, *metric information* and *sense*. Metric information refers to the distinction between a short and a long wall, irrespective of any other nongeometric property associated with the walls' surfaces, such as color, brightness, or scent. In geometry, *sense* refers to the distinction between left and right. Note, in fact, that even the simple use of purely geometric information does require an ability to combine different sources of information, i.e., metric information and sense. In fact, modularistic hypotheses based on the idea that animals lack a true ability to conjoin outputs of different modules in the absence of a language medium refers to the ability to conjoin information between (e.g., geometric and landmark information) and not within (e.g., metric properties and sense) different modules (see Spelke 2000, 2003; Spelke and Tsivkin 2001). The important point to stress is that in certain conditions animals might make use of a combination of nongeometric information and sense in order to reorient, without making any use of metric properties of the environment.

Consider the situation depicted in figure 5.3. In figure 5.3a the correct corner, A, can be distinguished from each one of the other three corners by using a combination of geometric information (metric plus sense) and featural information (blue color). In fact, corner A can be distinguished from corners C and D because it lacks any blue color, and it can be distinguished from corner B because it has a different metric arrangement of the short and long wall. The same is true even in figure 5.3b, when the correct corner A is localized between a blue and a white wall. However, in this case the correct corner (A) can be

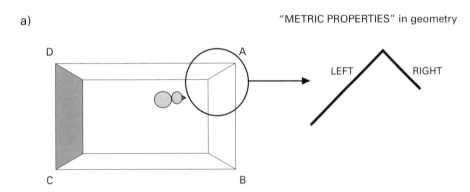

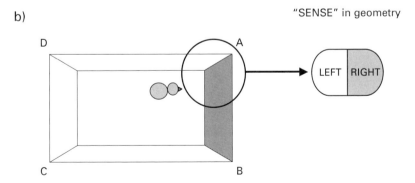

Figure 5.3
(Top) The information available at the correct corner, A, when the feature (blue wall) is far or near the wall. Animals can rely either on an association between metric properties and sense (panel a: short wall on the right and long wall on the left) or on an association between featural properties and sense (panel b: blue on the right and white on the left). Adapted from Sovrano and Vallortigara (2006).

distinguished from both its geometric equivalent (C) and its featural equivalent (B) without relying on the use of metric information. It suffices that the animal encodes the information that the correct corner is the corner with a white-blue arrangement (featural information) in which the blue is "on the right" (sense information). This combination of featural information and sense (without any reference to the metric of the environment) would suffice to disambiguate the problem, for corner A can now be distinguished easily from both corner C (because corner C lacks any blue color) and corner B (because in corner B the blue color, although present, is located in the wrong sense ordering).

We thus devised a test (figure 5.4) in which such a dissection of sense and metric information is made possible (Sovrano and Vallortigara 2006). Training is shown in figure 5.4 (left). At test (figure 5.4, right) the blue wall is dislocated from the AB to the CB wall (of course, the transformation also implies a change in size of the feature, which was accounted for experimentally by counterbalancing the two types of changes, from a large to a small blue wall and vice versa). As a result of the transformation, it would appear impossible for the animal to find a corner that matches featural and geometric information (sense and metric properties) as experienced during initial training (figure 5.4, left).

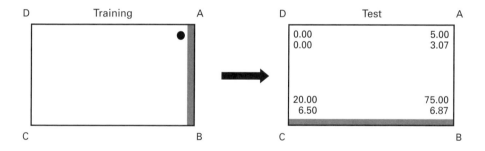

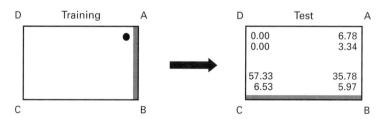

Figure 5.4
Schematic representation of an experiment in which chicks were first trained in the rectangular enclosure with the blue wall, and then tested after the displacement of the blue feature to an adjacent wall. See text for explanation. Adapted from Sovrano and Vallortigara (2006).

Let us consider the possible outcomes of the test. A first possibility is that animals simply match metric and sense information, and ignore featural information. If so, choices should be concentrated on corners A and C, and should appear equally distributed between the two corners. A second, complementary and opposite, possibility is that animals match featural information, ignoring geometric (metric and sense) information. If so, choice should be concentrated on corners B and C, and should appear equally distributed between these two corners. Alternatively, animals may consider both sources of information, geometric and nongeometric. If so, choices should again be concentrated along corners in the BC wall, because these are the only locations which possess the correct featural information. However, geometric information actually comprises two distinct aspects, metric properties and sense. Thus, there are two possibilities, or combinations of possibilities. If animals rely mainly on metric properties but tend to ignore sense as to featural information, then corner C should be preferred. This is because corner C possesses the same featural information (the blue color—even though with the wrong sense because the blue is on the left rather than on the right) and the same metrical arrangement of surfaces as during the initial training, i.e., long wall on the left and short wall on the right. If, on the contrary, animals rely mainly on the sense of the feature and tend to ignore metric properties of surfaces, then corner B should be preferred. This is because corner B possesses the same featural information, the blue color, with the same sense properties, blue on the right, as during the initial training, even though it does not possess the same metrical arrangement of surfaces—in this case the long wall is on the right and the short one on the left.

We tested young chicks in this task, using a large and a small environment (the same sizes used in previous work that has revealed effects on spatial reorientation in this species). The results (see figure 5.4) were striking: in the large enclosure chicks chose the corner that maintained the correct arrangement of the featural cue with respect to sense, whereas in the small enclosure they chose the corner that maintained the correct metric arrangement of the walls with respect to sense.

How can these results be explained? The key seems to be in the use of different associations with sense information in the two enclosures. In a large enclosure, animals may preferentially associate local featural information with sense information, whereas in a small enclosure animals may preferentially associate metric properties of the surfaces with sense information. Such different associations could be expected as those conveying more reliable information to the animal on the basis of visual (or other sensory) scanning of environments of different spatial scale. This is illustrated schematically in figure 5.5. If we assume that visual analysis of a corner (for instance, by head-direction cells) occurs at a fixed distance for the animal, then in a small environment (figure 5.5, bottom) the available visual information about the lengths of the surfaces may provide a reliable source of information for spatial reorientation. Thus, animals may rely on an association between the metric properties of the surfaces and the sense ("the correct corner has a short wall on the right and a long wall on the left"). In a large environment, however, vision of the full

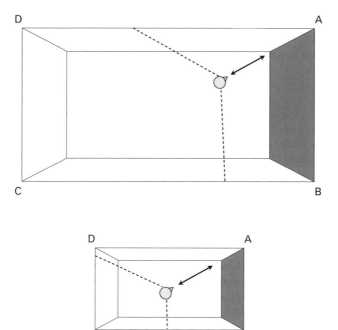

Figure 5.5
The information available to a chick looking to a corner from a fixed distance in a small enclosure (bottom), where metric information concerning surfaces is fully available, and in a large enclosure (top), where metric information is incomplete and featural information provides more reliable cues to reorient. Adapted from Sovrano and Vallortigara (2006).

spatial extent of the surfaces is prevented (figure 5.5, top) and can be obtained only through visual scanning by eye and head movements. Thus, animals may find it more convenient to rely on an association between the featural properties of the surfaces and the sense ("the correct corner has a blue feature on the right and a white feature on the left").

This hypothesis is not in contradiction to claims for a preference to use distal rather than proximal cues for reorientation, but provides a more precise account of the current findings with the rectangular task in large and small enclosures in a variety of species, as previously described.

It would be interesting to extend the investigation using our task in order to verify whether similar dissociation-association between metric properties, featural information, and sense could be observed in other species, in particular with children (see Nardini et al. 2008 for recent evidence that children use right-left sense of features in the blue-wall task). The evidence currently available suggests that the relative role of geometric and nongeometric (landmark) information can vary in different species, most likely because of differences in ecology and sense organs properties (see Brown and Braithwaite 2005).

Fish and birds can provide an interesting case in point. Although species of both classes have the capacity to integrate geometric and nongeometric information in the blue-wall task (chicks: Vallortigara et al. 2004; redtail splitfins: Sovrano et al. 2002), tests in which geometric and nongeometric cues provided contradictory information produced very different results: chicks seemed to be little affected by geometric cues and tended to rely mainly on local landmark information (Vallortigara et al. 1990), whereas redtail splitfins tended to rely mostly on the metric properties of the surfaces of the environment (Sovrano et al. 2003).

Recently we tested fish with the task developed by Sovrano and Vallortigara (2006) in order to verify whether the association between sense and metric vs. landmark information would follow different rules in different species (Sovrano et al. 2007). Results showed that in the large enclosure, fish chose the two corners with the feature, and preferred the one that maintained the correct arrangement of the featural cue with respect to geometric sense (i.e., left-right position). In contrast, in the small enclosure fish chose both the two corners with the features and the corner without any feature that maintained the correct metric arrangement of the walls with respect to sense. There were thus interesting differences with respect to data obtained in chicks. In the large enclosure chicks chose the corner that maintained the correct arrangement of the featural cue with respect to sense, whereas in the small enclosure they chose the corner that maintained the correct metric arrangement of the walls with respect to sense. Fish tested in the large tank also chose the corner that maintained the correct arrangement of the featural cue with respect to sense. However, in the small enclosure fish did not limit themselves to choosing the corner that maintained the correct metric arrangement of the walls with respect to sense among the two corners with the blue feature, but also chose quite clearly the corner in the geometric position lacking any featural cue.

All of this seems to suggest that, although the general hypothesis that in small spaces animals tend to link sense with metric properties of surfaces and in large spaces animals tend to link sense with local landmark cues appears to be quite correct, there seem to be species differences in the relative dominance of geometric and landmark information. Basically, it seems that for redtail splitfins geometric information is relatively more important than featural information than it is for chicks. This result confirms previous findings based on tests in which geometric and landmark cues provided contrasting information (e.g., Vallortigara et al. 1990 for chicks and Sovrano et al. 2003 for redtail splitfins). Perhaps such a difference could be expected considering that birds are highly visual animals with considerable spatial resolution capabilities; fish, in contrast, because of adaptation to an aquatic environment, show comparatively more reduced spatial resolution because of the spatial filtering produced by water.

There is recent evidence for species differences in the ability to deal with geometric and nongeometric information in birds. In contrast to domestic chicks and pigeons, wild-caught mountain chickadees (*Poecile gambeli*) do not spontaneously encode the geometry of an enclosure when salient features are present near the goal. Moreover, when trained without salient features they do encode geometric information, but this encoding is over-shadowed by features (Gray et al. 2005). The reason for these differences is unclear at present. One explanation could be that wild-caught birds have little experience with small enclosures and right corners, which are familiar to laboratory animals, thus leading to reliance on featural over geometric information. Somewhat the reverse could be true for small fish such as redtail splitfins that live in shallow, transparent water with pebbles and rich vegetation (Meyer et al. 1985; see also Burt de Perera 2004 for evidence of the use of geometric information in a species of blind fish that obviously cannot make any use of visual featural information).

Curiously, little research has been carried out on the influence of experience on the ability to process geometric information. Although modules need not be necessarily innate (Karmiloff-Smith 1992; see also Johnson, this volume; Sirois and Karmiloff-Smith, chapter 16, this volume), the issue of whether the ability to encode geometric information would require environmental triggering or some sort of experience with angled surfaces of different lengths appears to be quite interesting. Recent results obtained in my laboratory (Chiandetti and Vallortigara 2008) suggest, however, that at least domestic chicks may be predisposed to encode geometry (and see also Brown et al. 2007 for similar evidence in fish). We tested the navigational abilities of newborn domestic chicks hatched in the dark and reared soon after hatching in either a circular or rectangular cage. Later, chicks were trained in a rectangular enclosure with panels at the corners providing salient featural cues. Both circular-reared and rectangular-reared chicks proved identically able to learn the task. When tested after removal of the featural cues, both circular- and rectangular-reared chicks showed evidence of having spontaneously encoded geometric information. Moreover, when trained in a rectangular enclosure without any featural cue, chicks reared in rectangular, circular, or C-shaped cages proved to be equally able to learn and perform on geometry. These results suggest that effective use of geometric information for spatial reorientation does not require experience in environments with right angles and metrically distinct surfaces (see also Newcombe et al., chapter 6, this volume).

The Geometric Module in the Brain

The issue of whether or not the encoding of geometric information possesses the characteristics of a "module" (Fodor 1983) is still being debated (Cheng and Newcombe 2005; Newcombe 2005). On the one hand, as we have seen, comparative cognition research has suggested that conjoining of geometric and nongeometric information can be achieved in several species, irrespective of possession of a verbal language. On the other hand, a claim for a weaker version of modularity is supported by the observation of the "primacy" of geometric information over nongeometric information. The results obtained with chicks and fish suggest that even when nongeometric cues suffice for completely solving a spatial disorientation task, animals nonetheless encode purely geometric information from the distribution of large-scale spatial information. Such a primacy is understandable on ecological and evolutionary grounds.

A different strategy for assessing the extent to which the mechanisms that process geometric and nongeometric information are segregated would be to look at the neural bases of these processes. A first strategy we used to investigate this issue was to take advantage of the striking asymmetry of function between the left and right hemispheres in the avian brain (for a review see Vallortigara and Rogers 2005).

In animals with laterally placed eyes, such as most species of birds, there is a virtually complete decussation at the optic chiasm. In the optic nerves less than 0.1 percent of the fibers proceed to the ipsilateral side (Weidner et al. 1985). Since only a limited number of axons re-cross via the mesencephalic and thalamic commissures, the avian visual system is remarkably crossed. This means that information entering each eye is largely, though not completely (see Rogers and Deng 1999; Deng and Rogers 2002), processed by the contralateral side of the brain. Thus, by simply temporarily occluding one eye we can obtain some insights on lateralized functions of the avian brain.

In our experiments (see Vallortigara et al. 2004), chicks were trained binocularly in a rectangular enclosure with panels at the corners providing nongeometric cues (see figure 5.1c). When tested after removal of the panels, left-eyed chicks, but not right-eyed chicks, reoriented using the residual information provided by the geometry of the cage. When tested after removal of geometric information (i.e., in a square cage), both right- and left-eyed chicks reoriented using the residual nongeometrical information provided by the panels. When trained binocularly with only geometric information, at test left-eyed chicks reoriented better than right-eyed chicks. Finally, when geometric and nongeometric cues provided contradictory information (because of an affine transformation on the spatial distribution of panels), left-eyed chicks showed more reliance on geometric cues, whereas right-eyed chicks showed more reliance on nongeometric cues. The results suggest separate mechanisms for dealing with spatial reorientation, with the right hemisphere taking charge of large-scale geometry of the environment and with both hemispheres taking charge of local, nongeometric cues when available in isolation, but with a predominance of the left hemisphere when competition between geometric and nongeometric information occurs.

Little evidence is currently available on the extent to which these data obtained with the avian brain can be generalized to mammals, and to humans in particular. Clearly, birds are special in having complete decussation at the optic chiasm, lack of a callosum, and (relatively) reduced interhemispheric communication (Vallortigara 2000). Nonetheless, hemispheric differences quite like those reported here for chicks have been observed in rats. LaMendola and Bever (1997) tested rats in an eight-arm radial maze, the same five arms of which were always baited. Fewer errors (scored as returns to a baited arm which had already been visited, or entry of one of three arms that were never baited) were made when left whiskers were anesthetized and so only right whiskers were in use than when only left whiskers were in use. The dependence of this effect on a left-hemisphere involvement in the analysis of right-whisker input was confirmed by unilateral spreading depression of the left or right cortex, with left-hemisphere depression producing more errors in rats with both sets of whiskers in use. This left-hemisphere dominance was likely due to the fact that local nongeometric intramaze cues provided a unique and conspicuous label for each arm. When the maze was rotated, so that intramaze and extramaze cues were no longer in their usual relationship, a reversal in the relative performance of right- and left-whisker rats was observed; use of extramaze cues seems to favor dependence on a record based on the overall layout, or geometry, of the maze and thus dominance of the right hemisphere.

Some recent data may suggest dissociations along similar lines in humans. For instance, right hippocampal activation has been documented in taxi drivers asked to mentally navigate the streets of London (Maguire et al. 1997). Using the rectangular-room task, Pizzamiglio and colleagues (1998) showed that patients with right-brain damage with hemi-neglect are deficient in reorienting, though it proved difficult to establish a precise correlation between the site of the lesion and the deficit in the use of geometric or non-geometric information. More recently, however, Guariglia and colleagues (2000) found that in neglect patients, transcutaneous electrical neural stimulation significantly improved the ability to code geometric information, but was ineffective with nongeometric information. All this suggests the existence of separate systems for processing geometric and nongeometric information similar to those found in the avian brain.

It could be, therefore, that we are dealing with a very general and possibly ancient functional organization of the vertebrate brain to deal with the treatment of spatial information or, alternatively, with the fact that similar selective pressures produced, independently, analogous neural architectures in the avian and mammalian classes.

Further evidence for specific mechanisms dealing with geometric information in the brain arise from place-finding tasks, which are quite different from the reorientation tasks discussed here as the latter involve use of passive disorientation.

We investigated the abilities of young chicks to localize the central position of a closed environment in the absence of any external cues (Tommasi et al. 1997). After some days of training, during which food-deprived chicks were allowed to eat food that was buried under sawdust in the center of the floor of an arena, they developed a ground-scratching strategy to uncover the food in order to eat it. With training, chicks became more and more accurate in finding food, so that when they were eventually tested in the absence of any food, their pattern of ground scratching was concentrated in a very limited central area. We also showed that chicks were able to generalize among arenas of different shapes. For instance, when trained to find the center in a square arena and then tested in a triangular or circular one of nearly the same size, chicks searched in the central region of the novel arena.

We have also shown that when the environmental change involved a substantial modification in the size of the arena, as is the case for the transition from a square arena to another square arena of a larger size, the scratching bouts of chicks in the test (larger) arena were localized in two regions: the actual center of the test arena and (in part) at a distance from the walls that was equal to the distance from the walls to the center in the training (smaller) arena. Apparently, two behavioral strategies seem to be available to the chicks: encoding a goal location in terms of absolute distance and direction to the walls, and encoding a goal location in terms of ratios of distances (whatever their absolute values) from the walls. Tests carried out under monocular viewing (after binocular training) revealed striking asymmetries of brain function, encoding of absolute distance being predominantly a function of the left hemisphere and encoding of relative distance being predominantly a function of the right hemisphere (see Tommasi and Vallortigara 2001, 2004; Vallortigara 2006).

When training was performed in the presence of a conspicuous landmark, a red cylinder located at the center of the arena, animals searched at the central location even after the removal of the landmark (Vallortigara 2000). Apparently, domestic chicks seem to be able to use the geometrical relationships between the walls of the arena as well, though they were not explicitly trained to do so. Marked changes in the height of the walls of the arena produced some displacement in the spatial location of searching behavior, suggesting that chicks used the angular size of the walls to estimate distances within the arena (Tommasi and Vallortigara 2000). These results provide evidence that chicks are able to encode information regarding the absolute and relative distance of the food from the walls of the arena, and that they encode this large-scale spatial information even when orientation by a single landmark alone would suffice for food localization.

Encoding of large-scale information on the basis of the shape of the arena seems to depend upon hippocampal function (Tommasi et al. 2003). Domestic chicks with bilateral or unilateral lesions of the hippocampus were trained to search by ground-scratching for food hidden beneath sawdust in the center of a large enclosure; the correct position of food was indicated by a local landmark in the absence of any extra-enclosure visual cues. At test, the landmark was removed or displaced at a distance from its original position. Results showed that sham-operated chicks and chicks with a lesion of the left hippocampus searched in the center, relying on large-scale geometric information provided by the enclosure, whereas chicks with a lesion of either the right hippocampus or both hippocampi were completely disoriented (landmark removed) or searched close to the landmark shifted from the center (landmark displaced). These results indicate that encoding of geometric features of an enclosure occurs in the right hippocampus even when local information provided by a landmark would suffice to localize the goal, whereas encoding based on local landmark information seems to occur outside the hippocampus.

More direct confirmation for a role of the avian hippocampal formation in the encoding of geometric information comes from work carried out in pigeons with the rectangular-arena task. Bingman and colleagues (2006) trained homing pigeons (*Columba livia*) to locate a goal in one corner of a rectangular arena by either its shape (geometry) or the left–right configuration of colored features located in each corner (feature structure). Although control and hippocampal-lesioned pigeons were able to learn at a similar rate, the control birds made proportionally more geometric errors (i.e. choice based on geometric information) during acquisition. Moreover, on conflict probe trials, the control birds preferred geometrically correct corners, whereas the hippocampal-lesioned birds displayed a greater preference for the featurally correct corner. On geometry-only probe trials, both groups demonstrated an ability to identify the goal location. Thus, similar to what was found with chicks, hippocampal lesions in pigeons do not interfere with the encoding of featural information, but diminish the salience of geometric information. Interestingly, however, there seem to be species differences in the pattern of brain lateralization, for when faced with a conflict between geometric and nongeometric information, pigeons with a lesion to the left hippocampus seem to favor featural over geometrical cues (Nardi and Bingman 2007). It seems likely that this is due to a basic difference in the neural circuits involved in cerebral lateralization in the two species, the thalamofugal pathway in the chick and the tectofugal pathway in the pigeon (see reviews in Güntürkün 1997; Rogers 1996; Rogers and Andrew 2002; Vallortigara and Rogers 2005; Chiandetti et al. 2005).

Epilogue

It is apparent that the foundation of natural geometry, at least in its most basic aspects, is far removed from any strictly linguistic and cultural constraint (Dehaene et al. 2006) and is deeply rooted in phylogenetic history. Much remains to be investigated as to natural geometry in animals and human beings. First, the study of the development of these abilities and the role of experience and maturational factors is still in its infancy. Second, although we have plausible candidate regions in the brain for the treatment of geometric information, we know little about the specific neural mechanisms involved. Furthermore, we know virtually nothing about the brain regions involved in the integration of geometric and nongeometric cognition. I would guess that areas in the frontal cortex (or equivalent in animals with nonlaminated "cortex," such as birds) could be crucial. Some speculations could be advanced in this regard. It has been suggested that language, unique to humans, may be the device for assembling and coordinating the systems of core knowledge (Spelke 2003; Carruthers 2002). Perhaps a slightly different view could be put forward. Although I subscribe to the hypothesis that certain mechanisms that are usually regarded as part of the language abilities in humans do serve the function of integrating knowledge from different core-system modules, I believe they do so through computations that are not unique to language. The view I am pursuing is that these computations are best represented as cognitive precursors of language, shared by nonhuman animals, that probably served as the foundation on which the uniquely human computational capabilities have been built. Also, I believe that these computations are mostly instantiated into the frontal cortex (or its anatomical equivalent) in nonhuman animals, and for that reason they have been co-opted and used as precursors of the language faculty in our species. Preliminary work going on in my laboratory suggests, in fact, that the nidopallium caudolaterale, a brain area that is thought to be the avian equivalent of the mammalian prefrontal cortex (Güntürkün and Durstewitz 2000), may play a crucial role in the integration of geometric and nongeometric information.

Finally, the precise relationships between linguistic abilities unique of our species and possible limitations on geometrical cognition in nonhuman animals should be clarified. I would envisage that for natural geometry a story similar to that beautifully developed in these last years for the "number sense" (see Brannon and Terrace 1998; Dehaene 1997; Hauser et al. 2003; Rugani et al. 2007, 2008; see Brannon and Cantlon, chapter 10, this volume) will ultimately emerge (see also Spelke 2003). That is, animals probably possess a rudimentary sense of geometry that provides the foundation for the fully developed, and unique, human knowledge of geometry when it meets the possibility offered by the symbolic representations allowed by verbal language, which enable cognitive prostheses for spatial cognition such as maps, charts, and the like.

Acknowledgments

Financial support provided by the following institutions is gratefully acknowledged: MIUR (Ministero dell'Università e della Ricerca) Cofin 2004, grant number 2004070353_002 "Intel-lat"; MIPAF (Ministero delle Politiche Agricole e Forestali) "Ben-o-lat" via Dip. Sci. Zootecniche, University of Sassari; the Waltham Foundation; and Project EDCBNL (Evolution and Development of Cognitive, Behavioural and Neural Lateralization, 2006–2009), supported by the Commission of the European Communities within the framework of the specific research and technological development program "Integrating and Strengthening the European Research Area" (the "What It Means to be Human" initiative).

References

Biegler R, McGregor A, Healy SD (1999) How do animals "do" geometry? Anim Behav 57: F4–F8.

Bingman VP, Erichsen JT, Anderson JD, Good MA, Pearce JM (2006) Spared feature-structure discrimination but diminished salience of environmental geometry in hippocampal-lesioned homing pigeons (*Columba livia*). Behav Neurosci 120: 835–841.

Brannon EM, Terrace HS (1998) Ordering the numerosities 1 to 9 by monkeys. Science 282: 746–749.

Brown AA, Spetch ML, Hurd PL (2007) Growing in circles: Rearing environment alters spatial navigation in fish. Psychol Sci 18: 569–573.

Brown C, Braithwaite VA (2005) Effects of predation pressure on the cognitive ability of the poeciliid *Brachyraphis episcope*. Behav Ecol 16: 482–487.

Burgess N (2006) Spatial memory: How egocentric and allocentric combine. Trends Cogn Sci 10: 551–557.

Burt de Perera T (2004) Spatial parameters encoded in the spatial map of the blind Mexican cave fish, *Astyanax fasciatus*. Anim Behav 68: 291–295.

Carruthers P (2002) The cognitive functions of language. Behav Brain Sci 25: 657–726.

Cheng K (1986) A purely geometric module in the rat's spatial representation. Cognition 23: 149–178.

Cheng K, Newcombe NS (2005) Is there a geometric module for spatial orientation? Squaring theory and evidence. Psychon B Rev 12: 1–23.

Cheng K, Spetch ML (1998) Mechanisms of landmark use in mammals and birds. In: Spatial Representation in Animals (Healy S, ed), 1–17. Oxford: Oxford University Press.

Chiandetti C, Regolin L, Rogers LJ, Vallortigara G (2005) Effects of light stimulation in embryo on the use of position-specific and object-specific cues in binocular and monocular chicks. Behav Brain Res 163: 10–17.

Chiandetti C, Regolin L, Sovrano VA, Vallortigara G (2007) Spatial reorientation: The effects of space size on the encoding of landmark and geometry information. Anim Cogn 10: 159–168.

Chiandetti C, Vallortigara G (2008) Is there an innate geometric module? Effects of experience with angular geometric cues on spatial re-orientation based on the shape of the environment. Anim Cogn 11: 139–146.

Collett TS, Cartwright BA, Smith BA (1986) Landmark learning and visuo-spatial memories in gerbils. J Comp Physiol A 158: 835–851.

Dehaene S (1997) The number sense. Oxford: Oxford University Press.

Dehaene S, Izard V, Pica P, Spelke ES (2006) Core knowledge of geometry in an Amazonian indigene group. Science 311: 381–384.

Deipolyi A, Santos L, Hauser MD (2001) The role of landmarks in cotton-top tamarin spatial foraging: Evidence for geometric and non-geometric features. Anim Cogn 4: 99–108.

Deng C, Rogers LJ (2002) Factors affecting the development of lateralization in chicks. In: Comparative vertebrate lateralization (Rogers LJ, Andrew RJ, eds), 206–246. Cambridge: Cambridge University Press.

Fodor J (1983) The modularity of mind. Cambridge, MA: MIT Press.

Golob EJ, Taube JS (2002) Differences between appetitive and aversive reinforcement on reorientation in a spatial working memory task. Behav Brain Res 136: 309–316.

Gouteux S, Thinus-Blanc C, Vauclair J (2001) Rhesus monkeys use geometric and nongeometric information during a reorientation task. J Exp Psych Gen 130: 505–519.

Gray ER, Spetch ML (2006) Pigeons encode absolute distance but relational direction from landmarks and walls. J Exp Psych Anim B 32: 474–480.

Gray ER, Spetch ML, Kelly DM, Nguyen A (2004) Searching in the center: Pigeons (*Columba livia*) encode relative distance from walls of an enclosure. J Comp Psychol 118: 113–117.

Gray ER, Bloomfield LL, Ferrey A, Spetch ML, Sturdy CB (2005) Spatial encoding in mountain chickadees: features overshadow geometry. Biol Lett 1: 314–317.

Guariglia C, Coriale G, Cosentino T, Pizzamiglio L (2000) TENS modulates spatial reorientation in neglect patients. NeuroReport 11: 1945–1948.

Güntürkün O (1997) Avian visual lateralization: A review. NeuroReport 8: 3–11.

Güntürkün O, Durstewitz D (2000) Multimodal areas in the avian forebrain—blueprints for cognition? In: Brain evolution and cognition (Roth G, Wullimann M, eds), 431–450. Heidelberg: Spektrum Akademischer Verlag.

Hauser MD, Tsao F, Garcia P, Spelke ES (2003) Evolutionary foundations of number: Spontaneous representation of numerical magnitudes by cotton-top tamarins. P Roy Soc Lond B Bio 270: 1441–1446.

Hermer L, Spelke ES (1994) A geometric process for spatial reorientation in young children. Nature 370: 57–59.

Hermer L, Spelke ES (1996) Modularity and development: The case of spatial reorientation. Cognition 61: 195–232.

Hermer-Vazquez L, Moffet A, Munkholm P (2001) Language, space, and the development of cognitive flexibility in humans: The case of two spatial memory tasks. Cognition 79: 263–281.

Hupbach A, Nadel L (2005) Reorientation in a rhombic environment: No evidence for an encapsulated geometric module. Cognitive Dev 20: 279–302.

Kamil AC, Jones JJ (1997) The seed-storing corvid Clark's nutcracker learns geometric relationships among landmarks. Nature 390: 276–279.

Karmiloff-Smith A (1992) Beyond modularity: A developmental perspective. Cambridge, MA: MIT Press.

Kelly DM, Spetch ML (2001) Pigeons encode relative geometry. J Exp Psychol Anim B 27: 417–422.

Kelly DM, Spetch ML, Heth CD (1998) Pigeons (Columba livia) encoding of geometric and featural properties of a spatial environment. Journal Comp Psychol 112: 259–269.

LaMendola NP, Bever TG (1997) Peripheral and cerebral asymmetries in the rat. Science 278: 483–486.

Learmonth AE, Nadel L, Newcombe NS (2002) Children's use of landmarks: Implication for modularity theory. Psychol Sci 13: 337–341.

Learmonth AE, Newcombe NS, Huttenlocher J (2001) Toddlers' use of metric information and landmarks to reorient. J Exp Child Psychol 80: 225–244.

MacWhinney B (1991) The CHILDES project: Tools for analyzing talk. Hillsdale, NJ: Lawrence Erlbaum.

Maguire EA, Frackowiack RSJ, Frith CD (1997) Recalling routes around London: Activation of the right hippocampus in taxi drivers. J Neurosci 17: 7103–7110.

Meyer MK, Wischnath L, Foerster W (1985) Lebendgebärende Zierfishe: Arten der Welt. Melle: Mergus Verlag.

Nadel L, Hupbach A (2006) Cross-species comparisons in development: The case of the spatial "module." In: Attention and performance XXI (Johnson MH, Munakata Y, eds), 499–512. Oxford: Oxford University Press.

Nardi D, Bingman VP (2007) Asymmetrical participation of the left and right hippocampus for representing environmental geometry in homing pigeons. Behav Brain Res 178: 160–171.

Nardini M, Atkinson J, Burgess N (2008) Children reorient using the left/right sense of coloured landmarks at 18–24 months. Cognition 106: 519–527.

Newcombe NS (2005) Evidence for and against a geometric module: The roles of language and action. In: Action as an organizer of learning and development. Minnesota Symposia on Child Psychology, volume 33 (Rieser J, Lockman J, Nelson C, eds), 221–241. Mahwah, NJ: Lawrence Erlbaum.

Pizzamiglio L, Guariglia C, Cosentino T (1998) Evidence for separate allocentric and egocentric space processing in neglect patients. Cortex 34: 719–730.

Rogers LJ (1996) Behavioral, structural and neurochemical asymmetries in the avian brain: A model system for studying visual development and processing. Neurosci Biobehav R 20: 487–503.

Rogers LJ, Andrew RJ (2002) Comparative vertebrate lateralization. Cambridge: Cambridge University Press.

Rogers LJ, Deng C (1999) Light experience and lateralization of the two visual pathways in the chick. Behav Brain Res 98: 277–287.

Rugani R, Regolin L, Vallortigara G (2007) Rudimental numerical competence in 5-day-old domestic chicks: Identification of ordinal position. J Exp Psychol Anim B 33: 21–31.

Rugani R, Regolin L, Vallortigara G (2008) Discrimination of small numerosities in young chicks. J Exp Psychol Anim B 34: 388–399.

Sovrano VA, Vallortigara G (2006) Dissecting the geometric module: A sense-linkage for metric and landmark information in animals' spatial reorientation. Psychol Sci 17: 616–621.

Sovrano VA, Bisazza A, Vallortigara G (2001) Lateralization of response to social stimuli in fishes: A comparison between different methods and species. Physiol Behav 74: 237–244.

Sovrano VA, Bisazza A, Vallortigara G (2002) Modularity and spatial reorientation in a simple mind: Encoding of geometric and nongeometric properties of a spatial environment by fish. Cognition 85: B51–B59.

Sovrano VA, Bisazza A, Vallortigara G (2003) Modularity as a fish views it: Conjoining geometric and nongeometric information for spatial reorientation. J Exp Psychol Anim B 29: 199–210.

Sovrano VA, Bisazza A, Vallortigara G (2005) Animals' use of landmarks and metric information to reorient: Effects of the size of the experimental space. Cognition 97: 121–133.

Sovrano VA, Bisazza A, Vallortigara G (2007) How fish do geometry in large and in small spaces. Anim Cogn 10: 47–54.

Spelke ES (2000) Core knowledge. Am Psychol 55: 1233–1243.

Spelke ES (2003) What makes us smart. Core knowledge and natural language. In: Language in mind: Advances in the study of language and thought (Gentner D, Goldin-Meadow S, eds), 277–311. Cambridge, MA: MIT Press.

Spelke ES, Tsivkin S (2001) Initial knowledge and conceptual change: Space and number. In: Language acquisition and conceptual development (Bowerman M, Levinson S, eds), 70–91. Cambridge: Cambridge University Press.

Spetch ML, Cheng K, MacDonald SE, Linkenhoker BA, Kelly DM, Doerkson SR (1997) Use of landmark configuration in pigeons and humans: II. Generality across search tasks. J Comp Psychol 111: 14–24.

Tommasi L, Vallortigara G (2000) Searching for the center: Spatial cognition in the domestic chick (*Gallus gallus*). J Exp Psychol Anim B 26: 477–486.

Tommasi L, Vallortigara G (2001) Encoding of geometric and landmark information in the left and right hemispheres of the avian brain. Behav Neurosci 115: 602–613.

Tommasi L, Vallortigara G (2004) Lateralization of spatial cognition in the domestic chick (*Gallus gallus*): Sex- and task-related effects. Behav Brain Res 155: 85–96.

Tommasi L, Vallortigara G, Zanforlin M (1997) Young chickens learn to localize the centre of a spatial environment. J Comp Physiol A 180: 567–572.

Tommasi L, Gagliardo A, Andrew RJ, Vallortigara G (2003) Separate processing mechanisms for encoding geometric and landmark information in the avian brain. Eur J Neurosci 17: 1695–1702.

Vallortigara G (2000) Comparative neuropsychology of the dual brain: A stroll through left and right animals' perceptual worlds. Brain Lang 73: 189–219.

Vallortigara G (2004) Visual cognition and representation in birds and primates. In Vertebrate comparative cognition: Are primates superior to non-primates? (Rogers LJ, Kaplan G, eds), 57–94. Dordrecht: Kluwer Academic/Plenum Publishers.

Vallortigara G (2006) The cognitive chicken: Visual and spatial cognition in a non-mammalian brain. In: Comparative cognition: Experimental explorations of animal intelligence (Wasserman EA, Zentall TR, eds), 41–58. Oxford: Oxford University Press.

Vallortigara G, Rogers LJ (2005) Survival with an asymmetrical brain: Advantages and disadvantages of cerebral lateralization. Behav Brain Sci 28: 575–589.

Vallortigara G, Sovrano VA (2002) Conjoining information from different modules: A comparative perspective. Behav Brain Sci 25: 701–702.

Vallortigara G, Feruglio M, Sovrano VA (2005) Reorientation by geometric and landmark information in environments of different size. Developmental Sci 8: 393–401.

Vallortigara G, Zanforlin M, Pasti G (1990) Geometric modules in animals' spatial representation: A test with chicks. J Comp Psychol 104: 248–254.

Vallortigara G, Pagni P, Sovrano VA (2004) Separate geometric and non-geometric modules for spatial reorientation: Evidence from a lopsided animal brain. J Cognitive Neurosci 16: 390–400.

Vargas JP, Lopez JC, Salas C, Thinus-Blanc C (2004) Encoding of geometric and featural spatial information by goldfish (*Carassius auratus*). J Comp Psychol 118: 206–216.

Wang RF, Spelke ES (2002) Human spatial representation: Insights from animals. Trends Cogn Sci 6: 376–382.

Weidner C, Reperant J, Miceli D, Haby M, Rio JP (1985) An anatomical study of ipsilateral retinal projections in the quail using autoradiographic, horseradish peroxidase, fluorescence and degeneration technique. Brain Res 340: 99–108.

6 Is Cognitive Modularity Necessary in an Evolutionary Account of Development?

Nora S. Newcombe, Kristin R. Ratliff, Wendy L. Shallcross, and Alexandra Twyman

Our species has many distinctive characteristics, including upright posture, opposable thumbs, large brains, language, tool use, and many others. Arguably, one of the key characteristics of *Homo sapiens* is a developmental one: the extended proportion of our life span that comes before sexual maturity (Gould 1977). One of the crucial adaptive functions of this lengthy childhood is to allow for cognitive development. When a young organism must fend for itself, its interactions with the environment must be "good to go," and hence relatively preformed and inflexible. By contrast, human young can take their time, while protected by adults, to adapt to the environment in which they find themselves and to learn from the innovations and insights of prior generations. The same is true, albeit perhaps to a lesser extent, for other species in which there is a juvenile period before sexual maturity that is spent with mother, parents, or a band of adults.

Viewing it in this way, one might assume that an evolutionary approach to cognitive development would stress plasticity and learning, and might seek to relate interspecies differences to differences in the length of the juvenile age period. However, in reality, characterizing the nature of cognitive development has involved a repetitive struggle between nativism and empiricism, in which nativism has lately had a fairly dominant hand. For a while, Piaget's constructivism seemed to provide a way out of this opposition, but as Piaget's influence waned in the late 1970s and early 1980s (Gelman and Baillargeon 1983), a new nativism became the predominant mode of theorizing (e.g., Spelke et al. 1992). Alternative approaches appearing in the 1990s (Elman et al. 1996; Karmiloff-Smith 1992; Siegler 1998; Thelen and Smith 1994) may collectively be called emergentist theories because all of them suggest that there is significant developmental change, although there are differences as well as similarities among them (see chapters in Spencer et al., in press). However, nativism (under the banner of "core knowledge") has continued to be an attractive option for many cognitive developmentalists into the twenty-first century (Dehaene et al. 2006; Spelke 2000; Spelke and Kinzler 2007).

The persistence of nativism is a curious situation; all concerned, including individuals seen by others as unvarnished proponents of one side or the other, have professed support for the notion of *interactionism,* the idea that genetics and environment interact in complex and bidirectional ways to lead to development (Marcus 2004). However, nativism benefits from several advantages in the ongoing nature-nurture controversy. Chief among these advantages is the fact that it provides a simple and elegant story about how development and evolution fit together. In this way of thinking, adaptive pressures operate on a modular cognitive architecture (Cosmides and Tooby 1992). This brand of evolutionary psychology has in fact argued that evolution could *only* work if our cognitive organization is modular, because otherwise there would be no distinct target for adaptive pressures. For example, the adaptive value of fluently recognizing others leads to selection for modular face recognition abilities, the fact that living in social groups demands attention to equity in exchange leads to selection for a cheater detection module (Cosmides and Tooby 1989, 1992), and so on. Although modularity does not, strictly speaking, entail nativism (Barrett and Kurzban 2006; Fodor 2000; Karmiloff-Smith 1992), the two concepts are deeply intertwined in theorizing of this sort. In addition, innate origins are identified with modularity because they were in fact explicitly advanced as an attribute of a cognitive module in Fodor's original (1983) formulation of modularity.

The innate-module approach to the evolution and development of cognition is dramatically exemplified in recent proposals of an encapsulated geometric module that guides reorientation (Hermer and Spelke 1994, 1996). We are normally oriented to our spatial environment as we move through it, maintaining awareness of our position using both internal tracking mechanisms and relations to external landmarks. However, if we pass through a dark cave, or tumble down a hill, we may look around with very little idea of where we are, and need to reorient. Clearly, reorientation is an adaptive problem—the person who does not solve it will be unable to get home, avoid dangers, or find food. Experiments originally done with rats (Cheng 1986) and later done with human toddlers (Hermer and Spelke 1994, 1996) showed that reorientation was accomplished using information about the geometric shape of an enclosure. For example, in a rectangular space, after disorientation, searches for food or other objects concentrate on two geometrically congruent corners, for example, "long wall to left of short wall" (figure 6.1).

This pattern shows that geometric information is used to constrain likely search locations. Dramatically, when a prominent feature such as a colored wall or a corner panel potentially allows picking the correct spot, search remains evenly divided between the two geometrically congruent corners. The features are easy to notice and are used to guide search when there has been no disorientation. Hence, it seems that using geometric information to reorient is not only modular in the sense of making use of distinctive information uniquely relevant to the problem at hand (functional specialization) or in the sense of utilizing a specialized brain area (although there is some evidence there may be such an area; Epstein and Kanwisher 1998). Rather, it seems that this was a module in a very strong sense: encapsulated and unable to accept functionally relevant information.

Human adults, however, do use nongeometric information to reorient (Hermer and Spelke 1994, 1996). The transition from nonuse to use of nongeometric information, which

(a) Performance on task

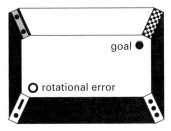

(b) Geometric information

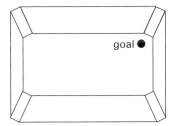

Figure 6.1
Geometric and featural (nongeometric) information in the relocation task (a) The task in a rectangular arena as seen from above. In attempting to relocate the goal after disorientation, subjects frequently commit the rotational error. This is the location at 180-degree rotation through the center from the correct location. (b) The geometric information is contained in the broad shape of the arena. The featural information is what is not shown: patterns on the panels, different brightnesses of walls, smells in the corner, and the like. When a "map" is used containing only geometric information, the goal and the rotational error cannot be distinguished. Adapted from Cheng and Spetch (1998).

takes place between the ages of five and six years (Hermer-Vazquez et al. 2001), poses an interesting issue for a nativist approach to cognition: How to account for developmental change? This challenge was answered by the suggestion that human language provides the tool for alteration of what would otherwise be a fundamental constraint on thought. When children acquire productive control of the terms "left" and "right," they become able to conjoin geometric and nongeometric information in a fashion unavailable in the absence of a symbolic system (Hermer-Vazquez et al. 2001). Interestingly, this research has been cited enthusiastically by proponents of culture- and language-based approaches to cognitive development (Haun et al. 2006; Levinson 2003).

The module-plus-language approach is, however, not the only way to conceptualize the evolution and development of a capacity for spatial reorientation. There are several difficulties with the hypothesis, including the facts that many nonhuman animals actually can use nongeometric information to reorient (see review by Cheng and Newcombe 2005), that human toddlers can use nongeometric information to reorient in larger and more ecologically valid spaces than those used in the original research (Learmonth et al. 2001, 2002), and that language does not appear to have a unique role in adult use of nongeometric information to reorient (Ratliff and Newcombe 2008). The main purpose in this chapter is to explore the promise of a different view of the relation of evolution and development, one more in the tradition of the plasticity-due-to-neoteny way of thinking. We argue both for a different view of orientation and reorientation and, more generally, for a different view of the relation between evolution and development than the currently popular one.

In the first section of the chapter, we outline an *adaptive combination* approach to spatial cognition and spatial development, and in the second section we review recent findings that support it (see Newcombe and Huttenlocher 2000, 2006, for more extended reviews of spatial development and this approach to it). In the third section, we critique two recent arguments for innate geometry: a demonstration that features alone cannot be used to reorient (Lee et al. 2006), and data on geometric concepts in the Munduruku (Dehaene et al. 2006). In the concluding section, we place the adaptive combination view in the framework of a prepared-learning approach to cognitive development and of an evolutionary approach to psychology that does not require cognitive modularity.

Adaptive-Combination Approach to the Development of Reorientation

People are frequently confronted with questions that require spatial estimation, such as "Which way should I head to get home from the library?" or "Where did I leave my cell phone?" There is considerable evidence for the use of multiple sources of information when we answer such questions. Cheng and colleagues (2007) review this evidence and theorizing, which includes several Bayesian models that show that such combination frequently maximizes the average accuracy of responses. Cheng and colleagues structure their review around three kinds of situations in which combination occurs, including when two or more currently available metric estimates (such as visual and haptic information; Ernst and Banks 2002) are combined, when current information is combined with the average of past experience (Kersten and Yuille 2003), and when current information is combined with categorical information that may or may not derive from past experience (Huttenlocher et al. 1991, 2000).

The overall thrust of the Cheng et al. (2007) review is that spatial conclusions are typically supported by various information sources whose use derives at least in part from experience. For example, recalibration of the relation of optic flow to distance traveled occurs when the relation is changed because one is walking on a treadmill that is itself moving, for example, pulled by a tractor (Rieser et al. 1995). Learning may work in one of two ways. First, it sometimes determines the relative weighting of the various information sources, with weightings affected by several factors, including the reliability of the source, how variably or inexactly it is coded, how perceptually salient it is, and how frequently it has been used in the past (e.g., Wang et al. 2005). Second, when two information sources lead to incompatible responses, learning may determine which of the sources will be preferentially relied on, in other words, it may shape a hierarchy of responses to be tried sequentially rather than production of an integrated estimate. In sum, the adaptive-combination approach involves the propositions that there are multiple sources of spatial information and that those sources are either integrated using weighting mechanisms or are hierarchically arranged in order of preference, and that those weightings and orderings are, at least in part, learned in the course of interaction with the spatial environment.

What happens when two information sources provide redundant information? In some cases both are learned, but in other cases, one of the two is ignored, or it is learned less easily or thoroughly than it would have been when presented alone. Classically, this phenomenon has been described either as *blocking* (when one information source has already been learned and prevents learning of a second source) or as *overshadowing* (when the two sources are presented concurrently, and the learning of either or both may be affected). Blocking and overshadowing seem to contradict the idea of adaptive combination, in that an information source is ignored even though it might contribute to increased precision of spatial estimation or even provide a way of estimating location when it would be otherwise impossible (as when the first source becomes perceptually unavailable, or unreliable). In addition, in terms of the geometric module hypothesis specifically, there are findings that show that learning distinctive features that mark a goal does not block learning of the geometry of an enclosure (Hayward et al. 2003; Pearce et al. 2001; Wall et al. 2004). One conclusion that could be drawn from such a lack of blocking effects is that the featural and geometric information are processed separately, perhaps in a fashion that might be called modular.

However, Miller and Shettleworth (2007) provide a nonmodular account of these findings on overshadowing and blocking, as well as one consistent with the adaptive combination approach. In doing so, they also bring order to the literature by explaining other findings that seem contradictory to overshadowing and blocking, in which learning one kind of information is easier or quicker or more robust when the other kind is present (e.g., Pearce et al. 2006) or in which blocking or overshadowing are sometimes observed (e.g., Gray et al. 2005). Miller and Shettleworth (2007) present an operant model related to the Rescorla-Wagner associative-learning model. In this account, features and geometry are both encoded on every trial, and the contingencies of one kind of information influence learning of the other kind and vice versa.

In summary, although many issues remain to be worked out in detail, there is growing evidence that spatial behavior typically depends on combining information from a variety of sources. This kind of theorizing is very different from that sometimes espoused in the literature, as, for example, when Wang and Spelke (2002) postulated that spatial behavior is determined completely by the geometric module for coping with reorientation, coupled with memory for viewpoint-specific representations of local sections of the environment that are related to each other through egocentric spatial updating. In fact, a recent critique of the Wang and Spelke argument by Burgess (2006) shows that egocentric and allocentric spatial representations coexist and interact in supporting spatial behavior, in general accord with the adaptive-combination point of view.

Recent Findings Supporting an Adaptive Combination to Reorientation

In this section we argue that the coexistence and interaction of various kinds of spatial information for reorientation, as postulated by the adaptive-combination view, is necessary to explain the data on development of the ability to reorient. Specifically, use of geometric and nongeometric information to reorient fluctuates systematically as a function of variables that affect the certainty with which the two kinds of information are encoded, their salience, and their cue validity. Such fluctuation could not be predicted by a modular theory. First, we examine fluctuation as a function of size of the enclosed space. Second, we discuss recent work on rearing and training effects. Third, we look at the effects of full enclosure as compared with a geometric outline that is only suggested by separated environmental elements, an issue that has the potential to shed light on the modularity issue but whose status is not yet empirically clear.

Room-Size Effects

In the literature on reorientation in human children, the first demonstration that very young children do sometimes use features as well as geometry to reorient, came from experiments by Learmonth and colleagues (2001). The contrast between the Learmonth et al. findings and those of the Spelke group were quickly shown to be due to the fact that the Learmonth et al. experiments were done in a room with quadruple the area of the Spelke group's experiments (Learmonth et al. 2002). The two papers by Learmonth and colleagues provide three challenges to the geometric module approach to the development of reorientation. First, children are using features as well as geometry by eighteen months, well before they control production of the terms "left" and "right" (and recall that acquisition of these linguistic terms is the only developmental mechanism postulated by the Spelke group). Second, a geometric module that only operated in extremely small spaces would not be very useful in our environment of adaptation; in fact, even the larger room used by Learmonth is quite small by the standards of the real world. Third, the modularity view cannot provide a cogent account of why the size of the space matters. The size of the experimental enclosure also appears to have a profound effect on nonhuman species, who have also shown a preference for using geometric information in small spaces but relying on nongeometric featural cues during reorientation in larger spaces (Sovrano et al. 2005; Vallortigara et al. 2005).

How does the adaptive-combination view account for the room-size effect? According to an adaptive-combination view, geometric information would be expected to predominate in studies where room shape is easily encoded with great certainty and low variability, as is true in most work so far, which has used fully enclosed spaces with a simple regular geometric shape such as a rectangle, triangle, or rhombus (an issue discussed in a later section of this chapter). In contrast, the nongeometric features are often likely encoded variably and with lower salience, for example, if they are small and mobile (Hermer and Spelke 1996, see experiments 3, 4 and 6; Gouteux et al. 2001). In terms of the room-size effect, an important variable is likely to be whether the features are distal or proximal. The further away a feature is located from an organism the greater the strength of encoding. Imagine movement around a local area. This movement creates very large variability in the location of a proximal feature. In contrast, movement creates only small variability in the location of distal features, according to an adaptive combination model (Nadel and Hupbach 2006; Newcombe and Ratliff 2007; O'Keefe and Nadel 1978).

Learmonth and colleagues (2008) explored how landmark proximity affects search patterns to produce the differences found between room sizes. They also examined the effect of the relative ease of moving around a space; smaller spaces constrict movement, which is known to lead to reduced spatial coding (for rats, see Foster et al. 1989; for children, see Acredolo 1978; Acredolo and Evans 1980; McComas and Dulberg 1997).[1] Children between three and six years of age performed the reorientation procedure of searching for a toy hidden in one of the four corners of a larger 8×12 foot rectangular room with one colored wall. Some of the children had their movements restricted by being placed within a small, centrally located 4×6 foot unfeatured rectangular area located within the larger room.

The results showed that at least three factors affect the age at which features are used to reorient. First, when the colored wall was more distal than it could be in the small room, children succeeded in using the feature to guide search at four years instead of six years, even when their movement was restricted. Second, the ability to move freely in the larger room also has an impact. When action is restricted, using features to reorient does not appear until four years, as compared to eighteen months when active movement is allowed (Learmonth et al. 2001). Third, when the toy was hidden in a corner of the unfeatured central enclosure—close to the child but far from the landmark—successful orientation did not occur until six years of age as compared to four years old when targets were placed adjacent to the distal colored-wall landmark. These variable ages of transition in use of a nongeometric feature suggest the overall inadequacy of a modularity-plus-language view.

Size of the experimental enclosure also changes reorientation strategies when a nongeometric feature, such as a colored wall, is displaced during testing from the location learned during training. When the learned geometry and feature locations are placed in conflict, fish (Sovrano et al. 2007) as well as chicks (Chiandetti et al. 2006; Sovrano and Vallortigara 2006) reorient by the geometry of a small enclosure, but the animals switch their search strategy in the larger spaces, relying on the current location of the nongeometric feature to reorient. Applying this conflict paradigm to identify the hierarchy of spatial cues used during adult reorientation, Ratliff and Newcombe (in press) found that the adults used geometric information to a greater degree in a small (4 × 6 foot) room whereas adults reoriented by the location of a feature in a larger (8 × 12 foot) room. Additionally, when training and testing occurred in rooms that were geometrically equivalent but of different sizes (the ratio of long to short walls remained constant although the room areas were different sizes, either large or small), reorientation behavior was consistently dominated by the feature location rather than the geometric shape of the room. Such search patterns suggest an adaptive approach to reorientation by means of integrating geometric and nongeometric information, depending on the certainty of encoding, reliability, and salience of the two types of spatial cues.

Effects of Training and Rearing

A core element of the adaptive-combination approach is the idea that spatial coding will be dynamically affected by experience—both recent experience (training effects) and early experience in a juvenile period (rearing effects). By contrast, the modularity-plus-language position has little room for such ideas, proposing instead that a fixed innately determined module can be changed only by the human capacity for linguistic encoding that can override the outputs of the module. There is considerable evidence for training effects, however, and some accumulating evidence for rearing effects. In this section we look at both issues.

Training Effects

Many training experiments have shown that flexibility of cue use can be achieved with both mature and juvenile participants, both human and nonhuman, if they have had the appropriate experience.

Pigeons   Pigeons flexibly use feature and geometric information, depending on the initial training experience (Kelly et al. 1998). All pigeons in these experiments were trained to find a hidden food source in an enclosed rectangular environment. One group of pigeons was trained with only geometric information while the other group was also trained with distinct feature information at each corner. The pigeons that had been initially trained with only geometric information were then retrained with the same feature information as the first group. During the test phase, the features were rotated 90 degrees so that the correct-feature corner was now in an incorrect geometric location. The pigeons that had been initially trained with features mainly selected the featurally correct corner, whereas the pigeons that had been initially trained with geometry divided the choices between the two geometrically correct corners and the correct-feature corners.

Pigeons and human adults   To extend this work, Kelly and Spetch (2004a, 2004b) trained pigeons and human adults with a two-dimensional schematic form of the reorientation task. A rectangle appeared with four landmarks at each corner of a computer screen. The pigeons and adults were divided into two groups; half were trained first only with geometric information, followed by geometric and feature information. The other half was trained first only with feature information, followed by geometric information. In the conflict trials, all of the adults chose the featurally correct corner, so the order of training had no effect. Thus, for schematic diagrams, feature information may be more salient than geometric information for human adults. For pigeons, in contrast to Kelly et al. (1998), the training order did not influence the choice on the conflict trials. All of the pigeons divided the search equally between the geometrically correct corners and the correct-feature corner., However, there was a difference in the training procedure. The pigeons in Kelly et al.'s (1998) experiment only received the feature and geometry training before the conflict trial. The pigeons in Kelly and Spetch's (2004b) experiment received the feature and geometry training followed by a geometry-only training session before the conflict test. One dose of geometry training, either before or after feature training, was enough to boost the use of geometric information for pigeons. Thus, it appears that the relative weightings of feature and geometry cues for pigeons can be quite malleable.

Human children   It also appears that the relative weighting of geometric and nongeometric information for children can be influenced by experience. As mentioned earlier in the chapter, children below the age of six are not normally able to use nongeometric cues to reorient in a small 4 × 6 foot room (Hermer and Spelke 1994, 1996). However, when given practice using nongeometric information, four- and five-year-old children can succeed at the task in the same size of enclosure (Twyman et al. 2007). These children were asked to practice the reorientation task in an equilateral triangle that had no distinctive geometric information. Each of the walls was a different color, so the children were given practice using nongeometric cues to reorient. Children were then tested in the small rectangular room and were able to reorient using both geometric and nongeometric cues. When children were given practice in the standard small rectangular room with the feature wall, a more subtle feature training task, these children were also able to conjoin geometric and nongeometric cues after a relatively small number of trials. Moreover, Learmonth and colleagues (2008) found that three-year-old children needed only four trials in a larger room with a feature—a situation in which they naturally use features as well as geometry—to show use of features in the small room, in which without prior experience they do not use features. Thus, it appears that practice with nongeometric cues, both salient and subtle, can influence the use of geometric and nongeometric information.

Rearing
Rearing experiments take the principles of training experiments one step further and dramatically display the flexibility of cue use. One of the first studies to demonstrate this flexibility was with wild-caught mountain chickadees (Gray et al. 2005). These birds live in forested areas lacking salient geometric cues, in contrast to the standard rearing

environment in a lab. The chickadees were trained to find food in the corner of an enclosed rectangle with one blue wall as the salient feature wall. When the target corner was adjacent to the feature wall, the chickadees did not encode the geometry of the enclosure. However, when the target corner was away from the feature wall, the chickadees did encode the geometry (figure 6.2). Thus, the use of geometric and nongeometric information depended on the proximity of the nongeometric, or featural, information to the target corner.

To further understand the effects of rearing, two groups of researchers used a laboratory version of the wild-caught chickadee experiment. Brown and colleagues (2007) reared convict cichlids *Archocentrus nigrofasciatus* in either a circular (lacking geometry) or rectangular tank (salient right angles). Unlike the chickadees, all of the fish encoded the geometry of the rectangle. However, there were still differences between the groups. Fish that had been reared in the circular tank more rapidly learned to use features than fish that had been reared in the geometry-rich rectangular tank. Further differences were revealed on conflict trials, where the feature wall was moved from a short wall to a long wall or vice versa, placing the learned geometry in conflict with the feature location. A conflict task reveals the hierarchy structure of the cues. Fish that had been reared in the circular

(a) Control Tests

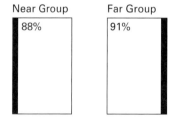

(b) Geometry Tests

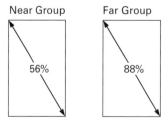

Figure 6.2
In this figure the data are presented as an average, with the correct corner in the top left position. From panel (a), both groups accurately selected the correct corner on probe trials where reinforcement was not available. The crucial test is in panel (b). Here, the near-feature group failed to encode geometry as they selected a geometrically equivalent corner at chance (50 percent). In contrast, the far-feature group encoded the geometry of the apparatus, performing above chance. Adapted from Gray et al. (2005).

tank chose the featurally correct corner more often than their rectangular-reared counterparts who more often chose a geometrically correct corner. Thus, the use of geometric and nongeometric information was influenced by the rearing environment of the convict cichlids.

Chiandetti and Vallortigara (2008) examined the influence of rearing environment on the performance of chicks in the reorientation task. This particular species is quite precocial, and hence experience might have less of an impact on the weighting of reorientation cues, compared to species with longer developmental periods. After hatching, chicks were placed in either a rectangular or circular cage for two days before training began on the third day of life. Whether training occurred in the presence or absence of features, all chicks encoded the geometry of the environment. But because the crucial conflict tests were not conducted, it remains unknown whether there may be a hierarchy of spatial cues related to rearing environment.

At this point we are just starting to understand some of the differences in the flexibility of use of geometric and nongeometric cues. There may be species-specific reasons why malleability is found in some cases, such as the children or the mountain chickadees, whereas a more crystallized pattern is found in other cases, such as the chicks or fish. It is also possible to look at these data as they relate to the developmental period. If one looks at the spectrum from precocial to altricial, it is possible that the amount of flexibility within the adaptive combination model may depend on where on this spectrum an organism lies. At the precocial end, we may find the chicks are "good to go" as soon as they hatch, indicating that their spatial navigation system may be crystallized early on. At the other end of the spectrum we might find that altricial species, such as humans, elephants, and hippopotamuses, with an elongated period of development, may be able to support a more flexible cognitive system, including spatial navigation as one example. Future research on species differences could prove to be worthwhile.

Inferred Geometric Information

Natural environments do not typically contain fully enclosed regular geometric spaces. The appeal of the geometric module hypothesis rests in part on the proposition that geometric aspects of the environment such as cliff faces and river courses are unlikely to change, whereas the coloration or texture of cliffs or rivers may change with the season or the weather (Gallistel 1990). Even though cliff faces or river courses are extended in space, however, they rarely delineate more than a portion of the area surrounding a person or animal, and what is delineated is done so in a complex and irregular way. In addition, many natural environments, such as open savannah areas, are fairly uniform except for discrete landmarks (Poucet 1993). These observations have several implications for the geometric module hypothesis. First, they suggest that the typical experiment conducted so far tests the role of geometry in reorientation at "industrial strength," namely when there is minimal uncertainty regarding the shape and when the geometry can easily be encoded from the ratio of long and short sides meeting at a right angle. Second, and following from the first point, they suggest that a crucial test of the geometric module hypothesis in an evolutionary-adaptive context is whether geometry can be used in cases where it must be inferred from fragmentary information, and if so, whether its strength is reduced when this is the case.

It appears that human adults can use geometry that is only suggested by the presence of separated landmarks marking the vertices of a geometric figure (Gouteux and Spelke 2001; Kelly and Bischof 2005), as can rats, as shown by Gibson and colleagues (2007b), although note that they changed the position and orientation of the arrays rather than disorienting the rats. However, nutcrackers do not use geometry defined in this way (Kelly 2005), which is a puzzling finding given that animals able to fly would appear to be particularly advantaged in discerning overall relations among separated aspects of the environment.

Kelly and Bischof (2005) have conducted several studies to examine the relative use of partial versus fully specified geometry. Human participants were presented with a nonimmersive three-dimensional-reorientation computer task. A rectangular room was displayed on the screen with uniquely colored and shaped landmarks in each corner. This environment contains two types of geometric information: fully specified surface information and partial information from a configuration of objects. The walls of the rectangle create a surface geometry. The relation between the landmarks also creates a rectangle and thus could be classified as configuration geometry. The weighting of surface and configuration geometry depended on the initial experience. Participants were trained with either surface geometry or configuration geometry, or both. At test, the surface and configuration geometry were placed in conflict (see figure 6.3). Participants who were presented with only one useful type of geometry weighted that category of geometry more heavily than the other type. For participants trained with both types of geometry, the searches were divided equally between surface and configuration geometry. Thus, the hierarchy of surface and configuration geometry depends on experience for adults, in accord with the adaptive combination view, but it was not clear that there was a preference for fully specified information over the configuration. However, this fact may be specific to use of human adults, of computerized testing, or of the training regime.

Do human children use geometry when overall shape is only partially specified? The answer to this question is not yet clear. Gouteux and Spelke (2001) found that children of three and four years need at least a set of partial extended surfaces, although not necessarily a closed figure, to use geometric information. Lee and Spelke (2008) found, similarly, that closed figures were necessary for four-year-olds to use geometric information, finding additionally that figures formed by flat lines were not used. In a series of investigations involving the use of maps (and so not directly relevant to the disorientation paradigm, although arguably still suggestive), Vasilyeva and Bowers (2006) found that the ability to infer geometric information from partial information improves markedly between the ages

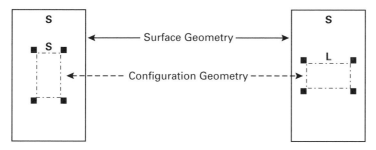

(a) Consistent Information   (b) Conflicting Information

Figure 6.3
Surface and configuration geometry. In the diagram, the large rectangle represents the fully specified surface geometry. The squares represent possible response locations. Imagine a rectangle connecting these points. Here, a second geometric relationship exists and this is called configuration geometry, as indicated by the dashed line. In panel (a), the two types of geometry agree with each other so that the small, S, and long, L, sides of the rectangles match. In panel (b), the relationship is now conflicting. Through this type of trial, the participant's bias for either surface or configuration geometry is revealed. For example, a participant may have been asked to learn that the top left square was correct in panel (a) during training. At test, in panel (b), the participant is asked to make a choice. If the preference is for surface geometry, then the participant will select the top left box. However, if the bias is for configuration geometry, then the participant selects the bottom left box. Original figure and caption, Kelly and Bischof (2005).

of three and six years. Similarly, Gibson et al. (2007a) found that children could not use the geometry of separated points on a computer screen to locate targets until six years of age. On the other hand, Garrad-Cole and colleagues (2001) found that children as young as eighteen to twenty-four months succeeded in using the geometry of four separated objects to define search (as well as in using featural information when available). Further studies using looking paradigms rather than search techniques showed sensitivity to the distances separating discrete objects in children as young as twelve to eighteen months (Lew et al. 2006) and even six to twelve months (Lew et al. 2005).

If one sets aside the studies of mapping or search on computer monitors and the studies using looking techniques, as being not directly relevant to search following disorientation, there is a straightforward contradiction between the studies of Gouteux and Spelke (2001) and Lee and Spelke (2008) on the one hand and that of Garrad-Cole et al. (2001) on the other hand. Cheng and Newcombe (2005) suggested two points of contrast: the use of a reference-memory task (Garrad-Cole et al. 2001) vs. a working-memory task (Gouteux and Spelke 2001), and the fact that experimental procedures with children were conducted by parents in Garrad-Cole et al.'s study. There may well be other differences, including the placement of the boxes with respect to a larger enclosing space (Lew et al. 2006). The whole question deserves a closer look, not only at methodological variables that might account for the discrepancy but also at the extent to which partial geometry is relied on compared to fully specified geometry and to features. The latter issue is key to the theoretical debate, because the adaptive-combination position clearly predicts that use of geometry should be weakened when its encoding would be expected to be more uncertain, and might strengthen as children learn more about the usefulness of such partial information.

Two Recent Arguments for Innate Geometry

So far, most of this chapter has concentrated on the adaptive-combination view of how organisms perform spatial reorientation tasks. Such a view is consistent with what we know about spatial functioning more generally—mobile animals seem to navigate using a wide variety of sources of relevant information. It is also consistent with plasticity approaches to evolution and development, as we discuss in more depth in the next and last section. However, the innate modularity approach to the evolutionary and developmental issues has maintained its popularity, despite critiques and empirical disconfirmations of many of its findings or predictions. In particular, two recent articles have advanced arguments for retaining this approach to spatial development. The first is directly relevant to the geometric module debate; the second is only indirectly relevant but is discussed here because of the considerable attention it received when it appeared.

Can Features Alone Be Used to Reorient?

Lee and colleagues (2006) asked what role landmarks might serve in four-year-olds' reorientation. Specifically, they asked whether landmarks would serve as reorientation cues or as beacons for an object's location. In order to probe this question, they placed three containers in an equilateral-triangle configuration in the center of a circular room. For the majority of their experiments across a series of trials they used two blue boxes (the indistinct containers) and one red cylinder (the distinct container) in which they hid a sticker. Their logic was that if children directly associated landmarks to locations, then they should only succeed when the object was hidden at the distinctive container. Children correctly found the target sticker when it was hidden at the cylinder whereas their searches were at chance when either of the two identical boxes covered the sticker (or stickers). From these search patterns, they concluded that children used the red cylinder only as a direct cue to an object's location. From their findings, they propose that "behavior following reorientation depends on two distinct processes: a modular reorientation process that is sensitive only to geometry and an associative process that directly links landmarks to goal locations" (p. 581).

These bold assertions are not, however, clearly supported by the experiments that Lee and colleagues conducted. Newcombe and colleagues (2007) pointed out that the small, movable landmarks placed on top of the targets used in Lee et al. may not be used because they lack the trustworthiness of large, stable landmarks and that, in addition, the area they defined was quite small. They suggested an alternative way to examine the use of features to reorient when associative processes can be ruled out, using an octagon with alternating short and long sides. If the octagon contains one colored wall, one examines the children's ability to discriminate among boxes located at three all-white corners that are geometrically congruent.

The first step is to examine reorientation in an octagonal space in which all of the walls are white, because no prior research has used such a complex geometry. Newcombe and colleagues (2006) found that two- and three-year-old children used the geometry of the space to guide their searches. Children were reliable in choosing boxes that bore a geometrically equivalent relationship (for example, long wall on the left connected to a short wall on the right) to the box where the target object, a toy duck, was hidden. These results provided the foundation for the critical test; reorienting in the octagon with one feature, a long red wall.

In the octagon with the red wall, Newcombe and colleagues (2007) found that three- and five-year-old children were able to reliably choose the correct corner in the cases in which children searched for the target in the unmarked, all-white corners (the target box did not border the red wall). Their correct searches were significantly greater than the average of the two other geometrically correct corners that bordered white walls. These results demonstrate that children in fact use features to reorient in a relatively large complex environment in a nonassociative fashion.

Geometric Principles among the Munduruku

The Munduruku are an Amazonian group who live in isolated villages and have little access to schools. Their language is reported to have few words for geometric or spatial concepts, they do not possess instruments for spatial measurement, and they do not use or draw maps to any great extent. Thus, if cultural or linguistic transmission were essential to the formation of basic geometric concepts, the Munduruku would be expected to perform poorly when asked about such fundamental concepts as parallelism or congruence. On the other hand, if the human mind comes equipped with the prerequisites for spatial thought, they would be expected to be able to recognize such concepts. Dehaene and colleagues (2006) evaluated geometric thinking among Munduruku children and adults by showing participants panels of six figures (using a solar-powered laptop). Five figures shared a key geometric characteristic that the other one lacked. For instance, there might be five pairs of parallel lines and one pair of nonparallel lines. Crucially, the five sets of parallel lines varied in several ways, such as their orientation and the distance between the paired lines. When asked to point out the "weird" or "ugly" image, the Munduruku reliably chose the geometrically odd figure, such as the nonparallel lines, as predicted by the "core knowledge" position (see figure 6.4a).

The results seem to show strong support for a hard-wired view of human cognitive ability, as was heavily stressed in media coverage of the study by outlets such as the *New York Times* (Bakalar 2006). However, some aspects of the data support plasticity (Newcombe and Uttal 2006). First, Dehaene and his colleagues tested American children and

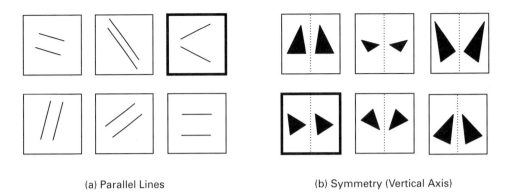

(a) Parallel Lines   (b) Symmetry (Vertical Axis)

Figure 6.4
Geometric principles among Americans and the Munduruku: perception of incongruent patterns. From among six images, participants select the incongruent tile (indicated here with a heavy border). In panel (a) both Americans and the Munduruku select the pair of lines that do not run parallel. In panel (b), there is a cultural difference for symmetry across a vertical axis. The above-chance performance of the Americans, as indicated by the heavy border, is not matched by the Munduruku. Adapted from Dehaene et al. (2006).

adults as a comparison group for their Amazonian sample, and they repeatedly found that American adults did better than Munduruku of any age, as well as better than American children. This improved performance shows us that culture, language, or education likely helps us build a more robust edifice on the foundation of our core intuitions. Second, the Munduruku performed particularly poorly on items involving geometric transformations (see figure 6.4b); the fact that American adults can cope well with such items is noteworthy because this ability is likely of practical importance to performance in science and technical disciplines. Third, Dehaene and colleagues also note, though they did not test, that it is possible that the geometric intuitions they assessed are acquired progressively during the first six years of life, that is, at ages younger than those they studied. Finer-grained study of geometric intuitions and mapping ability in Munduruku infants and very young children might show a progression of success, as has been found in previous studies of American infants and preschoolers, who often do *not* seem able to cope with some of the concepts with which the older American and Munduruku children showed success.

Plasticity and Modularity in Cognitive Development

Must we choose between plasticity and innate modularity, in an only slightly refreshed version of the nativist-empiricist debate? Perhaps not. Evolution and development have recently come together in the modern study of biology, in the form of evolutionary developmental biology, sometimes called evo-devo. The main ideas of this line of research are said to be innovation, modularity, plasticity, emergence, and inherency (Müller 2005).

This list of traits, and in particular the inclusion of modularity along with plasticity and emergence, points to the potential of this conceptual framework for allowing the formulation of integrated accounts of cognitive development that get beyond old dichotomies. Similarly, Barrett and Kurzban (2006) provide a road map to rapprochement when they write, "Emergentism should not be viewed as an alternative to an evolutionary approach. . . . In particular, the error is the view that proximate and ultimate causation are competitors" (p. 637). In other words, the ultimate causation created by adaptive pressures can be executed proximately in a variety of ways, and in particular, by endowing young organisms with prepared learning propensities rather than explicitly preformed representations (Greenough et al. 1987).

Consider the research area in which the notion of prepared learning was first proposed—the example of taste aversion and specific hungers. Some pairings of stimuli and consequences are far more easily learned than others. For example, specific tastes are more easily paired with nausea than with shock and audiovisual stimuli are more easily paired with shock than with nausea (Garcia and Koelling 1966). Conditioned taste aversion can be established even when there are long delays between the taste and the nausea (Garcia et al. 1966). These discoveries put learning in an evolutionary context without undermining the fact that real learning is occurring. Furthermore, the findings allow for specification of what initial structure really means. When investigators noted that rats deficient in some essential nutrient, such as thiamine, preferred to eat thiamine-rich diets to their usual fare, it was initially natural to postulate a "wisdom of the body" that recognized specifically what was lacking and sought it out. However, Rozin and Kalat (1971) showed that a general aversion to diets that create illness, such as those caused by vitamin deficiency or poisonous substances, leads to a general preference for novel food items in situations where only long-familiar foods are being consumed. There is no specific recognition of what substance is needed. Thus, an evolutionarily important goal (avoiding illness) can be reached by the provision of a general rule (try new foods if you feel bad when eating the usual ones) rather than specific knowledge (look for thiamine).

A similar but more recent example of the role of learning in understanding the evolution of development comes from Dukas's work on perceptual learning (see chapter 8, this volume). Whether or not it pays for an organism to specialize in recognizing camouflaged food items depends on the variety of foods in the environment: if food is plentiful and much of it is easily identified, then an investment in the perceptual learning required to find such food is ill advised. However, when camouflaged foods are the predominant sources of nutrition, perceptual learning is beneficial. In addition, when several camouflaged food sources are available, which prey a predator learns to recognize is a matter of chance, with the beneficial effect that specializations will vary across predators so that no one food source is as likely to be exhausted. In this case, an evolutionarily important goal (feeding) can be reached by the availability of a capacity for perceptual learning that occurs only in certain environments.

Is modularity required for a prepared-learning approach to cognitive development? The answer depends on one's definition of modularity. The kind of modularity that Müller had in mind when he included it on his list of attributes of an evo-devo approach is quite different from the kind of modularity stressed by Fodor (1983). As originally proposed by Fodor (1983), modularity was a strictly defined concept requiring the demonstration of several attributes, notably encapsulation from other informational sources and associated resistance to change, and was said to characterize sensory input more than central processes. However, the term "modularity" quickly came to refer simply to the idea that there may be neural and functional specialization for processes such as face or place recognition (Epstein and Kanwisher 1998; Kanwisher et al. 1997) and that evolution worked by selection pressure on such specializations (Cosmides and Tooby 1992). Unfortunately, subsequent authors have often been quite unclear about what they have in mind when they use the term. Newcombe and Ratliff (2007) argued that encapsulation is central to a clear definition of modularity and that when researchers simply mean neural specialization, they should say so, rather than using one term to mean many different things. Barrett and Kurzban (2006) disagree, saying that encapsulation as well as various other criteria are unimportant to modularity, and instead suggest that "module" is one way of talking about the simple fact of functional specialization.

In summary, we have argued in this chapter against the idea that evolution can only work to create cognitive advances by affecting selection for innately based and encapsulated modules. It might do so, but it need not. Instead, and more consistent with the existence of a lengthy juvenile period that itself may have overall evolutionary value, our species may have been subject to selection pressures for prepared learning that enables flexible accommodation to the vast array of environmental niches in which we have been able to live successfully. Such preparation would include starting points for learning as well as powerful learning algorithms, and that initial equipment may lead to emerging cognitive and neural specialization.

Note

1. Foster and colleagues (1989) found that completely preventing movement of the rats affected place cell firing. However, place cells do fire in the absence of self-motion when rats are moved passively (Gavrilov et al. 1998), which disrupts proprioceptive cues but leaves vestibular signals as the only reliable cue (Stackman et al. 2003).

References

Acredolo LP (1978) Development of spatial orientation in infancy. Dev Psychol 14: 224–234.

Acredolo LP, Evans D (1980) Developmental change in the effects of landmarks on infant spatial behavior. Dev Psychol 16: 312–318.

Bakalar N (2006) Mastering the geometry of the jungle (or doin' what comes naturally). New York Times, January 24, F3.

Barrett HC, Kurzban R (2006) Modularity in cognition: Framing the debate. Psychol Rev 113: 628–647.

Brown AA, Spetch ML, Hurd, PL (2007) Growing in circles: Rearing environment alters spatial navigation in fish. Psychol Sci 18: 569–573.

Burgess N (2006) Spatial memory: How egocentric and allocentric combine. Trends Cogn Sci 10: 551–557.

Cheng K (1986) A purely geometric module in the rat's spatial representation. Cognition 23: 149–178.

Cheng K, Newcombe NS (2005) Is there a geometric module for spatial orientation? Squaring theory and evidence. Psychon B Rev 12: 1–23.

Cheng K, Shettleworth SJ, Huttenlocher J, Rieser JJ (2007) Bayesian integration of spatial information. Psychol Bull 133: 625–637.

Cheng K, Spetch ML (1998) Mechanisms of landmark use in mammals and birds. In: Spatial representations in animals (Healy S, ed), 4. Oxford: Oxford University Press.

Chiandetti C, Regolin L, Sovrano VA, Vallortigara G (2006) Spatial reorientation: The effects of space size on the encoding of landmark and geometry information. Anim Cogn 10: 159–168.

Chiandetti C, Vallortigara G (2008) An innate geometric module? Effects of experience with angular geometric cues on spatial reorientation based on the shape of the environment. Anim Cogn 11: 139–146.

Cosmides L, Tooby J (1989) Evolutionary psychology and the generation of culture II. Case study: A computational theory of social exchange. Ethol Sociobiol 10: 51–97.

Cosmides L, Tooby J (1992) Cognitive adaptations for social exchange. In: The adapted mind (Barkow JH, Cosmides L, Tooby J, eds), 163–228. New York: Oxford University Press.

Dehaene S, Izard V, Pica P, Spelke E (2006) Core knowledge of geometry in an Amazonian indigene group. Science 311: 381–384.

Elman J, Bates E, Johnson M, Karmiloff-Smith A, Parisi D, Plunkett K (1996) Rethinking Innateness: A connectionist perspective on development. Cambridge, MA: MIT Press.

Epstein R, Kanwisher N (1998) A cortical representation of the local visual environment. Nature 392: 598–601.

Ernst MO, Banks MS (2002) Humans integrate visual and haptic information in a statistically optimal fashion. Nature 415: 429–433.

Fodor JA (1983) The modularity of mind. Cambridge, MA: MIT Press.

Fodor JA (2000) Replies to critics. Mind Lang 15: 350–374.

Foster T, Castro C, McNaughton B (1989) Spatial selectivity of rat hippocampal neurons: dependence on preparedness for movement. Science 244: 1580–1582.

Gallistel CR (1990) The organization of learning. Cambridge, MA: MIT Press.

Garcia J, Ervin FR, Koelling RA (1966) Learning with prolonged delay of reinforcement. Psychon Sci 5: 121–122.

Garcia J, Koelling RA (1966) Relation of cue to consequence in avoidance learning. Psychon Sci 4: 123–124.

Garrad-Cole F, Lew AR, Bremner JG, Whitaker CJ (2001) Use of cue configuration geometry for spatial orientation in human infants (*Homo sapiens*). J Comp Psychol 115: 317–320.

Gavrilov VV, Wiener SI, Berthoz A (1998) Discharge correlates of hippocampal complex spike neurons in behaving rats passively displaced on a mobile robot. Hippocampus 8: 475–490.

Gelman R, Baillargeon R (1983) A review of some Piagetian concepts. In: Handbook of child psychology, volume 3 (Flavell JH, Markman EM, eds), 167–230. New York: Wiley.

Gibson BM, Leichtman MD, Kung DA, Simpson MJ (2007a) Use of landmark features and geometry by children and adults during a two-dimensional search task. Learn Motiv 38: 89–102.

Gibson BM, Wilks TJ, Kelly DM (2007b) Rats encode the shape of an array of discrete objects. J Comp Psychol 121: 130–144.

Gould SJ (1977) Ontogeny and phylogeny. Cambridge, MA: Harvard University Press.

Gouteux S, Spelke ES (2001) Children's use of geometry and landmarks to reorient in an open space. Cognition 81: 119–148.

Gouteux S, Thinus-Blanc C, Vauclair J (2001) Rhesus monkeys use geometric and nongeometric information during a reorientation task. J Exp Psychol Gen 130: 505–519.

Gray ER, Bloomfield LL, Ferrey A, Spetch ML, Sturdy CB (2005) Spatial encoding in mountain chickadees: Features overshadow geometry. Biol Lett 1: 314–317.

Greenough WT, Black JE, Wallace CS (1987) Experience and brain development. Child Dev 58: 539–559.

Haun DBM, Rapold CJ, Call J, Jazen G, Levinson SC (2006) Cognitive cladistics and cultural override in hominid spatial cognition. P Natl Acad Sci USA 103: 17568–17573.

Hayward A, McGregor A, Good MA, Pearce JM (2003) Absence of overshadowing and blocking between landmarks and the geometric cues provided by the shape of a test arena. Q J Exp Psychol B 56: 114–126.

Hermer L, Spelke E (1994) A geometric process for spatial reorientation in young children. Nature 370: 57–59.

Hermer L, Spelke E (1996) Modularity and development: The case of spatial reorientation. Cognition 61: 195–232.

Hermer-Vazquez L, Moffet A, Munkholm P (2001) Language, space, and the development of cognitive flexibility in humans: The case of two spatial memory tasks. Cognition 79: 263–299.

Huttenlocher J, Hedges LV, Duncan S (1991) Categories and particulars: Prototype effects in estimating spatial location. Psychol Rev 98: 352–376.

Huttenlocher J, Hedges LV, Vevea JL (2000) Why do categories affect stimulus judgment? J Exp Psychol Gen 129: 220–241.

Kanwisher N, McDermott J, Chun M (1997) The fusiform face area: A module in human extrastriate cortex specialized for the perception of faces. J Neurosci 17: 4302–4311.

Karmiloff-Smith A (1992) Beyond Modularity: A Developmental perspective on cognitive science. Cambridge, MA: MIT Press.

Kelly DM (2005) Use of geometric and featural cues in avian species. Paper presentation at the American Association for the Advancement of Science, Washington, D.C.

Kelly DM, Bischof WF (2005) Reorienting in images of a three-dimensional environment. J Exp Psychol Hum Perc Perform 31: 1391–1403.

Kelly DM, Spetch ML (2004a) Reorientation in a two-dimensional environment: I. Do adults encode the featural and geometric properties of a two-dimensional schematic of a room? J Comp Psychol 118: 82–94.

Kelly DM, Spetch ML (2004b) Reorientation in a two-dimensional environment: II. Do pigeons (*Columba livia*) encode the featural and geometric properties of a two-dimensional schematic of a room? J Comp Psychol 118: 384–395.

Kelly DM, Spetch ML, Heth CD (1998) Pigeons' (*Columba livia*) encoding of geometric and featural properties of a spatial environment. J Comp Psychol 112: 259–269.

Kersten D, Yuille A (2003) Bayesian models of object perception. Curr Opin Neurobiol 13: 150–158.

Learmonth A, Nadel L, Newcombe NS (2002) Children's use of landmarks: Implications for modularity theory. Psychol Sci 13: 337–341.

Learmonth A, Newcombe NS, Huttenlocher J (2001) Toddler's use of metric information and landmarks to reorient. J Exp Child Psychol 80: 225–244.

Learmonth A, Newcombe NS, Sheridan M, Jones M (2008) Action and reorientation ability: The role of restricted movement at 3 and 5 years. Dev Sci 11: 414–426.

Lee SA, Shusterman A, Spelke ES (2006) Reorientation and landmark-guided search by young children. Psychol Sci 17: 577–582.

Lee SA, Spelke ES (2008) Children's use of geometry for reorientation. Dev Sci, in press.

Levinson SC (2003) Space in language and cognition. Cambridge: Cambridge University Press.

Lew AR, Foster KA, Bremner JG (2006) Disorientation inhibits landmark use in 12–18 month-old infants. Infant Behav Dev 29: 334–341.

Lew AR, Foster KA, Bremner JG, Slavin S, Green M (2005) Detection of geometric but not topological, spatial transformation in 6- to 12-month-old infants in a visual exploration paradigm. Dev Psychol 29: 31–42.

Marcus G (2004) The birth of the mind. New York: Basic Books.

McComas J, Dulberg C (1997) Children's memory for locations visited: Importance of movement and choice. J Motor Behav 29: 223–230.

Miller NY, Shettleworth SJ (2007) Learning about environmental geometry: An associative model. J Exp Psychol Anim B 33: 191–212.

Müller GB (2005) Evolutionary developmental biology. In: Handbook of evolution: The evolution of living systems (including hominids), volume 2 (Wuketits F, Ayala FJ, eds), 87–115. Weinheim: Wiley.

Nadel L, Hupbach A (2006) Cross-species comparisons in development: The case of the spatial "module". In: Attention and Performance XXI (Johnson MH, Munakata Y, eds), 499–512. Oxford: Oxford University Press.

Newcombe NS, Huttenlocher J (2000) Making space: The development of spatial representation and reasoning. Cambridge, MA: MIT Press.

Newcombe NS, Huttenlocher J (2006) Development of spatial cognition. In: Handbook of child psychology, 6th ed. (Damon W, Lerner R, eds), volume 2: Perception, cognition, and language (Kuhn D, Siegler R, eds), pp 734–776. Hoboken: Wiley.

Newcombe NS, Jones M, Shallcross W (2007) How are geometric and featural information used to reorient in a complex space? In: Symposium, "Spatial representation in young children: How is geometric and non-geometric location information processed?" Society for Research in Child Development, Boston, MA (March).

Newcombe NS, Jones M, Shallcross W, Ratliff KR (2006, November). Combining featural and geometric information in reorientation. Paper presented at the 47th annual meeting of the Psychonomic Society, Houston, TX.

Newcombe NS, Ratliff KR (2007) Explaining the development of spatial reorientation: Modularity-plus-language versus the emergence of adaptive combination. In: The emerging spatial mind (Plumert J, Spencer J, eds), pp 53–76. New York: Oxford University Press.

Newcombe NS, Uttal DH (2006) Whorf versus Socrates, round 10. Trends Cogn Sci 10: 394–396.

O'Keefe J, Nadel L (1978). The hippocampus as a cognitive map. Oxford: Oxford University Press.

Pearce JM, Ward-Robinson J, Good M, Fussel C, Aydin A (2001) Influence of a beacon on spatial learning based on the shape of the test environment. J Exp Psychol Anim B 27: 329–344.

Pearce JM, Graham M, Good MA, Jones PM, McGregor A (2006) Potentiation, overshadowing, and blocking of spatial learning based on the shape of the environment. J Exp Psychol Anim B 32: 201–214.

Poucet B (1993) Spatial cognitive maps in animals—New hypotheses on their structure and neural mechanisms. Psychol Rev 100: 163–182.

Ratliff KR, Newcombe NS (2008) Is language necessary for human spatial reorientation? Reconsidering evidence from dual task paradigms. Cognitive Psychol, 56: 142–163.

Ratliff KR, Newcombe NS (in press) Reorienting when cues conflict: Evidence for an adaptive combination view. Psychol Sci.

Rieser JJ, Pick HL, Ashmead DH, Garing AE (1995) Calibration of human locomotion and models of perceptual-motor organization. J Exp Psychol Hum Perc Perform 21: 480–497.

Rozin P, Kalat JW (1971) Specific hungers and poison avoidance as adaptive specializations of learning. Psychol Rev 78: 459–486.

Siegler RS (1998) Children's thinking, 3rd ed. Upper Saddle River, NJ: Prentice Hall.

Sovrano VA, Bisazza A, Vallortigara G (2005) Animals' use of landmarks and metric information to reorient: Effects of the size of the experimental space. Cognition 97: 122–133.

Sovrano VA, Bisazza A, Vallortigara G (2007) How fish do geometry in large and in small spaces. Anim Cogn 10: 47–54.

Sovrano VA, Vallortigara G (2006) Dissecting the geometric module: A sense-linkage for metric and landmark information in animals' spatial reorientation. Psychol Sci 17: 616–621.

Spelke ES (2000) Core knowledge. Am Psychol 55: 1233–1243.

Spelke ES, Breinlinger K, Macomber J, Jacobson K (1992) Origins of knowledge. Psychol Rev 99: 605–632.

Spelke ES, Kinzler KD (2007) Core knowledge. Dev Sci 10: 89–96.

Spencer J, Thomas M, McClelland J (in press) Towards a new grand theory of development? Connectionism and dynamic systems theory reconsidered. Oxford: Oxford University Press.

Stackman RW, Golob EJ, Bassett JP, Taube JS (2003) Passive transport disrupts directional path integration by rat head direction cells. J Neurophysiol 90: 2862–2874.

Thelen E, Smith LB (1994) A dynamic systems approach to the development of cognition and action. Cambridge, MA: MIT Press.

Twyman A, Friedman A, Spetch ML (2007) Penetrating the geometric module: Catalyzing children's use of landmarks. Dev Psychol 43: 1523–1530.

Vallortigara G, Feruglio M, Sovrano VA (2005) Reorientation by geometric and landmark information in environments of different size. Dev Sci 8: 393–401.

Vasilyeva M, Bowers E (2006) Children's use of geometric information in mapping tasks. J Exp Child Psychol 95: 255–277.

Wall PL, Botly LCP, Black CK, Shettleworth SJ (2004) The geometric module in the rat: Independence of shape and feature learning in a food finding task. Learn Behav 32: 289–298.

Wang HB, Johnson TR, Sun YL, Zhang JJ (2005) Object location memory: The interplay of multiple representations. Mem Cognition 33: 1147–1159.

Wang RF, Spelke ES (2002) Human spatial representation: Insights from animals. Trends Cogn Sci 6: 376–382.

III QUALITIES AND OBJECTS

The three chapters in this section summarize research regarding how learning and attention affect the perception and categorization of objects and object properties.

In chapter 7, Daniel Osorio examines color perception in chicks as a model for various aspects of object cognition, including the abilities to generalize and categorize, and to do so flexibly with changes in task or context. (The flexible adaptation of perception to task demands is also considered by Reuven Dukas (chapter 8) and by Robert L. Goldstone, Alexander Gerganov, David Landy, and Michael Roberts (chapter 9). Osorio points out that chicks can make extremely fine color discriminations. He asks whether their aptitude for discrimination interferes with their ability to treat different colors as equivalent, an essential component of generalization. The question of whether or not chicks can generalize is also important because it intersects with a question that is raised across different cognitive domains: To what extent is language a prerequisite for cognitive behaviors (in this case for the ability to form categories)? (See also chapters 5 and 6, by Giorgio Vallortigara and Alexandra Twyman, respectively, for similar considerations in the space domain, and chapter 10, by Elizabeth M. Brannon and Jessica F. Cantlon, in the number domain.) Osorio surveys previous research and theory on generalization in humans and pigeons, and describes his research showing that chicks can generalize, and that they do so in a manner consistent with a flexible Bayesian model. (For additional discussion of Bayesian models, see chapter 13, by Paul W. Glimcher).

In chapter 8, Reuven Dukas examines the evolutionary biology of limited attention, covering research with humans, monkeys, and jays (and referring to research with other species), and also discussing computational modeling efforts. He explores the questions of why evolutionary change has not expanded attentional capacity so that limited-attention problems are eliminated, and discusses how perceptual learning and the development of expertise can counteract deficits due to limited attention. Regarding learning, chapter 8 fits well with the topics of generalization and perceptual learning covered in chapters 7 and 9. Dukas summarizes research and modeling efforts concerning the trade-offs involved in allocating attention to prey vs. to predators; these trade-offs arise because of limited attention. Both eating and avoiding being eaten are necessary for survival and animals must find a way to allocate the limited attention at their disposal to best balance these demands. Dukas shows that animals allocate their attention flexibly to few or many targets depending on the salience of the targets. The theme of flexibility reoccurs in the two other chapters in this section. Dukas closes his chapter by briefly summarizing the emerging exciting research on both the evolution of attention capacities and genetic variations in attention networks.

In chapter 9, Goldstone, Gerganov, Landy, and Roberts argue that our perceptual systems flexibly and readily adapt to the tasks an individual must accomplish, forming new perceptual feature detectors as needed. They summarize empirical research and modeling efforts showing that task requirements constrain the features used for perception and categorization: conjunctions of features can be unitized if a task can be accomplished more efficiently by doing so, or they can be differentiated if a task requires attention to individual features. They describe a flexible model, the "conceptual and perceptual learning by unitization and segmentation" (CPLUS) model, which can build detectors via either differentiation or unitization while building connections between the detectors and categories. Goldstone and colleagues emphasize human learning and development and describe research showing that perceptual features can be altered by experience.

Taken together, the chapters in this section cover an impressive array of research on attention and learning in a number of different species, accomplished by means of tasks whose range reaches from foraging to conjunctive categorization. The chapters in this section show how new answers to questions essential for understanding cognition are generated when research with adult humans is complemented by research with chicks, jays, and developing humans as well as by computational modeling efforts.

7 Color Generalization by Birds

Daniel Osorio

Color vision is important for object recognition, because under different viewing conditions the chromaticity (hue and saturation) of an object is more stable than its brightness. Even so, the spectrum reflected from a given surface alters substantially with changes in illumination and with specular effects such as gloss. At the same time a change in pigmentation (object color) may or may not give information about biologically relevant properties such as the food value of an object. In some circumstances accurate judgment of color may be essential, as when a bird chooses between potential mates, or when it has to distinguish edible insect prey from a toxic species. On the other hand a fruit might remain edible as it ripens from yellow to red, but be inedible when it is green or brown. Given that the relevance of a color difference between two surfaces depends on both the objects of interest and the viewing conditions, it is interesting to ask whether animals are able to learn about how stimuli vary so as to make the effective use of sensory information for object recognition.

More broadly there is a widely held view that human concepts and categories are dictated by language (Whorf and Carrol 1956; Kay and Kempton 1984; Davidoff 2001). It follows from this argument that language is essential for perceptual categorization—that is, the ability to make sharp distinctions on a continuum of stimuli (Harnad 1987; Davidoff 2001). This focuses interest on how nonhuman species classify objects (Herrnstein and Loveland 1964). Pigeons have been successfully trained to classify objects ranging from tree leaves (Cerella 1979) to human faces and works of art (Watanabe et al. 1995; Troje et al. 1999), but the complexity of leaves, faces, and paintings makes it difficult to understand how they are recognized (Aust and Huber 2006). By comparison with color one can investigate generalization with well-defined stimuli on a low-dimensional perceptual continuum.

This chapter starts with background information on bird color vision, and goes on to look at how birds generalize from familiar to novel colors, especially how they use information about variation among familiar stimuli, and what they learn in the initial encounter with a novel stimulus. Historically, most work on object recognition and sensory generalization by animals has used pigeons, and I compare some of the findings on pigeons with our own more recent work on poultry chicks. We find that week-old poultry chicks learn color quickly and accurately. Presumably the ability to make fine discriminations is advantageous, but it means that the chicks may face difficulties when it is beneficial to treat relatively diverse colors as equivalent—to make a perceptual category. We can therefore investigate how these birds generalize between stimuli that they can easily discriminate.

The relationship between discrimination and generalization has long been a focus of work on animal perception (Lashley and Wade 1946; Hull 1947; Blough 1969; Honig and Urcuioli 1981; Ham and Osorio 2007). Matters would be straightforward if the perceived magnitude of a large stimulus were lawfully related to the discrimination threshold—specifically, if any two stimuli that differ by a given number of just noticeable differences (jnd's) appear equally distinct. Metrics (or laws) for large stimulus differences have been proposed since the nineteenth century (Stevens 1957) and have been applied to color (Schrödinger 1920; Wyszecki and Stiles 1982). If these metrics are valid, then judgments of similarity between stimuli (a process of generalization) should depend on processes that also set the discrimination threshold. Conversely, generalization and categorization may be quite distinct from discrimination. Whereas discrimination thresholds are probably fixed by low-level phenomena such as noise in receptors (Vorobyev and Osorio 1998), it would be beneficial for judgments of similarity to be more flexibly matched to a particular task or ecological context (Nosofsky 1992). To distinguish between these possibilities it is helpful to understand color metrics and, more generally, what we mean by color vision in animals.

Defining Color and Color Differences for Animals

The concepts and language that refer to color come from human subjective experience, but they strongly influence work on animal color vision. For example, the existence of conscious color sensations (or qualia) such as red or blue suggests that color is represented separately from other sensory qualities (Lueck et al. 1989; Stoerig 1998). Self-evidently it is difficult to demonstrate that animals experience qualia, and this has led to debate about the definition of color vision for nonhuman species; there are three main views on this. The first and simplest definition refers to the ability to discriminate lights by their spectral composition. Single-celled algae and jellyfish, whose "eyes" do not produce a focused image, use the spectrum to orient themselves toward or away from a light. This phototactic behavior is often described as wavelength-specific behavior, in contrast to "true" color vision (Menzel 1979; Kelber et al. 2003). Innate color preferences are also treated as wavelength-specific behaviors: for example, when a butterfly selects a specific leaf color for egg laying, or a firefly locates the bioluminescence of a potential mate (Menzel 1979; Kolb and Scherer 1982; Booth et al. 2004). Workers such as Menzel (1979) offer a different definition, and suggest that color vision entails the ability to learn. This view reflects the influence of von Frisch (1914), who demonstrated that bees can learn the color of a food source, and carries the implication that there is a central representation of color where learning can take place. Finally, Stoerig (1998) uses a still more "cognitive" criterion by arguing that conscious experience is a requirement for color vision.

Regardless of the definition of color vision, color discrimination depends upon having more than one spectral type of photoreceptor. The outputs of different receptor types are compared by mechanisms (such as opponent neurons) that give chromatic signals. These signals are sensitive to the spectral composition of a light, but relatively insensitive to its overall intensity. Given that receptors ultimately determine whether a stimulus can be detected, it is often helpful to specify chromaticity in terms of receptor excitations (figures 7.1, 7.2; Macleod and Boynton 1979; Kelber et al. 2003). The properties of cones in the avian retina were poorly known until about 1980 (figure 7.1; Hart and Hunt 2007). Instead much work with pigeons used the monochromatic spectrum as the metric for evaluating color perception (Guttman and Kalish 1956; Honig and Urcuioli 1981). Wavelength is well defined, but the wavelength discrimination function ($\Delta\lambda/\lambda$) is not uniform across the spectrum, so that a given wavelength difference does not equate to a consistent level of discriminability (figure 7.2c). Moreover, in avian receptor space (figure 7.2a) the monochromatic locus curves sharply at 550 nm, so that color differences do not even increase monotonically with wavelength separation. Unfortunately, studies of color generalization by pigeons often used wavelengths around 550 nm (Hanson 1959; Honig and Urcuioli 1981).

To investigate the relationship between discrimination and generalization a well-defined metric is important. It is possible to use the $\Delta\lambda/\lambda$ function, or to rescale data (such as generalization curves) so that they can be fitted by a common function (Shepard 1965).

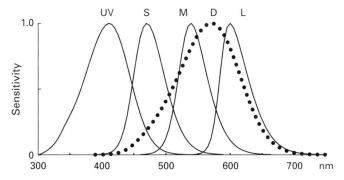

Figure 7.1
Estimated spectral sensitivities of chicken cone photoreceptors that were used for modeling color signals (pigeon receptors are similar). In common with most birds chickens have five types of cones (Hart and Hunt 2007). These are known as UV or violet (UV/VS), short (S), medium (M), and long (L) wavelength single cones, and double cones (D). Colored oil droplets sharpen the spectral sensitivities of the S, M, and L single cones. There is evidence that the UV, S, M, and L single cones give tetrachromatic color vision, whereas the double cones (D) give an avian luminance signal (Osorio et al. 1999b; Goldsmith and Butler 2005; Jones and Osorio 2004; Cuthill 2006). For the experiments that are described in this chapter the illumination was filtered with a cut-off at about 480 nm to exclude the UV receptor. Excluding the fourth receptor simplifies the task of producing color stimuli with commercial media such as inkjet printers.

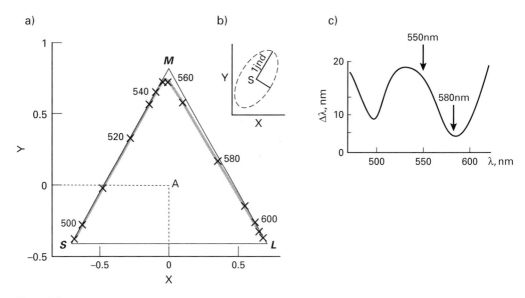

Figure 7.2
Representation of chromaticity and color differences for birds. (a) A chromaticity diagram for chicken S, M, and L single cones. Color loci are given by the formula: $X = \sqrt{\frac{1}{2}}(l-s)$; $Y = \frac{2}{3}(m - \frac{1}{2}(l-s))$, where l, m and s are normalized responses of the L, M, and S cones such that $l + m + s = 1$, and for the illuminant $l = m = s$ (Osorio et al. 1999a). A spectrally flat reflector is by definition achromatic and lies at the origin (A). The triangle corresponds to the gamut of colors that can be achieved with positive receptor excitation, and the gray line corresponds to the monochromatic locus, with wavelengths indicated at 10 nm intervals from 490 nm – 620 nm (x). The monochromatic line is close to the edges of the color triangle because of the small overlap between L and S receptor spectral sensitivities (see figure 7.1). Note that Euclidean distances between monochromatic lights vary in a complicated way with their spectral separation; this potentially complicates the interpretation of studies that define stimuli in terms of wavelength. (b) The locus of colors that are just noticeably different (jnd) from a given stimulus (S) form an ellipse. If color thresholds are set by noise in photoreceptors, then loci plotted in a space whose axes are determined by receptor excitations produce threshold ellipses that are approximately uniform across the X, Y space (Vorobyev and Osorio 1998; Kelber et al. 2003; Goldsmith and Butler 2003, 2005). It follows that a given vector corresponds to a fixed number of jnd's. Schrödinger (1920) proposed that the perceived magnitude of suprathreshold difference is proportional to the (minimum) number of jnd's separating two colors (Wyszecki and Stiles 1982; see also Ham and Osorio 2007). (c) The wavelength discrimination function ($\Delta\lambda$ vs. λ) for pigeons (adapted from Honig and Urcuioli 1981). As predicted from the chromaticity diagram, wavelength discrimination at 580 nm is finer than at 550 nm. This difference arises because L and S cones are insensitive to 550 nm light, whereas at 580 nm both L and M cones respond (see figure 7.1). The minimum value of $\Delta\lambda$ of about 5 nm can be compared to the threshold for ten-day-old chicks in our studies, which is at least tenfold smaller (unpublished observations; see also figure 7.6b).

Even so, uncertainty about the underlying metric remained a concern in early work on color generalization by pigeons (Guttman and Kalish 1956; Shepard 1965; Blough 1969; Honig and Urcuioli 1981). It is interesting that in studies of pigeons, the extent of generalization measured on a wavelength scale varied substantially less than would be expected from the wavelength discrimination function (figures 7.2 and 7.4; see Shepard 1965). As I shall discuss, this observation suggests that generalization of suprathreshold color differences is independent of discrimination.

Photoreceptor spectral sensitivities have now been measured for many species of bird, including poultry (Bowmaker and Knowles 1977; Govardovskii and Zueva 1977; Kelber et al. 2003; Hart and Hunt 2007), which makes it possible to relate perceptual measures of color difference to photoreceptor responses (Vorobyev and Osorio 1998; Vorobyev et al. 1998). Nearly all birds have four types of single cones, which have relatively narrow spectral sensitivities, and also double cones, whose sensitivity approximates that of the human long-wavelength (red) cone (figure 7.1). There is evidence that birds use their single cones for tetrachromatic color vision, whereas the double cones, which are most numerous, serve an avian luminance system that is analogous to the magnocellular system of primates (Osorio et al. 1999b,c; Goldsmith and Butler 2003, 2005; Jones and Osorio 2004). Also, we have shown that color discrimination thresholds can be predicted by a model that assumes that these thresholds are set by chromatic (i.e., opponent) mechanisms whose performance is limited by noise in photoreceptors (Vorobyev and Osorio 1998). One can therefore define colors in terms of receptor excitations, and specify color differences relative to the discrimination threshold (figures 7.1, 7.2). This is helpful in distinguishing roles of low- and high-level processes in perception of color difference (Ham and Osorio 2007).

Color Vision in Poultry Chicks

The experiments described here used male poultry chicks, which are obtained from a commercial hatchery and then housed and trained in pairs. In training, which starts a week after hatching, the chicks are placed in a 0.4 m × 0.3 m arena with paper food containers scattered across the floor (figure 7.3a, 7.3b). Normally there are eight food containers, four each of two colors. One color (S_+) contains chick crumbs, and the other (S_-) is empty. The chicks are trained for six six-minute sessions over three days, with about twenty pairs of chicks used in each experimental cohort. Chicks learn to peck at the containers to extract food crumbs, and to recognize rewarded containers. During training, the S_+ containers are replenished at one-minute intervals. Even though lost time (< five seconds) is the only cost of selecting the S_- stimuli, the chicks become highly selective, directing close to 100 percent of pecks to the rewarded color.

Stimulus colors, defined in terms of photoreceptor excitations (figures 7.1, 7.2), are printed onto the food containers with an inkjet printer. Colors are embedded in a random tiling of 2×6 mm rectangles (which is easily resolved by the chicks). The pattern normally consists of, on average, 70 percent achromatic (gray) background tiles and 30 percent chromatic tiles of the stimulus color (indicated in the figures by a black cross; Osorio et al. 1999c). The mean brightness of the background and stimulus colors are set to be equal for the double cones (i.e., isoluminant; see Jones and Osorio 2004). To prevent the chicks from using brightness rather than chromatic information, the intensity of the tiles is randomized with a uniform distribution and contrast range of 30 percent.

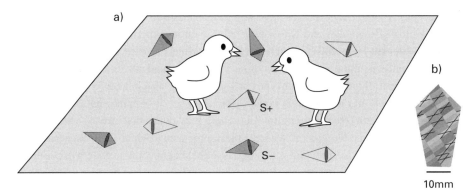

Figure 7.3
Testing color vision of poultry chicks. (a) In our experiments, week-old male poultry chicks are trained in pairs to obtain food from paper food containers, eight of which scattered across the floor of a 0.4 m × 0.3 marena. Normally there are four containers of one color (S+) and four of a different color (S-), all with the same mean intensity, which has the same brightness as the arena floor. S+ contains chick crumbs and S- identifies empty food containers. See text for further details. (b) The food containers are printed by a standard inkjet printer with a random tiling of 2 mm × 6 mm rectangles (easily resolved by the chicks). The pattern normally consists of (on average) 70 percent achromatic (gray) background tiles and 30 percent chromatic tiles of the stimulus color (here indicated by X-shaped black crosses (see text and Osorio et al. 1999c). The mean brightness of the background and stimulus colors are set to be equal for the double cones, and the intensities of the tiles is randomized (see text).

After training, the chicks are tested "in extinction" by presenting them with empty food containers for the familiar (S+ and S- colors) and novel colors. As I shall explain, the birds' color preferences are not stable, but change as a result of testing. For this reason chicks are never tested more than twice. Each test lasts about a minute, and we score ten selections by the two birds (that is, an average of five per bird). This first test reveals the stimulus preferences that are established during training. The second test then shows what is learned about the novel stimuli in the first test.

Accurate Color Recognition

Chicks learn the color of the small paper food containers quickly and accurately (figure 7.3). When they are trained with a single S+ color and are then tested for a single two-minute period without a reward they clearly prefer S+ to novel colors that differ by the equivalent of less than 2 nm on the monochromatic locus at 580 nm (figures 7.2, 7.4; Osorio et al. 1999a). We have not directly compared accuracy in this generalization task to the discrimination threshold, but chicks can readily learn to discriminate colors that differ by the equivalent of 0.5 nm on the monochromatic locus at 580 nm (see figure 7.6). By comparison, the chicks' memory of achromatic brightness and of contrast is poor (Osorio et al. 1999a; unpublished observations). This difference in the accuracy of memory

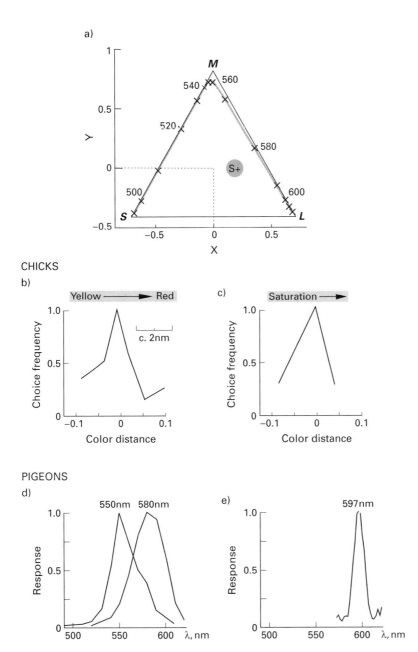

Figure 7.4
Generalization of color by chicks and pigeons following training to a single S₊ (Osorio et al. 1999a). (a–c) Color preferences for chicks trained to obtain food from containers printed with color S₊, which has a hue corresponding to light of about 580 nm (a), but is unsaturated (Osorio et al. 1999a). After training (see text) chicks were presented with novel colors that differed either predominantly in "hue" (b) or saturation (c). On a first encounter, there is a clear preference for the familiar color over novel colors that differ by the equivalent of <2 nm on the monochromatic locus at 580 nm (cf. figure 7.2c). (d–e) Wavelength generalization by pigeons from experiments by Guttman and Kalish (1956) (d), and Blough (1975) (e) is broader than that for chicks (b). Also, despite the large differences in the discrimination threshold (figure 7.2a, 7.2c) generalization over wavelength found by Guttman and Kalish (c) is roughly equal at 550 nm and 580 nm (arrows in figure 7.2c; see also Shepard 1965; Honig and Urcuioli 1981).

for chromatic as opposed to achromatic signals probably reflects their reliability in natural viewing conditions; brightness varies much more according to illumination, so there is no value in learning its precise value for object recognition.

In birds, fine wavelength discrimination is favored by the colored oil droplets in their cones (figure 7.1; Vorobyev 2003). Even so, the chicks' memory for color is impressive, if only because casual observation suggests that humans could not match them. This accuracy may reflect the importance of color (as opposed to shape) for object recognition in these animals. In addition, generalization by the chicks is finer than that reported for pigeons in a conventional operant apparatus (figure 7.4; Guttman and Kalish 1956; Blough 1969, 1975). As we discuss in the final section, this difference in performance could either reflect a species difference, or the nature of the experimental task.

It is easy to see why a precise memory might be beneficial in some circumstances, but often the colors of natural food items—such as fruit, seeds and insects—vary. There could also be a problem with failures of color constancy when objects are viewed under different types of illumination (Brainard and Freeman 1997; Vorobyev et al. 1998). It is therefore worth asking how the birds cope when colors vary—either when different colors offer the same reward, or when the birds compare stimuli that differ in value (such as S_+ vs. S_-). Before describing our findings on how chicks generalize when they have learned about more than color, it is useful to outline current understanding of this subject.

Models of Stimulus Generalization by Animals

When an animal has learned about a stimulus or stimuli on a perceptual dimension x, a generalization curve is defined by the relative strength of response (R) as a function of x (figures 7.4, 7.5, 7.6). For a single stimulus, the curve is usually centered on the stimulus value and may be either exponential (pointed), or rounded (figures 7.4, 7.5; Shepard 1965, 1987; Blough 1969).

Two main types of model have been advanced to account for behavioral generalization on perceptual continuums. One type of model proposes that generalization primarily reflects mechanistic constraints. Pavlov (1927) suggested that any stimulus produces a distributed response in the nervous system, and the overlap of neural responses between stimuli determines the extent of generalization between them. This idea was formalized by Spence (1937) and Hull (1943), and the basic model has since been extended to account for a range of experimental data and in response to insights provided by neural network models of the brain (Enquist and Arak 1993, 1998; Ghirlanda and Enquist 1999, 2003; McLaren and Mackintosh 2002; Cheng 2002). In essence, these mechanistic models postulate some type of internal representation, or map, of the perceptual space; the specific form of the generalization curve depends on how signals spread across this neural map. Models of this kind often imply a close relationship between the extent of generalization

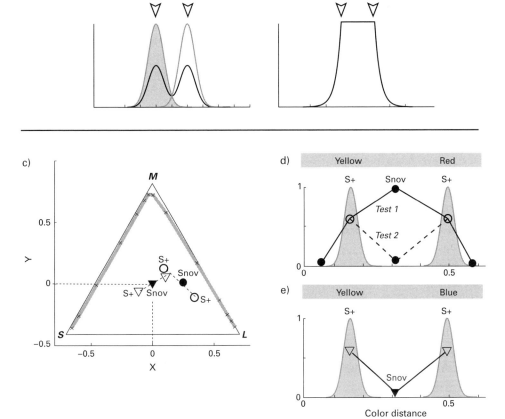

Figure 7.5
Models of generalization by animals trained to two S_+ and a diagrammatic summary of experimental findings for chicks (Jones et al. 2001; Baddeley et al. 2001). (a) A model that treats each sample independently (gray curves), with the overall generalization curve given by linear summation of curves to the separate samples (Spence 1937; Kalish and Guttman 1957, 1959; Blough 1969). (b) A Bayesian model predicts exponential generalization from a single S_+, and flat interpolation between two examples with exponential decay beyond them (Shepard 1987; Tenenbaum and Griffiths 2001). (c) Loci of S_+ pairs *i* (open circles) and *iv* (open triangles) described in the text. Pair *i* (red and yellow) lay on a "hue axis," pair *iv* (blue and yellow) were complementary, lying equal and opposite distances from the achromatic point. Control subjects were trained to a single color. A test compared preferences of chicks for the S_+ and novel colors that lay at an intermediate hue (filled circle) or at the achromatic point (filled triangle). (d) For S_+ pair *i* (open circles in c) the intermediate orange is strongly preferred compared to the prediction of figure 7.5a. The model outlined in (b) predicts flat interpolation, but a full Bayesian model that takes account of stimulus uncertainty could account for this prototype effect, where an intermediate is preferred to exemplars (Jones et al. 2001; Baddeley et al. 2001). There is a similar preference for intermediates with S_+ blue and green (intermediate turquoise), or blue and red (intermediate purple). (e) For S_+ pair *iv* (open triangles in c) there is no interpolation. Instead the preference for the intermediate achromatic color is consistent with the prediction of (a). These observations imply that chicks will not establish a color category between these complementary colors (see also Jones et al. 2001; Baddeley et al. 2001).

and the sensory discrimination threshold (figure 7.2; Hull 1947; Blough 1969; Honig and Urcuioli 1981).

An alternative type of model proposes that generalization is best understood as a process that takes account of how the value of a given stimulus is expected to vary as a function of x (Blough 1969; Shepard 1987). An animal may readily discriminate a novel stimulus S_{nov} from a familiar one S_+, and then estimate the probability that they share common properties. The strength of the response to S_{nov} relative to S_+, and hence the observed generalization curve, would depend on how the response strength is related to the probability of a given outcome, for example, as described by the matching law (Herrnstein 1961).

Shepard (1987) described a probabilistic model for generalization from a single stimulus value, which Tenenbaum and Griffths (2001) expressed in a Bayesian form that can be extended to multiple stimulus values. The model proposes that the brain entertains multiple hypotheses about the true relationship between value and the stimulus parameter x. These hypotheses are summed with weightings that are proportional to their probability of being consistent with observations and/or prior assumptions. New observations alter the weightings. For a single known value, and given general assumptions about the properties of natural objects, Shepard's model predicts exponential generalization curves, such as those observed in pigeons (figures 7.4, 7.5b; Shepard 1965; Blough 1969). In the presence of noise, the curves will develop "shoulders," and hence appear Gaussian (Shepard 1987; Jones et al. 2001). If there are multiple exemplars of S_+ that have equal value, then there should be a flat generalization curve across the region of perceptual space bounded by the known examples, with exponential boundaries (figure 7.5b; Tenenbaum and Griffiths 2001). A sharply demarcated uniform region of this kind is, in effect, a perceptual category (Harnad 1987).

Generalization with Multiple S_+ Colors

As we have mentioned, the chicks' high fidelity to a single S_+ color raises the question of how they use information from multiple examples (figure 7.5a,b; Jones et al. 2001). Generalization from multiple examples is relevant to natural behavior because an animal will rarely encounter identical stimuli twice. Also, different theoretical models make distinguishable predictions for multiple stimuli. The reader may also refer to the older literature that tested pigeons with two or more S_+ colors (Kalish and Guttman 1957, 1959; Blough 1969), and found limited support for Spence's (1937) and Hull's (1943) theoretical predictions about interactions between generalization curves.

Our experiments used two S_+ colors. There were four S_+ pairs, which to the human eye were (*i*) red and yellow, (*ii*) blue and green, (*iii*) blue and red, and (*iv*) blue and yellow (figure 7.5c illustrates the loci of pairs *i* and *iv*; see also Jones et al. 2001). Each pair of colors had approximately equal discriminability. Experimental controls had a single S_+, which was one or other of the training colors. After training, a single test of less than one minute compared preferences for S_+ colors with S_{nov} colors that were either intermediate between S_+ colors in the receptor space (figure 7.5c) or lay beyond the range delimited by S_+ colors.

The main finding was that for S_+ pairs *i–iii* the preference for intermediate S_{nov} colors— namely (*i*) orange, (*ii*) turquoise, and (*iii*) purple—was greater than that predicted by summing the generalization curves for a single S_+ (figures 7.5a, 7.5d; Spence 1937; Hull 1943; Kalish and Guttman 1959; Blough 1969; Jones et al. 2001). In addition, for S_+ pair *i* (red and yellow), chicks did not extrapolate to S_{nov} colors outside the range delimited by these S_+ colors (other training conditions were not tested in this way). These observations suggest that the chicks interpolate over the range delimited by known examples (as opposed to having a general preference for novelty), which is the result predicted by the Bayesian model of generalization (Shepard 1987; Jones et al. 2001; Tenenbaum and Griffiths 2001).

Interestingly, the birds did not interpolate between blue and yellow (pair *iv*), which were complementary colors (figures 7.5a, 7.5c, 7.5e; Jones et al. 2001). Instead the preference for the intermediate, gray, was low and at the level predicted by summing generalization curves for the controls. This raises the possibility that innate rules affect the probability of two separate stimuli being assigned to a continuum (or category). Such a rule would be in reasonable accord with the properties of natural objects in that there are many examples of fruit that ripen from green through yellow to red or to purplish colors, whereas classes of object that range between complementary colors (i.e., through gray) are unusual.

Differential Training and Peak-Shift

After an animal is trained differentially with S_+ and an unrewarded S_- it is commonly found that the peak of the generalization curve is displaced from S_+ in the direction away from S_- (figure 7.6a; Hanson 1959; Friedman and Guttman 1965; Weiss and Weissman 1992; Ghirlanda and Enquist 2003). This phenomenon, known as peak-shift, recently has attracted attention as a basis for the evolution of "exaggerated" animal display signals such as peacock tails (Enquist and Arak 1993, 1998).

Models that assume interaction between separate generalization curves (figure 7.5a; Spence 1937) either predict no peak-shift (e.g., for exponential generalization curves, figure 7.5b) or predict that the magnitude of the displacement of the peak away from S_+ should increase as the separation of S_+ from S_- falls (Ghirlanda and Enquist 1999, 2003). Experimentally peak-shift has been observed (on the wavelength axis) in pigeon color vision with S_+ at 550 nm (but see figure 7.2), when there is also a marked narrowing of the generalization curve (Hanson 1959; Friedman and Guttman 1965; Weiss and Weissman 1992).

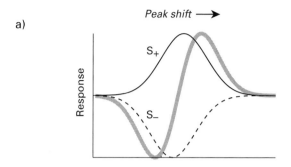

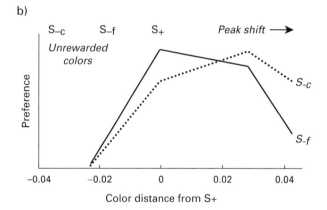

Figure 7.6
The effect of the difference between positive and unrewarded stimulus colors on peak shift (adapted from Baddeley et al. 2007). (a) Peak-shift is a displacement of the preferred stimulus away from S_. If there is a linear interaction between the generalization curves to S$_+$ and S$_-$, then the peak shift should increase as the separation between S$_+$ and S$_-$ decreases (Spence 1937; Hanson 1959; Ghirlanda and Enquist 2003). (b) For poultry chicks, varying the separation of S$_+$ from S$_-$ has the opposite effect on peak-shift from that predicted by Spence (1937). Preferences are given by the number of times a given stimulus was selected during a test. There is a clear peak-shift—that is, displacement of the preference away from S$_-$—but contrary to the predictions of many models the shift is *smaller* after chicks have learned a fine color discrimination, S$_{-f}$, than a coarse discrimination, S$_{-c}$. Note that S$_{-f}$ is readily discriminated from S$_+$ when the color distance is 0.02 units in the XY color space, which corresponds to a wavelength difference of about 0.5 nm at 580 nm (see figure 7.2). An interpretation of this effect is that when fine differences are known to be important, chicks make finer scale distinctions between stimuli so that generalization curves are narrowed (Baddeley et al. 2007).

In our experiments on peak-shift, chicks were trained to make either a fine or a coarse color discrimination (Baddeley et al. 2007). For the coarse condition, the color difference between S$_+$ and the unrewarded color (S$_{-c}$) was double that in the fine condition (S$_{-f}$). Even with S$_{-c}$ the differences between S$_+$ and S$_-$ were very much smaller than those used by Hanson (1959) in his tests of pigeons. For instance, in the experiments that tested peak-shift along a hue axis, the difference between S$_+$ and S$_{-f}$ was equivalent to a wavelength of <1 nm at 580 nm (figure 7.6). We also tested a saturation axis, where the S_- colors were more saturated than S_+ so that any peak-shift was toward gray.

After training there was a single test where the chicks had a choice between four colors: S_{-f}, S_+, and two novel colors. Relative to S_+, these novel colors lay opposite the S_- stimuli (i.e., in the direction of peak-shift). All chicks could readily discriminate S_{-f} from S_+. The main finding was that the peak-shift was smaller in the S_{-f} than in the S_{-c} treatment (figure 7.6b; Baddeley et al. 2007). This effect of separation on peak-shift is inconsistent with Hanson's (1959) observations on pigeons and is contrary to models that predict the extent of peak-shift from the overlap between the separate S_+ and S_- generalization curves (figures 7.5a, 7.6a; Spence 1937; Hull 1943; Ghirlanda and Enquist 1999).

The finding that small color differences give smaller peak-shifts than large differences is reminiscent of the observation in pigeons that generalization curves narrow after differential training (Hanson 1959; Friedman and Guttman 1965). Similarly, we found that when chicks learn a fine discrimination, this reduces the extent of generalization on an orthogonal axis in color space (Baddeley et al. 2007). The implication of these observations is that the extent of generalization and peak-shift is scaled to match the current signal properties (Nosofsky 1992). If differences between profitable and unprofitable stimuli are small, then the range over which the animal generalizes to novel stimuli is correspondingly small.

Stimulus Generalization and Learning

The comparisons of preferences for S_+ with novel colors (S_{nov}) that we have described (figures 7.4, 7.5, 7.6) refer to a single test that lasts about a minute, and takes place about an hour after the final training session (but increasing the interval up to forty-eight hours has little effect). During the initial test, at least for male chicks, there is no change in preferences for S_+ compared to S_{nov} colors (unpublished observations). However, when chicks are re-tested after about an hour (and up to twenty-four hours), with no intervening training, there is always a marked decline in the preference for S_{nov} compared to S_+. This decline in relative preference for the novel stimulus results in a sharpening of the generalization curve for a single S_+ (Osorio et al. 1999a), a collapse of the interpolation effect between two S_+ colors (figure 7.5d), and a reduction in peak-shift (Baddeley et al. 2007, experiment 4).

Hull (1947) drew attention to studies of generalization by rats and humans from a single S_+, which found that responses to novel stimuli are more labile (susceptible to extinction) than were responses to familiar stimuli. Hull pointed out that this effect shows that the subjects can discriminate familiar from novel stimuli, so that generalization is not simply a failure of discrimination (Lashley and Wade 1946). Our observations confirm that animals generalize between stimuli that are easily discriminated, and reinforce the point that generalization is a specialized process.

The labile response to S_{nov} compared to S_+ means that the animal is learning more quickly about S_{nov} than about S_+. This effect is intuitively reasonable, because the predicted value of the novel stimulus is not based upon direct experience, and hence has a lower confidence than the prediction about S_+. One interpretation is that the chicks pay more attention to novel stimuli than to familiar objects (Pearce and Hall, 1980). Bayesian models of learning allow the level of confidence to control the rate of learning (Dayan et al. 2000; Dayan and Yu 2003; Courville et al. 2006). Such effects are known where confidence about a stimulus is experimentally controlled (Körding and Wolpert 2004), or where an event has several possible causes (Dayan and Yu 2003), but to our knowledge this effect has not been considered in accounts of stimulus generalization by animals. Nor do I know of models of sensory generalization that explicitly allow for different rates of learning about known and novel stimuli.

Conclusion: Color Generalization by Chicks and Pigeons

Color and pattern attracts the attention of chicks, which have innate preferences for small contrasting objects and for orange over blue (Osorio et al. 1999b; Miklosi et al. 2002; Ham and Osorio 2007). When they are faced with the task of extracting food from objects that resemble seed pods or insect prey, chicks learn color accurately. However, precision alone does not guarantee efficient foraging, and it is interesting to ask how animals deal with the range of circumstances that they may encounter. For example, bees trade accuracy for speed as required by the demands of a task (Chittka et al. 2003, Dyer and Chittka 2004). Ideally the process of generalization should take account of how properties of objects vary. The complexity and diversity of ways in which natural objects vary mean that it will be impossible to apply a fixed model, and that the animal should constantly update its internal model of how stimuli vary. Probabilistic models of decision making and learning suggest how an ideal system should behave to meet these requirements (Dayan et al. 2000; Tenenbaum and Griffiths 2001; Chater et al. 2006). Our observations on chicks suggest that such models are likely to be applicable to sensory generalization in animals.

It is interesting that our findings on chicks, differ substantially from those of comparable studies of pigeons (figures 7.2, 7.4, 7.5; review Honig and Urcuioli 1981); especially for generalization from two S_+ or with S_+ and S_- colors (Kalish and Guttman 1957, 1959; Hanson 1959; Friedman and Guttman 1965; Blough 1969). The differences mean that the experimental data from pigeons can be interpreted to support different theoretical accounts of generalization (Honig and Urcuioli 1981; Ghirlanda and Enquist 2003) from those that we favor for chicks. One possible reason for the discrepancy is that pigeons, when feeding, use color less than chicks. Pigeons view the region below and in front of the head, where they normally look for food, with the so-called red field on the retina, which has an unusually high density of long wavelength single cones (figure 7.1). Color discrimination in the red field is probably inferior to that in the remainder of the visual field (Remy and Emmerton 1989; Vorobyev and Osorio 1998).

Another possible reason for the difference between chicks and pigeons is that the specific task is important. In unpublished work we found that if, over a period of five days, chicks view either edible or distasteful food crumbs on either red or blue plates, they do not learn which plate has the edible food. One is not surprised that an animal learns more readily about an object upon which it feeds than about the background upon which the object is found. In operant training of pigeons, experimental stimuli (such as colored lights) are usually quite distinct from the reward, and they may learn less easily. At the same time, experimental procedures with pigeons typically involve extinction tests run over a number of days that are interleaved with training. This method would overlook labile generalization phenomena that we find in chicks, such as the interpolation between two S_+ colors (figure 7.5). Finally, it may be that the young age and restricted experience of the chicks lead to differences in generalization behavior as compared to that of adult pigeons. Regardless of the explanation, the differences between experimental observations from chicks and pigeons draw attention to the way in which sensory judgments may depend not only on low-level constraints such as photon noise in photoreceptors but also on the specific nature of the task to hand.

References

Aust U, Huber L (2006) Picture-object recognition in pigeons: Evidence of representational insight in a visual categorization task using a complementary information procedure. J Exp Psychol Anim B 32: 190–195.

Baddeley RJ, Osorio D, Jones CD (2001) Colour generalization by domestic chicks. Behav Brain Sci 24: 654–655.

Baddeley RJ, Osorio D, Jones CD (2007) Generalization of color by chickens: Experimental observations and a Bayesian model. Am Nat 169: S27–S41.

Blough DS (1969) Generalization gradient shape and summation in steady-state tests. J Exp Anal Behav 12:91–104.

Blough DS (1975) Steady state data and a quantitative model of generalization and discrimination. J Exp Psychol Anim B 1: 3–21.

Booth D, Stewart AJA, Osorio D (2004) Colour vision in the glow-worm *Lampyris noctiluca* (L.) (Coleoptera: Lampyridae): Evidence for the green-blue chromatic mechanism. J Exp Biol 207: 2373–2378.

Bowmaker JK, Knowles A (1977) The visual pigments and oil droplets of the chicken retina. Vision Res 17: 755–764.

Brainard DH, Freeman WT (1997) Bayesian color constancy. J Opt Soc Am A 14: 1393–1411.

Cerella J (1979) Visual classes and natural categories in the pigeon. J Exp Psychol Hum Perc Perform 5: 68–77.

Chater N, Tenenbaum JB, Yuille A (2006) Probabilistic models of cognition: Conceptual foundations. Trends Cogn Sci 10: 287–291.

Cheng K (2002) Generalization: Mechanistic and functional explanations. Anim Cogn 5: 33–40.

Chittka L, Dyer AG, Bock F, Dornhaus A (2003) Bees trade off foraging speed for accuracy. Nature 424: 388.

Courville AC, Daw ND, Touretzky DS (2006) Bayesian theories of conditioning in a changing world. Trends Cogn Sci 10: 294–300.

Cuthill IC (2006) Color perception. In: Bird coloration, volume 1: Mechanisms and measurement (Hill GE, McGraw KJ, eds), 3–40. Cambridge MA: Harvard University Press.

Davidoff J (2001) Language and perceptual categories. Trends Cogn Sci 5: 382–387.

Dayan PS, Kakade S, Montague PR (2000) Learning and selective attention. Nat Neurosci 3: 1218–1223.

Dayan P, Yu AJ (2003) Uncertainty and learning. IETE J Res 49: 171–182.

Dyer AG, Chittka L (2004) Bumblebees (*Bombus terrestris*) sacrifice foraging speed to solve difficult colour discrimination tasks. J Comp Physiol A: 190: 759–763.

Enquist M, Arak A (1993) Selection of exaggerated male traits by female aesthetic senses. Nature 361: 446–448.

Enquist M, Arak A (1998) Neural representation and the evolution of signal form. In: Cognitive ecology: The evolutionary ecology of information processing and decision making (Dukas R, ed), 21–87. Chicago: University of Chicago Press.

Friedman H, Guttman N (1965) Further analysis of the various effects of discrimination training on stimulus generalization gradients. In: Stimulus generalization (Mostofsky DI, ed), 255–267. Palo Alto: Stanford University Press.

Frisch, K von (1914) Der Farbensinn und Formensinn der Biene. Zool Jahrb Allg Zool 35: 1–188.

Ghirlanda S, Enquist M (1999) The geometry of stimulus control. Anim Behav 58: 695–706.

Ghirlanda S, Enquist M (2003) A century of generalization. Anim Behav 66: 15–36.

Goldsmith TH, Butler BK (2003) The roles of receptor noise and cone oil droplets in the photopic spectral sensitivity of the budgerigar, *Melopsittacus undulatus*. J Comp Physiol A 189: 135–142.

Goldsmith TH, Butler BK (2005) Color vision of the budgerigar *Melopsittacus undulatus*: Hue matches, tetrachromacy, and intensity discrimination. J Comp Physiol A 19: 933–951.

Govardovskii VI, Zueva LV (1977) Visual pigments of chicken and pigeon. Vision Res 17: 537–543.

Guttman N, Kalish HI (1956) Discriminability and stimulus generalization. J Exp Psychol 51: 79–88.

Ham AD, Osorio D (2007) Colour preferences and colour vision in poultry chicks. P Roy Soc Lond B Bio 271: 1941–1948.

Hanson HM (1959) Effects of discrimination training on stimulus generalization. J Exp Psychol 58: 321–334.

Harnad S (1987) Categorical perception: The groundwork of cognition. New York: Cambridge University Press.

Hart NS, Hunt DM (2007) Avian visual pigments: Characteristics, spectral tuning, and evolution. Am Nat 169: S7–S26.

Herrnstein RJ (1961) Relative and absolute strength of response as a function of frequency of reinforcement. J Exp Anal Behav 4: 267–272.

Herrnstein RJ, Loveland DH (1964) Complex visual concept in the pigeon. Science 146: 549–551.

Honig WK, Urcuioli PJ (1981) The legacy of Guttman and Kalish (1956): Twenty-five years of research on stimulus generalization. J Exp Anal Behav 36: 405–445.

Hull CL (1943) Principles of behaviour. New York: Appleton Century Crofts.

Hull CL (1947) The problem of primary stimulus generalization. Psychol Rev 54: 120–134.

Jones CD, Osorio D (2004) Discrimination of oriented visual textures by poultry chicks. Vision Res 44: 83–89.

Jones CD, Osorio D, Baddeley RJ (2001) Color categorization by domestic chicks. P Roy Soc Lond B Bio 268: 2077–2084.

Kalish HI, Guttman N (1957) Stimulus generalization after equal training on two stimuli. J Exp Psychol 53:139–144.

Kalish HI, Guttman N (1959) Stimulus generalization after training on three stimuli: A test of the summation hypothesis. J Exp Psychol 57: 268–272.

Kay P, Kempton W (1984) What is the Sapir-Whorf hypothesis? Am Anthropol 86: 65–79.

Kelber A, Vorobyev M, Osorio D (2003) Animal colour vision—behavioural tests and physiological concepts. Biol Rev 78: 81–118.

Kolb G, Scherer C (1982) Experiments on wavelength specific behavior of *Pieris brassicae* L. during drumming and egg-laying. J Comp Physiol A 149: 325–332.

Körding KP, Wolpert DM (2004) Bayesian integration in sensorimotor learning. Nature 427: 244–247.

Lashley KS, Wade M (1946) The Pavlovian theory of generalization. Psychol Rev 53: 72–87.

Lueck CJ, Zeki S, Friston KJ, Deiber MP, Cope P, Cunningham VJ, Lammertsma AA, Kennard C, Frackowiak RS (1989) The colour centre in the cerebral cortex of man. Nature 340: 386–389.

Macleod DI, Boynton RM (1979) Chromaticity diagram showing cone excitation by stimuli of equal luminance. J Opt Soc Am 69: 1183–1186.

McLaren IPL, MacKintosh NJ (2002) Associative learning and elemental representation: II. Generalization and discrimination. Anim Learn Behav 30: 177–200.

Menzel R (1979) Spectral sensitivity and color vision in invertebrates. In: Handbook of sensory physiology, volume VII/6A (Autrum H, ed), 503–580. Berlin: Springer-Verlag.

Miklósi A, Gonda ZS, Osorio D, Farzin A (2002) The effects of the visual environment on responses to colour by domestic chicks. J Comp Physiol A 188: 135–140.

Nosofsky RM (1992) Similarity scaling and cognitive process models. Annu Rev Psychol 43: 25–53.

Osorio D, Jones CD, Vorobyev M (1999a) Accurate memory for color but not pattern contrast in chicks. Curr Biol 9: 199–202.

Osorio D, Miklósi A, Gonda ZS (1999b) Visual ecology and perception of coloration patterns by domestic chicks. Evol Ecol 13: 673–689.

Osorio D, Vorobyev M, Jones CD (1999c). Colour vision of domestic chicks. J Exp Biol 202: 2951–2959.

Pavlov IP (1927) Conditioned reflexes (GV Anrep, transl.) Oxford: Clarendon.

Pearce JM, Hall G (1980) A model for Pavlovian learning: Variations in the effectiveness of conditioned but not of unconditioned stimuli. Psychol Rev 87: 532–552.

Remy M, Emmerton J (1989) Behavioral spectral sensitivities of different retinal areas in pigeons. Behav Neurosci 103: 170–177.

Schrödinger E (1920) Grundlinien einer Theorie der Farbenmetric im Tagessehen. Ann Phys 63: 81–520.

Shepard RN (1965) Approximation to uniform gradients of generalization by monotone transformations of scale. In: Stimulus generalization (Mostofsky DI, ed), 94–110. Palo Alto: Stanford University Press.

Shepard RN (1987) Towards a universal law of generalization for psychological science. Science 237: 1317–1323.

Spence KW (1937) The differential response in animals to stimuli varying in a single dimension. Psychol Rev 44: 430–444.

Stevens SS (1957) On the psychophysical law. Psychol Rev 64: 153–181.

Stoerig P (1998) Wavelength information processing versus color perception: Evidence from blindsight and color-blind sight. In: Color vision: Perspectives from different disciplines (Backhaus WGK, Kliegl R, Werner JS, eds), 131–147. Berlin: Walter de Gruyter.

Tenenbaum JB, Griffiths TL (2001) Generalization, similarity, and Bayesian inference. Behav Brain Sci 24: 629–641.

Troje NF, Huber L, Loidolt M, Aust U, Fieder M (1999) Categorical learning in pigeons: The role of texture and shape in complex static stimuli. Vision Res 39: 353–366.

Vorobyev M (2003) Coloured oil droplets enhance colour discrimination. P Roy Soc Lond B Bio 270: 1255–1261.

Vorobyev M, Osorio D (1998) Receptor noise as a determinant of colour thresholds. P Roy Soc Lond B Bio 265: 351–358.

Vorobyev M, Osorio D, Bennett ATD, Marshall NJ, Cuthill IC (1998) Tetrachromacy, oil droplets and bird plumage colours. J Comp Physiol A 183: 621–633.

Watanabe S, Sakamoto J, Wakita M (1995). Pigeons' discrimination of paintings by Monet and Picasso. J Exp Anal Behav 63: 165–174.

Weiss SJ, Weissman RD (1992) Generalization peak shift for autoshaped and operant key pecks. J Exp Anal Behav 57:127–143.

Whorf BL, Carrol JB (1956) Language, thought and reality: Selected writings of Benjamin Lee Whorf. Cambridge, MA: MIT Press.

Wyszecki G, Stiles WS (1982) Color science. New York: Wiley.

8 Evolutionary Biology of Limited Attention

Reuven Dukas

When we direct our whole attention to any one sense, its acuteness is increased.
—Charles Darwin, 1872

Cognition may be defined as the set of traits concerned with the acquisition, retention, and use of information that help an individual survive and reproduce. As with most other biological characteristics, it is reasonable to assume that a given cognitive trait is a product of evolution by natural selection. The two basic conditions allowing the evolution of a given cognitive trait are, first, genetically based variation in that trait among individuals within a species and, second, such genetic variation must be associated with variation in fitness, defined as the lifetime reproductive success of an individual (Dukas 2004b). Evolutionary analyses have been instrumental in advancing scientific knowledge on other classes of biological traits such as anatomy and morphology (Futuyma 2005). Similarly, further testing of evolutionary-based predictions about cognitive traits can help us understand many of the remaining unresolved issues pertaining to brain and behavior.

In this chapter I examine attention from an evolutionary perspective. I focus on limited attention, which means that the brain can process information only at some finite rate. My evolutionary-based approach to studying limited attention can readily be linked to traditional cognitive analyses of attention, which indicate that there are three distinct networks of attention identified by anatomy and function. These three networks deal with (1) alerting, defined as achieving an alert state and sustaining attention; (2) orienting, meaning focusing on a selected set of information; and (3) executive control, involving the resolution of conflict among responses (Posner and Petersen 1990; Fan et al. 2002). Limited attention relates to the orienting network. In fact, as I shall elaborate, limited attention is the reason individuals have to orient to a restricted set of information at any given time.

Much of the chapter will focus on my work relating limited attention to fitness. I will then review evidence indicating genetically based individual variation in attention, discuss the evolution of attentional capacities, and suggest promising lines for future research.

Limited Attention

The animal brain is capable of integrating vast amounts of information perceived by a variety of sense organs with extensive information stored in memory and acting upon this knowledge in ways that enhance fitness (Dukas 2004b). Although the brain appears very powerful, its power is not unlimited. As expected from first principles, all major cognitive abilities are subjected to obvious limitations. The rate of acquiring new information (learning rate) is limited; long-term memory is imperfect, meaning that potentially relevant information may be forgotten; working memory has a very small capacity; and the rate of information the brain can process at any given time is restricted (Dukas 1998; Marois and Ivanoff 2005). I refer to the last constraint as limited attention.

A few lines of evidence support the notion of limited attention. First, in primates, approximately 60 percent of the neocortex is devoted to vision (Van Essen et al. 1992; Barton 1998). Even so, only 0.02 percent of the information perceived by the eyes and 1 percent of the information transmitted from the eyes to the brain by the optic nerve is attended to at any given time (Van Essen et al. 1992; Van Essen and Anderson 1995). That is, the information bottleneck is in the processing of information by the visual cortex and not in either sensing the information or transmitting it from the eyes to the brain (Clark and Dukas 2003). Second, the amount of attention devoted to a secondary task, and performance on that task, are negatively correlated with the amount of attention necessary for successful completion of a primary task. For example, Rees and colleagues (1997) instructed human subjects to focus on a linguistic task (the primary task) presented at the center of a computer display, which also included moving stimuli at its periphery. Performance measures and the results of brain imaging (fMRI) indicated that subjects devoted less attention to the peripheral moving stimuli when the primary task was difficult (detecting bisyllabic words in a sequence of successive single-word presentations) than when it was easy (detecting words printed in upper-case letters). Finally, the third line of evidence for limited attention involves extensive and well-replicated data from electrophysiological recordings in monkeys and brain imaging in humans. When subjects face difficult detection tasks, focusing attention on either a specific stimulus or a specific location (figure 8.1) is associated with enhanced response of the neurons that process that stimulus or location.

Furthermore, simultaneous behavioral tests reveal that focused attention is associated with higher detection probability than divided attention (Moran and Desimone 1985; Kastner and Ungerleider 2000; Muller et al. 2006). For example, when human subjects were instructed to report whether items in two successive images slightly differed in shape, color, or speed, they performed better when informed which attribute would differ between the images than when told that any of the three attributes may differ (figure 8.2).

Simultaneous brain imaging indicated that the enhanced performance was associated with heightened neuronal activity in the specific brain region processing the anticipated attribute (Corbetta et al. 1990a, 1990b).

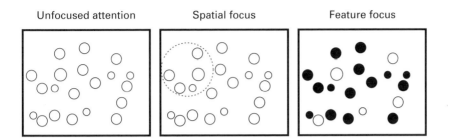

Figure 8.1
The effect of unfocused vs. focused attention on the ease of detecting a cryptic target. All three panels contain the same target and background items at identical spatial configurations. The target in all three panels is the same circle, which is slightly larger than all the other circles. The target detection task is most difficult under the unfocused-attention condition. The target detection is easier if the subject is instructed to focus his or her attention either only on the dotted circle in the spatial attention panel or on the white circles in the feature focus panel. The target circle, which is at the middle right side of the large circle in the spatial attention panel, appears in the same location in all three panels.

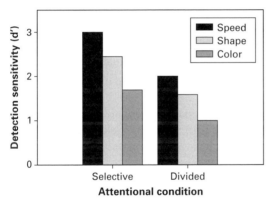

Figure 8.2
Sensitivity (d′), which is a corrected measure of the frequency of correct detection of slight differences in shape, color, or speed between two successive images, was significantly higher under the selective- than divided-attention condition ($P < 0.001$). Data from Corbetta et al. (1990b).

The Optimal Allocation of Attention

The data indicating that limited attention constrains performance raise a fundamental functional question. How do animals choose what information to attend to at any given time? To answer this question, Dukas and Ellner (1993) integrated mechanistic information from cognitive neuroscience with a theoretical model based on evolutionary principles. The prey model (Stephens and Krebs 1986) simply assumes that animals have evolved feeding strategies that maximize fitness. In its simplest form, the model assumes that foragers attempt to maximize their net rate of energy intake, which is the amount of energy assimilated from food items consumed minus the energy expended to acquire and handle these food items, over the time it takes to search for and handle the items (Stephens and Krebs 1986).

The attentive prey model of Dukas and Ellner (1993) extends the simple prey model by assuming that foragers have only a certain probability of detecting a given prey type they encounter, where encounter means physical proximity to prey. The probability of detecting prey is positively correlated with prey conspicuousness, defined as the degree of dissimilarity between the prey and its surrounding background. Finally, the probability of detecting a given prey type is also positively correlated with the amount of attention devoted to that prey.

Suppose foragers encounter several equally profitable food types. In this case, the simple prey model predicts that the foragers should search for and feed on all types. Predictions of the attentive prey model, however, depend on prey conspicuousness. For conspicuous prey, the prediction is identical to that of the simple prey model: foragers should search for all prey types. On the other hand, for inconspicuous (cryptic) prey, the attentive prey model predicts that foragers should focus their search on a single prey type and ignore all others. This pair of predictions is intuitively appealing because it agrees with our everyday routines. To maximize our productivity, we typically divide attention among a few easy tasks that can be successfully accomplished simultaneously. We prefer, however, to focus our full attention on a single challenging task at any given time, knowing that we cannot execute any other task simultaneously without severely diminishing performance.

Computer simulations using realistic foraging parameters indeed illustrate that animals searching for conspicuous prey types would benefit from searching for all types simultaneously, but that animals searching for cryptic prey types would gain more from searching only for a single type at any given time (figure 8.3).

The attentive prey model explains well the phenomenon of search image, which implies that animals searching for cryptic food focus their search on one prey type while bypassing other types. Search image had been well documented in a variety of species but poorly explained (Tinbergen 1960; Dawkins 1971; Pietrewicz and Kamil 1979; Blough 1991; Reid and Shettleworth 1992; Bond and Kamil 1999).

Search image has received considerable attention because such behavior by predators can help maintain large variation in the visual appearance of animals and plants. Suppose that a predator focuses attention on a common morph of a certain prey species. Individuals belonging to a distinct, rare morph of that species could suffer lesser predation and hence gain higher fitness than the common morph (Clark 1962; Endler 1988). Although the prediction that selective attention by predators helps maintain phenotypic variation is theoretically feasible, no field data exist to support it. The only existing evidence agreeing with that prediction is a laboratory study using blue jays (*Cyanocitta cristata*) as predators and computer-simulated moths as "prey" (Bond and Kamil 2002). A few alternative mechanisms, including chance or divergent selection imposed by a few predator species with

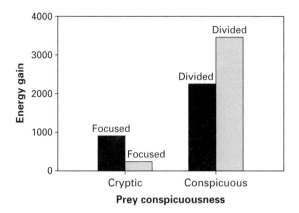

Figure 8.3
The net rate of energy intake of a simulated forager encountering items of three distinct food types with identical conspicuousness. Simulations were conducted for each of the four combinations of conspicuousness (cryptic or conspicuous prey) and attention (focused or divided attention). That is, the forager could either focus attention on searching for one food type during the session or divide attention among all three types at the same time. All three food types had identical densities, net energy content, and handling time. Data from Dukas and Ellner (1993).

distinct perceptual abilities, can also maintain prey polymorphism. Thus it is still unknown whether selective attention by predators helps maintain phenotypic variation of prey in nature (Abrams 2000; Dukas 2004a).

In the foregoing discussion of the attentive prey model, I focused on the special simple case of foragers encountering a few prey types all similar in their profitability. What should foragers do if they encounter several cryptic food types that vary in profitability? For this case, the attentive prey model predicts that the foragers should focus their search on the single most profitable type while tuning out all other types (Dukas and Ellner 1993). We can generalize this prediction into the intuitive prediction that individuals should focus attention on the most valuable information at any given time, where the value of information is independently quantified as its potential effect on fitness. Sometimes, however, animals may have to focus on some valuable information while ignoring other potentially important information in order to successfully execute a task. I will discuss such a case in the following section.

The attentive prey model (Dukas and Ellner 1993) was based mostly on literature from monkeys and humans. To evaluate the model's general relevance, Dukas and Kamil (2001) tested the major assumption of the model, that foragers engaged in the difficult task of searching for cryptic prey have lower foraging success when they search for more than one distinct prey type simultaneously.

The experiment involved blue jays trained to search for and peck at cryptic targets presented at random locations on a computer monitor equipped with infrared sensors.

The most relevant part of the study involved comparisons between jays' performance in three types of daily sessions. Session A consisted of fifty trials each including target type A appearing at a random location on a background type *A*, on which target A was cryptic. Session B consisted of 50 trials each including target type B appearing at a random location on a background type *B*, on which target B was cryptic. Finally, session A/B consisted of random presentations of twenty-five trials with target type A and 25 trials with target type B each appearing at a random location on a background type *A/B*, on which either target was cryptic. Each trial in all three sessions was preceded with the presentation of a start signal at which jays had to peck for initiating the trial. The start signal included an image of target A in session A, target B in session B, and targets A and B in session A/B. Hence both the start key and experience throughout the session indicated to jays which target(s) could appear in the successive trials. That is, the jays could focus their attention on searching for a single type in session A and in session B, but they had to divide their attention between searching for either target type in session A/B.

As predicted, the average rate of target detection was significantly lower when jays divided their attention between searching for the two cryptic target types in each trial than when they focused attention on searching for a single type per trial (figure 8.4).

That is, when the jays were forced under experimental manipulation to divide their attention while performing a difficult search task, their performance on a task related to foraging success was lower than under the focused attention condition (Dukas and Kamil 2001). Because foraging success is tightly linked to fitness, one may argue that limited attention has fitness costs. I will elaborate on that issue below.

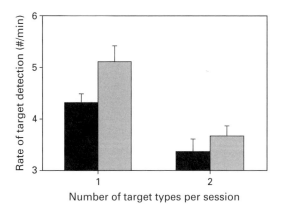

Figure 8.4
The rate of target detection by blue jays in experimental sessions in which they searched for only one of two cryptic target types, and in sessions in which they searched for the two targets simultaneously. The black and gray bars depict target types A and B respectively. Target detection rate was significantly higher when the jays focused attention on a single target type ($P < 0.001$). From Dukas and Kamil (2001).

Fitness Costs of Limited Attention

So far I have focused on the issue of how to optimally allocate limited attention in order to maximize fitness. Often, however, the optimal allocation of attention might imply that animals cannot devote sufficient attention to a secondary task with large effects on fitness. The most ubiquitous case experienced by the majority of animals is that of balancing feeding and antipredatory behavior (Lima and Dill 1990; Lima 1998). Some minimum level of feeding is necessary to avoid imminent death by starvation and ample feeding is typically necessary for reproduction. Most animals, however, are vulnerable to predation while they feed. Thus they must somehow decide about the optimal allocation of attention between searching for food and looking out for predators. Is a more challenging food search task, which requires more attention, associated with lesser attention devoted to approaching predators?

Consider a blue jay perched on a tree trunk and searching for highly camouflaged insects. At the same time, there is a slight chance that a predator such as a hawk may be swiftly approaching. We simulated this setting in the laboratory, but for ethical and practical reasons, we used two target types and no predators (Dukas and Kamil 2000). Each daily session consisted of fifty trials and each trial included a 500 ms presentation of a single target, either a caterpillar, which appeared at a random location within a circle at the center of the computer monitor at a frequency of 0.5 per trial, or a cryptic moth, which could appear at a random location within one of two peripheral ellipses at a frequency of 0.25 per ellipse each trial. The difficulty of the peripheral task always remained the same. The central task, however, could be either easy, when the caterpillar was conspicuous, or difficult, when the caterpillar was cryptic. We predicted that, in center-easy sessions, the jays would devote attention to both the center and periphery, but that under the center-difficult condition, the jays would focus much of their attention on the central circle, because they could detect a target there at a frequency of 0.5 compared to only 0.25 for each peripheral ellipse. Consequently, we predicted that the frequency of detecting the peripheral target would be lower under the center-difficult than center-easy sessions.

The results strongly agreed with this prediction: the jays were almost three times less likely to detect the peripheral target in the center-difficult than center-easy sessions (figure 8.5a). In agreement with the prediction, the frequency of detecting the central target was similar in the two session types (figure 8.5a). This suggested that by changing the amount of attention devoted to the central task, the jays could maintain high detection rates of the central target at the cost of missing many more peripheral targets in the center-difficult than center-easy sessions. Data on detection latencies (figure 8.5b) indicated that the differences in frequency of target detection were not caused by an alternative strategy such as successive allocation of attention to the center and then periphery (Dukas and Kamil 2000).

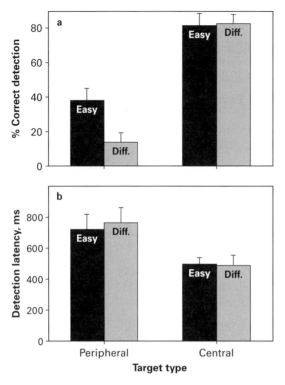

Figure 8.5
(a) The percentage of correct detection (mean + 1 SE) of the peripheral target was significantly higher during the center-easy (dark bars) than center-difficult (gray bars) sessions, but correct detection of the central target was similar in either session type. (b) The average detection latency of the peripheral target was similar during the center-easy (dark bars) and center-difficult (gray bars) conditions. Detection latency of the central target was also similar during the center-easy and center-difficult conditions. From Dukas and Kamil (2000).

The laboratory test with blue jays allowed us to critically test for the cost of limited attention. As already mentioned, however, mortality owing to limited attention is probably ubiquitous because the majority of animals must constantly balance the two competing tasks of feeding while avoiding predation. Several studies, though not critically testing for limited attention, indeed suggest that mortality owing to limited attention is common. Male moths (*Spodoptera littoralis*) walking toward pheromone-emitting fertile females were much less likely to freeze in response to the sound of predatory bats (Skals et al. 2005). Similarly, female wolf spiders (*Schizocosa uetzi*) were twice as likely to be caught by a simulated predator when attending to a male's courtship display than when resting (Hebets 2005). Finally, a few fish studies documented either lesser responses to approaching predators when feeding than resting or lower foraging efficiency after encountering a model predator (Milinski and Heller 1978; Metcalfe et al. 1987; Krause and Godin 1996). Although highly suggestive, many of the above cases may be at least partially explained

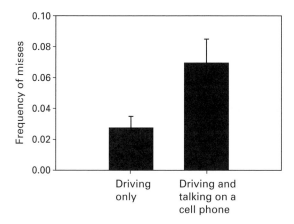

Figure 8.6
The cost of limited attention in human drivers. Dividing attention between talking on a cell phone and driving increases the likelihood of missing red lights in controlled experiments of simulated driving. Data from Strayer and Johnston (2001).

by changes in motivation rather than limited attention. For example, the male moths chasing females might notice the bat sound but choose to keep the chase in spite of the looming danger.

Another animal increasingly experiencing the cost of limited attention is the modern human driver, who stubbornly attempts to control a vehicle while simultaneously operating some electronic device such as cell phone, Blackberry, laptop, GPS or iPod. Many studies have clearly documented that dividing attention between driving and using an electronic gadget such as a cell phone increases drivers' reaction time and reduces the probability of responding to hazards (Strayer and Johnston 2001; Barkana et al. 2004; Horrey and Wickens 2006). For example, subjects in a simulated driving task were instructed to brake in response to random presentations of red lights flashed at a computer monitor.

Compared to control subjects who paid full attention to the simulated driving task, subjects who were engaged in a cell phone conversation missed the red lights more than twice as often (figure 8.6) and their responses to red lights were about 10 percent slower (Strayer and Johnston 2001).

Why Is Attention Limited?

If limited attention is associated with increased mortality in a variety of animals including humans, why have not we all evolved higher attentional capacities? Clark and Dukas (2003) addressed this issue by quantifying the optimal allocation of attention and the optimal attentional capacity in animals facing the common task of balancing foraging and antipredatory behavior. The basic idea underlying the model is that attentional capacity, in addition to its obvious benefits, also has a cost, assumed to be increased energetic expenditures necessary to support a larger brain. With realistic parameters, the model indicates that a relatively low attentional capacity combined with successive allocation of focused attention constitute an optimal strategy that balances the need to process high rates of information flow and the cost of building and maintaining brain tissue (Clark and Dukas 2003; Dukas 2004a).

How Do Animals Cope with Limited Attention?

Whereas it is established that limited attention is a central constraint influencing animal cognition and behavior, a few features may allow animals to reduce potentially adverse effects of limited attention. First, brain lateralization, which is ubiquitous among vertebrates, implies that the right and left brain hemispheres specialize on distinct tasks (Rogers and Andrew 2002). Recent studies in domestic chicks (*Gallus domesticus*) and fish (*Girardinus falcatus*) examined the effects of lateralization on performance by comparing lateralized and less lateralized individuals that were generated via either environmental manipulation or artificial selection. In both the domestic chicks and fish studies, the more lateralized individuals performed better in dual tasks involving foraging while attending to predators (Rogers et al. 2004; Dadda and Bisazza 2006a) and foraging while attending to harassing males (Dadda and Bisazza 2006b). It thus appears that one of a few advantages of brain lateralization is enhanced performance on tasks requiring the simultaneous division of attention between important tasks.

Second, another way animals can cope with limited attention is by learning what to attend to. For example, individuals that have to detect either cryptic food items or hidden ambushing predators may learn over time where such items are most likely to be located. They can then focus much of their attention on the most relevant locations in the visual field at any given time to maximize the use of their limited attention (Shaw and Shaw 1977; Dukas 2002). A functionally similar though distinct mechanism, termed "inhibition of return," allows animals to ignore recently rewarded locations or features in settings in which such locations or features are not typically rewarded successively (Posner et al. 1985; Shepherd and Platt, chapter 14, this volume). Finally, in humans, many tasks that are attention-demanding while executed by novice individuals require little attention from experts. For example, people learning how to drive focus their attention on operating the vehicle and negotiating traffic whereas experienced drivers typically find that these tasks require almost no conscious attention and hence they can devote more attention to concurrent tasks such as conversing with a passenger (LaBerge and Samuels 1974; Dukas 2002).

Genetically Based Individual Variation in Attention

The beginning of the third millennium has seen tremendous advancements in the technology enabling powerful, fast, and cheap genetic analyses. The genetic revolution is rapidly penetrating into all biological disciplines, including cognitive neuroscience (Plomin et al. 2003; Craig and Plomin 2006). Research on genetic variation associated with attentional networks is still in its early stages. Not surprisingly, the first few genes to be targeted have been well-known genes involved in a variety of cognitive functions (see Butcher et al. 2006). For example, allelic variation in the *dopamine D4 receptor* gene (DRD4) and *monoamine oxidase a* (MAOA) was associated with variation in executive attention (Fossella et al. 2002). Furthermore, fMRI scans revealed that subjects with DRD4 and MAOA alleles associated with better performance on the executive attention task had more activation in the anterior cingulate than subjects possessing the inferior alleles (Fan et al. 2003). Similarly, the ε4 allele of the *apolipoprotein E* (APOE) gene, which is well known for its association with susceptibility to late-onset Alzheimer's disease (Raber et al. 2000; Smith 2000), has also been linked to deficits in visual attention as well as learning and memory in nondemented middle-aged carriers (Greenwood et al. 2000, 2005). The overall frequency of ε4 among Western Europeans and North Americans is 13.5 percent, but ε4 frequencies greatly vary among populations (Raber et al. 2000; Smith 2000).

The early results from studies on the genetic basis of attentional networks already establish that there is ample genetically based individual variation in attentional abilities. It is likely, though, that there are hundreds of genes involved in controlling attention, and that most of these genes also influence other cognitive abilities (Greenspan 2001; Butcher et al. 2006; Savitz et al. 2006). Ultimately, then, we will have to possess a large data base on the genetic networks underlying attention and other cognitive functions in order to understand the selective forces that have acted on attentional networks.

The Evolution of Attentional Capacities

There has been relatively little research on the evolutionary biology of attention as well as other cognitive abilities. Two difficulties encountered in work on the evolution of a cognitive trait is the absence of a fossil record and the difficulty of quantifying a given trait. The first obstacle can be overcome by employing alternative techniques, including comparative research such as the fruitful work on spatial memory in a few taxa of birds and mammals (Gaulin and Fitzgerald 1986; Krebs et al. 1989; Sherry et al. 1989; Lucas et al. 2004; Pravosudov et al. 2006) and experiments involving evolution by artificial selection (Tolman 1924; Mery and Kawecki 2002). The other major problem of quantification can be alleviated by conducting multiple tests and including proper controls to verify that observed species differences in a cognitive trait are not caused merely by distinct responses to the general experimental settings (e.g., Shettleworth and Westwood 2002; Jones and Healy 2006). In sum, although evolutionary research on attention is feasible, such work is in its infancy.

Conclusions and Prospects

Research indicates that limited attention is a relevant biological trait influencing animal fitness and that there is genetically based individual variation in attentional capacities. Our knowledge on the effect of limited attention on fitness could be enhanced from two lines of research. First, the critical work on limited attention has been conducted in the laboratory. It is important that we extend that work to quantify the effects of limited attention on either foraging success or antipredatory behavior in natural settings. Second, we have to quantify the cost of possessing a certain attentional ability as well as any other cognitive trait (Dukas 1999; Clark and Dukas 2003; Mery and Kawecki 2005). Such knowledge will help us understand the trade-offs that have influenced the evolution of observed cognitive abilities.

Work on the genetic networks underlying attention could gain significantly from further development of classical model systems for attention research. Fruit flies and mice have proved instrumental in research on the neurogenetics of learning and memory because they are more accessible than humans for experimentation and genetic manipulation (Tang et al. 1999; Bucan and Abel 2002; Tully et al. 2003). Similarly, recent work on attention in fruit flies and mice seems promising for neurogenetics work on attention (Swinderen and Greenspan 2003; Han et al. 2004).

We still know little about key issues, including the evolution of attentional abilities and whether behavioral and ecological differences among species are associated with differences in attentional abilities. The former topic may be addressed through artificial-selection experiments using fruit flies or mice (see Swinderen and Greenspan 2003; Han et al. 2004). The latter issue is somewhat more challenging. First, one should identify a group of closely related species that on the basis of their natural history and behavior are predicted to possess distinct attentional abilities. Second, we have to develop robust tests of attentional abilities that can be used for between-species comparisons. The attention network test developed for humans may be a good starting point (Fan et al. 2002). Finally, we must also envision some nonattention cognitive tests in which we would predict no significant differences between the same set of species tested for differences in attentional abilities.

Acknowledgments

I thank Lynn Nadel, Mary Peterson, and Luca Tommasi for organizing "The New Cognitive Sciences" workshop; staff of the Konrad Lorenz Institute for superb hospitality; and Luca Tommasi and Lauren Taylor for comments on the manuscript. My research has been supported by the Natural Sciences and Engineering Research Council of Canada, Canada Foundation for Innovation, Ontario Innovation Trust, and the National Institute of Health (USA).

References

Abrams PA (2000) Character shifts of prey species that share predators. Am Natur 156: S45–S61.

Barkana Y, D Zadok, Y Morad, I Avni (2004) Visual field attention is reduced by concomitant hands-free conversation on a cellular phone. Am J Ophthalmol 138: 347–353.

Barton RA (1998) Visual specialization and brain evolution in primates. P Roy Soc Lond B Bio 265: 1933–1937.

Blough P (1991) Selective attention and search images in pigeons. J Exp Psychol Anim B 17: 292–298.

Bond AB, AC Kamil (1999) Searching image in blue jays: Facilitation and interference in sequential priming. Anim Learn Behav 27: 461–471.

Bond AB, AC Kamil (2002) Visual predators select for crypticity and polymorphism in virtual prey. Nature 415: 609–613.

Bucan M, Abel T (2002) The mouse: Genetics meets behaviour. Nat Rev Gen 3: 114–123.

Butcher LM, JKJ Kennedy, R Plomin (2006) Generalist genes and cognitive neuroscience. Curr Opin Neurobiol 16: 145–151.

Clark B (1962) Balanced polymorphism and the diversity of sympatric species. In: Taxonomy and geography (Nichols D, ed) 47–70. Oxford: Systematics Associations.

Clark CW, R Dukas (2003) The behavioral ecology of a cognitive constraint: Limited attention. Behav Ecol 14: 151–156.

Corbetta M, S Miezin, GL Dobmeyer, GL Shulman, SE Petersen (1990a) Attentional modulation of neural processing of shape, color, and velocity in humans. Science 248: 1556–1559.

Corbetta M, S Miezin, GL Dobmeyer, GL Shulman, SE Petersen (1990b) Selective and divided attention during visual discrimination of shape, color, and speed: Functional anatomy by positron emission tomography. J Neurosci 11: 2383–2402.

Craig I, R Plomin (2006) Quantitative trait loci for IQ and other complex traits: Single-nucleotide polymorphism genotyping using pooled DNA and microarrays. Genes Brain Behav 5: 32–37.

Dadda M, Bisazza A (2006a) Does brain asymmetry allow efficient performance of simultaneous tasks? Anim Behav 72: 523–529.

Dadda M, Bisazza A (2006b) Lateralized female topminnows can forage and attend to a harassing male simultaneously. Behav Ecol 17: 358–363.

Darwin C (1872) The expression of the emotions in man and animals. 3rd ed. Oxford: Oxford University Press.

Dawkins M (1971) Shifts of 'attention' in chicks during feeding. Anim Behav 19: 575–582.

Dukas R (1998) Constraints on information processing and their effects on behavior. In: Cognitive ecology (Dukas R, ed) 89–127. Chicago: University of Chicago Press.

Dukas R (1999). Costs of memory: Ideas and predictions. J Theor Biol 197: 41–50.

Dukas R (2002) Behavioural and ecological consequences of limited attention. Philos T Roy Soc Lond B 357: 1539–1548.

Dukas R (2004a) Causes and consequences of limited attention. Brain Behav Evol 63: 197–210.

Dukas R (2004b) Evolutionary biology of animal cognition. Annu Rev Ecol Evol Syst 35: 347–374.

Dukas R, Ellner S (1993) Information processing and prey detection. Ecology 74: 1337–1346.

Dukas R, Kamil AC (2000) The cost of limited attention in blue jays. Behav Ecol 11: 502–506.

Dukas R, Kamil AC (2001) Limited attention: The constraint underlying search image. Behav Ecol 12: 192–199.

Endler JA (1988) Frequency-dependent predation, crypsis and aposomatic coloration. Philos T Roy Soc Lond B 319: 505–523.

Fan J, Fossella J, Sommer T, Wu Y, Posner MI (2003) Mapping the genetic variation of executive attention onto brain activity. P Natl Acad Sci USA 100: 7406–7411.

Fan J, McCandliss BD, Sommer T, Raz A, Posner MI (2002) Testing the efficiency and independence of attentional networks. J Cognitive Neurosci 14: 340–347.

Fossella J, Sommer T, Fan J, Wu Y, Swanson JM, Pfaff DW, Posner MI (2002) Assessing the molecular genetics of attention networks. BMC Neurosci 3: 14–24.

Futuyma DJ (2005) Evolution. Sunderland, MA: Sinauer.

Gaulin SJC, Fitzgerald RW (1986) Sex-differences in spatial ability: An evolutionary hypothesis and test. Am Natur 127: 74–88.

Greenspan RJ (2001) The flexible genome. *Nat Rev Genet* 2: 383–387.

Greenwood P, Sunderland T, Friz J, Parasuraman R (2000) Genetics and visual attention: Selective deficits in healthy adult carriers of the e4 allele of the apolipoprotein E gene. P Natl Acad Sci USA 97: 11661–11666.

Greenwood PM, Lambert C, Sunderland T, Parasuraman R (2005) Effects of apolipoprotein E genotype on spatial attention, working memory, and their interaction in healthy, middle-aged adults: Results from the National Institute of Mental Health's BIOCARD study. Neuropsychology 19: 199–211.

Han CJ, O'Tuathaigh CM, Koch C (2004) A practical assay for attention in mice. In: Cognitive neuroscience of attention (Posner MI, ed) 294–312. New York: Guilford Press.

Hebets EA (2005) Attention-focusing interactions among signals in multimodal communication: Evidence from the courtship behavior of *Schizocosa uetzi* (Araneae: Lycosidae). Behav Ecol 16: 75–82.

Horrey WJ, Wickens CD (2006) Examining the impact of cell phone conversations on driving using meta-analytic techniques. Hum Factors 48: 196–205.

Jones C, Healy S (2006) Differences in cue use and spatial memory in men and women. P Roy Soc Lond B Bio 273: 2241–2247.

Kastner S, Ungerleider LG (2000) Mechanisms of visual attention in the human cortex. Annu Rev Neurosci 23: 315–341.

Krause J, Godin JGJ (1996) Influence of prey foraging posture on flight behavior and predation risk: predators take advantage of unwary prey. Behav Ecol 7: 264–271.

Krebs JR, Sherry DF, Healy SD, Perry VH, Vaccarino AL (1989) Hippocampal specialization in food-storing birds. P Natl Acad Sci USA 86: 1388–1392.

LaBerge D, Samuels SJ (1974) Toward a theory of automatic processing in reading. Cognitive Psychol 6: 293–323.

Lima SL (1998) Nonlethal effects in the ecology of predator-prey interactions. BioScience 48: 25–34.

Lima SL, Dill LM (1990) Behavioral decisions made under the risk of predation: A review and prospectus. Can J Zool 68: 619–640.

Lucas JR, Brodin A, de Kort SR, Clayton NS (2004) Does hippocampal size correlate with the degree of caching specialization? P Roy Soc Lond B Bio 271: 2423–2429.

Marois R, Ivanoff J (2005) Capacity limits of information processing in the brain. Trends Cogn Sci 9: 296–305.

Mery F, Kawecki TJ (2002) Experimental evolution of learning ability in fruit flies. P Natl Acad Sci USA 99: 14274–14279.

Mery F, Kawecki TJ (2005) A cost of long-term memory in *Drosophila*. Science 308: 1148.

Metcalfe NB, Huntingford FA, Thorpe JE (1987) Predation risk impairs diet selection in juvenile salmon. Anim Behav 35: 931–933.

Milinski M, Heller R (1978) Influence of a predator on the optimal foraging behaviour of sticklebacks (*Gasterosteus aculeatus* L.). Nature 275: 642–644.

Moran J, Desimone R (1985) Selective attention gates visual processing in the extrastriate cortex. Science 229: 782–784.

Muller MM, Andersen S, Trujillo NJ, Valdes-Sosa P, Malinowski P, Hillyard SA (2006) Feature-selective attention enhances color signals in early visual areas of the human brain. P Natl Acad Sci USA 103: 14250–14254.

Pietrewicz A, Kamil AC (1979) Search image formation in the blue jay (*Cyanocitta cristata*). Science 204: 1332–1333.

Plomin R, Defries JC, Craig IW, McGuffin P, eds (2003) Behavioral genetics in the postgenomic era. Washington: American Psychological Association.

Posner MI, Petersen SE (1990) The attention system of the human brain. Annu Rev Psychol 13: 25–42.

Posner MI, Rafal RD, Choate LS, Vaughan J (1985) Inhibition of return: Neural basis and function. Cognitive Neuropsych 2: 211–228.

Pravosudov V, Kitaysky A, Omanska A (2006) The relationship between migratory behaviour, memory and the hippocampus: An intraspecific comparison. P Roy Soc Lond B Bio 273: 2641–2649.

Raber J, Wong D, Yu GQ, Buttini M, Mahley RW, Pitas RE, Mucke L (2000) Apolipoprotein E and cognitive performance. Nature 404: 352–354.

Rees G, Frith CD, Lavie N (1997) Modulating irrelevant motion perception by varying attentional load in an unrelated task. Science 278: 1616–1619.

Reid PJ, Shettleworth SJ (1992) Detection of cryptic prey: Search image or search rate? J Exp Psychol Anim B 18: 273–286.

Rogers LJ, Andrew R (2002) Comparative vertebrate lateralization. Cambridge: Cambridge University Press.

Rogers LJ, Zucca P, Vallortigara G (2004) Advantages of having a lateralized brain. P Roy Soc Lond B Bio 271: S420–S422.

Savitz J, Solms M, Ramesar R (2006) The molecular genetics of cognition: Dopamine, COMT and BDNF. Genes Brain Behav 5: 311–328.

Shaw ML, Shaw P (1977) Optimal allocation of cognitive resources to spatial locations. J Exp Psychol Hum Percept Perform 3: 201–211.

Sherry DF, Vaccarino AL, Buckenham K, Herz RS (1989) The hippocampal complex of food-storing birds. Brain Behav Evol 34: 308–317.

Shettleworth SJ, Westwood RP (2002) Divided attention, memory, and spatial discrimination in food-storing and nonstoring birds, black-capped chickadees (*Poecile atricapilla*) and dark-eyed juncos (*Junco hyemalis*). J Exp Psychol Anim B 28: 227–241.

Skals N, Anderson P, Kanneworff M, Lofstedt C, Surlykke A (2005) Her odours make him deaf: Crossmodal modulation of olfaction and hearing in a male moth. J Exp Biol 208: 595–601.

Smith JD (2000) Apolipoprotein E4: An allele associated with many diseases. Ann Med 32: 118–127.

Stephens DW, Krebs J (1986) Foraging theory. Princeton, NJ: Princeton University Press.

Strayer DL, Johnston WA (2001) Driven to distraction: Dual-task studies of simulated driving and conversing on a cellular telephone. Psychol Sci 12: 462–466.

Swinderen BV, Greenspan RJ (2003) Salience modulates 20–30 Hz brain activity in *Drosophila*. Nat Neurosci 6: 579–586.

Tang YP, Shimizu E, Dube GR, Rampon C, Kerchner GA, Zhuo M, Liu G, Tsien JZ (1999) Genetic enhancement of learning and memory in mice. Nature 401: 63–69.

Tinbergen L (1960) The natural control of insects on pinewoods I. Factors influencing the intensity of predation by songbirds. Arch Neerl Zool 13: 265–343.

Tolman EC (1924) The inheritance for maze-learning ability in rats. J Comp Psychol 4: 1–18.

Tully T, Bourtchouladze R, Scott R, Tallman J (2003) Targeting the CREB pathway for memory enhancers. Nat Rev Drug Discov 2: 267–277.

Van Essen DC, Anderson CH (1995) Information processing strategies and pathways in the primate visual system. In: An introduction to neural and electronic networks (Zornetzer SF, Davis JL, Lau C, McKenna T, eds), 45–76. San Diego: Academic Press.

Van Essen DC, Anderson CH, Felleman DJ (1992) Information processing in the primate visual system: An integrated systems perspective. Science 255: 419–423.

9 Learning to See and Conceive

Robert L. Goldstone, Alexander Gerganov, David Landy, and Michael E. Roberts

Human concept learning depends upon perception. Our concept of "car" is built out of perceptual features such as "engine," "tire," and "bumper." However, recent research indicates that the dependency works both ways. We see bumpers and engines in part because we have acquired "car" concepts and detected examples of them. Perception both influences and is influenced by the concepts that we learn. We have been exploring the psychological mechanisms by which concepts and perception mutually influence one another, and building computational models to show that the circle of influences is benign rather than vicious.

Perceptual Learning Is "Early" Neurologically, Functionally, and Developmentally

An initial suggestion that concept learning influences perception comes from a consideration of the differences between novices and experts. Experts in many domains, including radiologists, wine tasters, and Olympic judges, develop specialized perceptual tools for analyzing the objects in their domains of expertise. Much of training and expertise involves not only developing a database of cases or explicit strategies for dealing with the world but also tailoring perceptual processes to more efficiently represent the world (Gibson 1991). Tuning one's perceptual representation to the environment is a risky proposition. Once a perceptual representation has been altered, it affects all "downstream" processes that act as consumers of this altered representation. It makes sense to adapt perceptual systems slowly and conservatively. However, the payoffs for perceptual flexibility are also too enticing to forego. They allow an organism to respond quickly, efficiently, and effectively to stimuli without dedicating on-line attentional resources. Instead of strategically determining how to use an unbiased perceptual representation to fit one's needs, it is often easier to rig up a perceptual system to give task-relevant representations, and then simply leave this rigging in place without strategic control. Perceptual learning is early in several senses: neurological, functional, and developmental.

Neurological Evidence

Several sources of evidence point to expertise influencing perceptual processing at a relatively early stage of processing. First, electrophysiological recordings show enhanced electrical activity at about 164 milliseconds after the presentation of dog or bird pictures to dog and bird experts, but only when they categorized objects within their domain of expertise (Tanaka and Curran 2001). A similar early electrophysiological signature of expertise is found with fingerprint experts when they are shown upright fingerprints, but is delayed when the fingerprints are inverted (Busey and Vanderkolk 2005). Interestingly, the timing and form of this expertise-related activity is similar to the pattern found when people are presented with faces, a stimulus domain in which, arguably, almost all people are experts (Gauthier et al. 2003).

Second, prolonged practice with a subtle visual categorization results in much improved discrimination, but the improvements are highly specific to the trained orientation (Notman et al. 2005). This profile of high specificity of training is usually associated with changes to early visual cortex (Fahle and Poggio 2002). Practice in discriminating small motions in different directions significantly alters electrical brain potentials that occur within 100 milliseconds of the stimulus onset (Fahle 1994). These electrical changes are centered over the primary visual cortex, suggesting plasticity in early visual processing. Karni and Sagi (1993) find evidence, based on the specificity of training to eye (interocular transfer does not occur) and retinal location, that is consistent with early, primary visual cortex adaptation in simple discrimination tasks. In the auditory modality, training in a selective attention task produces differential responses as early in the sensory processing stream as the cochlea (Puel et al. 1988). This amazing degree of top-down modulation of a peripheral neural system is mediated by descending pathways of neurons that project from the auditory cortex all the way back to olivocochlear neurons, which in turn project to outer hair cells within the cochlea (Suga and Ma 2003).

Third, expertise can lead to improvements in the discrimination of low-level simple features, as with the documented sensitivity advantage that radiologists have over novices in detecting low-contrast dots in X-rays (Sowden et al. 2000). Fourth, imaging techniques have succeeded in identifying brain regions associated with the acquisition of expertise. Expertise for visual stimuli as eclectic as butterflies, cars, chess positions, dogs, and birds has been associated with an area of the temporal lobe known as the fusiform face area (Bukach et al. 2006). The identification of a common brain area implicated in many domains of visual expertise suggests the promise of developing general theories and models of perceptual learning. This is the main purpose of our work.

Several other pieces of auxiliary evidence point to experience having early effects on perception, where "early" is operationalized neurologically in terms of a relatively small number of intervening synapses connecting a critical brain region to the external world. Experience making fine tactile discriminations influences primary somatosensory cortices. Monkeys trained to make discriminations between slightly different sound frequencies develop larger somatosensory cortex representations for the presented frequencies than control monkeys (Recanzone et al. 1993). Similarly, monkeys learning to make a tactile discrimination with one hand develop a larger cortical representation for that hand than for the other hand (Recanzone et al. 1992). Elbert and colleagues (1995) measured brain activity in the somatosensory cortex of violinists as their fingers were lightly touched. There was greater activity in the sensory cortex for the left hand than the right hand, consistent with the observation that violinists use their left-hand fingers considerably more than their right-hand fingers.

Functional Evidence

In terms of functional evidence, experience often exerts an influence before other putatively early perceptual processes have been completed. Peterson and Gibson (Peterson 1994; Peterson and Gibson 1994; Peterson et al. 1991) found that the organization of a scene into figure and ground is influenced by the visual familiarity of the contours. Their participants were more likely to respond that familiar, compared to unfamiliar, forms were figural elements occluding the background. This effect was not found when flipping the scenes upside down eliminated familiarity, but was found regardless of whether the familiar object was black or white. Interpreting the familiar region as a figure was found even when the unfamiliar regions had the strong Gestalt organization cue of symmetry. Peterson and Lampignano (2003) found direct evidence that the acquired familiarity of a shape successfully competes against Gestalt cues such as partial closure to determine the organization of a scene into figure and ground.

Consistent with an influence of training that occurs relatively early in the information-processing stream, perceptual organizations that are natural according to Gestalt laws of perception can be overlooked in favor of perceptual organizations that involve familiarized materials. Behrmann and colleagues (1998) found that judgments about whether two parts had the same number of humps were faster when the two parts belonged to the same object rather than different objects. Further work found an influence of experience on subsequent part comparisons. Two fragments were interpreted as belonging to the same object if they had co-occurred many times in a single shape (Zemel et al. 2002). As shown in figure 9.1, object fragments that are not naturally grouped together because they do not follow the Gestalt law of good continuation (according to which there is an inherent tendency to see a line continuing its established direction) can nonetheless be perceptually joined if participants are familiarized with an object that unifies the fragments.

Developmental Evidence

Perceptual learning is also "early" in the developmental sense. Many of the most striking changes to our perceptual systems occur in the first two years of life. Infants are surprisingly adept at adapting their perceptual systems to statistical regularities in their environment. Needham and Baillargeon (1998, see also Needham 1999; Needham et al. 2005)

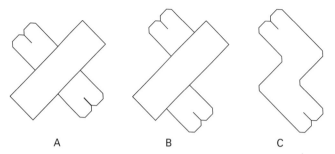

A   B   C

Figure 9.1
Images used by Zemel et al. (2002). Object fragments that are not naturally grouped together because they do not follow the Gestalt law of good continuation (panel B) can nonetheless be perceptually joined if participants are familiarized with an object that unifies the fragments (panel C). Figure courtesy of Zemel and colleagues.

found that exposing infants to single or paired objects tended to lead the infants to parse subsequent events in terms of these familiarized configurations. As shown in figure 9.2, infants initially exposed to a cylinder abutting a rectangular box showed relatively long looking times, suggesting surprise, if one of the objects subsequently moved separately from the other. This surprise occurred even though the natural perceptual cue of minima of curvature (which would segment a scene into parts at negative minima of curvature on silhouette edges) (Hoffman and Richards 1984) would suggest a plausible division between the cylinder and box.

Paul Quinn and his colleagues (Quinn and Schyns 2003; Quinn et al. 2006) were interested in further pursuing the question of whether infants, like adults, can perceive objects in terms of familiarized parts rather than the parts given by default perceptual organizations. They contrasted familiarity-based segmentations with segmentations derived from one of the Gestalt perceptual laws of organization, good continuation. In figure 9.3, the shapes in the "familiarization" set are all ambiguous, interpretable as either a polygon combined with an overlapping circle or as a closed figure consisting of both straight lines and curves combined with a three-quarter-circle "Pac-man" shape.

The former interpretation is consistent with good continuation. Consistent with this law, three-to-four-month-old infants tend to see the shapes in the "familiarization" set as containing a circle and a polygon. The evidence for this is that when the infants are subsequently presented with the full and three-quarters circle, they look at the full circles 39 percent of the time and three-quarters circles 61 percent of the time (Quinn et al. 2006), shown as path A in figure 9.3. Prior base-line experiments showed that this looking preference was not due to a general preference for the Pac-man shape; when infants were not first shown either the prefamiliarized or familiarized shapes, there was no reliable tendency for infants to preferentially look at the Pac-man shape. Together with many other experiments on visual shape perception, this first result suggests that infants have a novelty preference—a preference to look at unfamiliar objects—and that the Pac-man shape seems

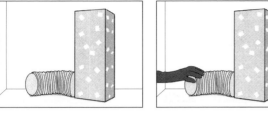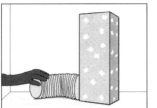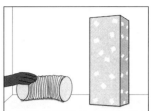

Move-Apart Event

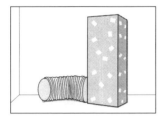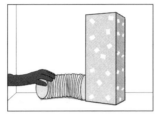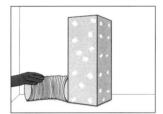

Move-Together Event

Figure 9.2
Stimuli from Needham and Baillargeon (1998). Infants exposed to a cylinder juxtaposed with a rectangular box showed relatively long looking times (suggesting surprise) if one of the objects moved separately from the other, as depicted in the move-apart event in the top panel. Figure courtesy of Needham and Baillargeon.

novel because, although it is present in the familiarized shapes, it is not the natural segmentation for infants to make. Their natural segmentation, like that of adults, is to obey follow the law of good continuation and interpret the ambiguous complexes as containing circles.

A second condition suggests that the infants' segmentations can be altered by prior learning. For some infants, looking at the "familiarization" shapes was preceded by looking at the "prefamiliarization" shapes shown in figure 9.3. These "prefamiliarization" shapes consist of the Pac-man shape combined with a polygon. Habituation trials directly after infants saw the "prefamiliarization" shapes show that the infants interpreted these forms as containing the Pac-man shape, rather than a partially covered circle, as indicated by their tendency to look at the novel-seeming circle 56 percent of the time when it was presented next to a Pac-man shape. This tendency to preferentially look at the circle continued to be found even after the "familiarization" stimuli were shown to infants (path B in figure 9.3). This strongly suggests that the "familiarization" shapes are now interpreted as containing Pac-men rather than circles, and thus circles seem novel and worth more extended scrutiny. Taken together, these results indicate that early in development, children are predisposed to learn shapes from their environments and then interpret their environment in terms of these learned shapes.

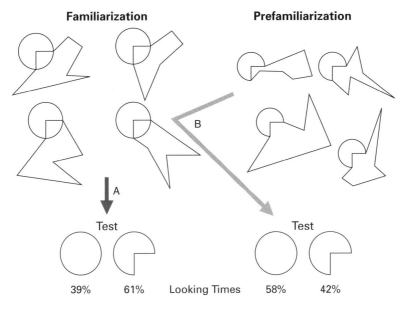

Figure 9.3
When three- to four-month-old infants are familiarized with figures consisting of a complex polygon superimposed on a circle, they tend to look more at the three-quarter-circle "Pac-man" type of shape than at the full circle. However, when they are prefamiliarized with polygons superimposed with the three-quarters "Pac-man," they tend to look more at the full circle.

Perceptual Learning via Unitization

Perceptual learning is powerful because it is not only early in the above three senses, but also, unlike a reflex, is task-dependent. This combination of properties allows perception to be both fast and useful. The nature and degree of perceptual learning is typically closely tied to the task, goals, and knowledge of the observer. Although perceptual learning may occur without awareness (Watanabe et al. 2001), it is more common for researchers to report learning that depends upon both the objective frequency and subjective importance of the physical feature (Sagi and Tanne 1994; Shiu and Pashler 1992). For example, altering the color of target objects in a visual search paradigm from training to transfer tasks does not influence performance unless the training task requires encoding of color (Logan et al. 1996). Our empirical research has been focused on the particular mechanisms by which perceptual processes are modified by experience and tasks. One result of category learning is to create perceptual units that combine stimulus components useful for the categorization. Such a process is one variety of the more general phenomenon of unitization, by which single functional units are constructed that are triggered when a complex configuration arises (Goldstone 1998, 2000). In the next section, the complementary process, dimension differentiation, will be described. Although unitization and dimension differentiation seem to be contradictory processes, we will argue on computational grounds that they reflect the same mechanism of determining useful perceptual building blocks for representing patterns.

Cattell (1886) invoked the notion of perceptual unitization to account for the advantage found for identifying tachistoscopically presented words relative to nonwords. Unitization has also been posited in the field of attention, where researchers have claimed that shape components of often-presented stimuli with practice become processed as a single functional unit (LaBerge 1973). Shiffrin and Lightfoot (1997) report evidence from the slopes of the lines relating the number of distracter elements to response time in a feature search task. When participants learned a conjunctive search task in which three line segments were needed to distinguish the target from distracters, impressive and prolonged decreases in search slopes were observed over twenty hour-long sessions. These prolonged decreases were not observed for a simple search task requiring attention to only one component. The authors concluded that conjunctive training leads to the unitization of the set of diagnostic line segments, resulting in fewer required comparisons.

Our own experiments (Goldstone 2000) have explored unitization from a complementary perspective. First, our experiments reflect our primary interest in the influence of category learning on unitization, under the hypothesis that a unit will tend to be created if the parts that make up the unit frequently co-occur, and if the unit is useful for determining a categorization. Second, we use a new method for analyzing response-time distributions to assess the presence of unitization.

Whenever the claim for the construction of new units is made, two objections must be addressed. First, perhaps the unit existed in people's vocabulary before categorization training. Our stimuli are designed to make this explanation unlikely. Each unit to be sensitized is constructed by connecting five randomly chosen curves. There are ten curves that can be sampled, yielding 10^5 possible different units. As such, if it can be shown that a subject can be sensitized to any randomly selected unit, then an implausibly large number of vocabulary items would be required under the constraint that all vocabulary items are fixed and a priori. The second objection is that no units need be formed; instead, people analytically integrate evidence from the five separate curves to make their categorizations. However, this objection will be untenable if participants, at the end of extended training, are faster at categorizing the units than would be expected by the analytic approach.

In our experiments the categorization task was designed so that evidence for five components must be received before certain categorization responses are made. That is, it was a conjunctive categorization task. The stimuli and their category memberships are shown in figure 9.4.

Each of the letters refers to a particular segment of one "doodle." Each doodle was composed of five segments, with a semicircle below the segments added to create a closed figure. To correctly place the doodle labeled "ABCDE" into category 1, all five components, "A," "B," "C," "D," and "E," must be processed. For example, if the right-most

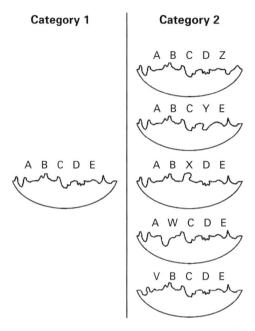

Figure 9.4
Stimuli used by Goldstone (2000). Each letter represents a particular stimulus segment, and each stimulus is composed of five segments. To categorize the item represented by "ABCDE" as belonging to Category 1, it is necessary to process information associated with each of the segments.

component were not attended, then "ABCDE" could not be distinguished from "ABCDZ," which belongs in category 2. Only the complete five-way conjunction suffices to accurately categorize "ABCDE." If unitization occurs during categorization, then, with training, the stimulus "ABCDE" may become treated functionally like a single component. If this occurs, then participants should be able to quickly respond that this stimulus belongs to category 1. So a pronounced decrease in the time required to categorize the conjunctively defined stimulus "ABCDE" was taken as initial evidence for unitization.

For improvement in the conjunctive task to be taken as evidence for unitization, two important control conditions are necessary. First, it is important to show that tasks that do not require unitization do not show comparable improvements. To this end, a control task was included that allows participants to categorize the item "ABCDE" by attending to only a single component rather than a five-way conjunction. This was done by having category 2 contain only one of the five category 2 doodles shown in figure 9.4, randomly selected for each participant. This "One" (component) condition should not result in the same speed-up over training as the "All" (components) condition where five components must be attended. If it does, then the speed-up can be attributed to a simple practice effect rather than unitization. Second, it is important to show that stimuli that cannot be unitized also do not show comparable speed-ups. For this control condition, it was necessary to attend a five-way conjunction of components, but the ordering of the components within the stimulus was randomized. That is, "ABCDE" and "CEBDA" were treated as equivalent. In this "Random" condition, a single template cannot serve to categorize the "ABCDE" stimulus and unitization should therefore not be possible.

The results from the experiment were suggestive of unitization. The results in figure 9.5 reflect only the correct responses to the category 1 doodle "ABCDE."

The horizontal axis shows the amount of practice over a 1.5-hour experiment. The condition where all components were necessary for categorization and where they were combined in a consistent manner to create a coherent image showed far greater practice effect than the others. This dramatic improvement suggests that the components are joined to create a single functional unit to serve categorization. Particularly impressive speed-ups were found when and only when unitization was possible and advantageous.

This paradigm also provides stronger evidence for unitization. The alternative to the unitization hypothesis is that responses in the "All" task are obtained by integrating evidence from five separate judgments of the type required in the "One" task. In arguing against this analytic account, a highly efficient version of the analytic account was devised so that it could be observed whether it still predicted response times that were too slow. The first advantage given to the analytic model was fully parallel processing; "All" responses were made by combining five "One" responses, but evidence for these five "One" responses was assumed to be obtained simultaneously. Second, the analytic model was given unlimited capacity; identifying one component was not slowed by the need to identify another component. In obtaining predictions from this charitably interpreted

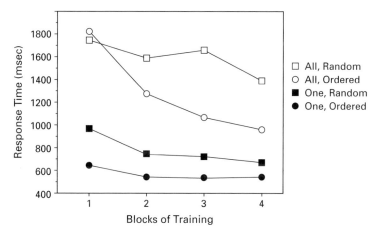

Figure 9.5
Results from Goldstone (2000). The most pronounced improvement was observed when all components were required for a categorization ("All"), and the components were always in the same positions ("Ordered").

analytic model, it is important to remember that the "All" task is a conjunctive task; to categorize ABCDE as a category 1 item with the required 95 percent categorization accuracy, all five components must be identified. Also, there is intrinsic variability in response times, even in the simple task where only one component must be identified. An analytic model of response times can be developed that predicts what the "All" task response-time distribution should be, given the "One" task distribution. After training, a distribution of response times in the "One" task can be empirically determined. To derive the analytic model's predictions, one can randomly sample five response times from this distribution. The maximum of these five times, rather than the average, is selected because no response can be made to the conjunction until all components have been recognized. We can repeat this selection process several times to create a distribution of the maximums, and this yields the predicted response-time distribution for the "All" task. Fortunately, there is an easier, more formal way of obtaining the predicted distribution. The "One" task response-time distribution is converted to a cumulative response-time distribution, and each point on this distribution is raised to the fifth power. If the probability of one component's being recognized in less than 400 msec is 0.2, then the probability of all five components' being recognized in less than 400 msec is 0.2 raised to the fifth power, assuming sampling independence.

A replication of the experiment shown in figure 9.4 was conducted that included the "Ordered All" and "One" tasks. Only four research assistants participated as participants, but unlike in the 1.5-hour experiment described previously, each participant was given fourteen hour-long training sessions. The results, shown in figure 9.6, are only for category 1 responses on the final day of the experiment.

These results indicate violations of the analytic model. Naturally, the "One" task was the fastest (most shifted to the left) according to the cumulative response-time distributions. The analytic model's predictions are shown by the curve labeled "One^5," which is obtained simply by raising each point on the "One" curve to the fifth power. For two of the four participants, the actual "All" distribution was faster than the analytic model's predictions for all regions of the distribution. For all four participants, the fastest 30 percent of response times for the "All" task were faster than predicted by the analytic model, even though all participants were achieving accuracies greater than 95 percent. Although the advantage of the "All" over the "One^5" distribution may not look impressive, the entire distributions were significantly different by a Kolmogorov-Smirnoff test for all participants except the participant C.H. Why were the violations of the analytic model restricted to the fast response times? A likely possibility is that a range of strategies was used for placing ABCDE into category 1 in the "All" task. On trials where a participant used the analytic strategy, the charitably interpreted analytic model would be expected to underestimate observed response times, given the implausibility of pure parallel, unlimited capacity processing. However, on trials where participants used the single constructed unit to categorize ABCDE, violations of the analytic model are predicted. On average, the unit-

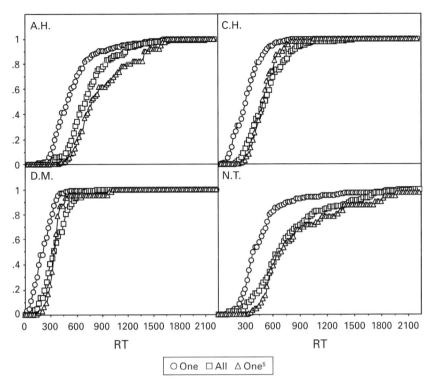

Figure 9.6
The cumulative response time distributions for the four participants taken from the last session of the experiment. The "One" and "All" distributions were empirically obtained. The "One⁵" distribution is obtained by raising each point along the "One" distribution to the fifth power, and represents the analytic model's predicted cumulative distribution for the "All" task. Violations of this analytic model occur when the "All" task's distribution is shifted to the left of the analytic model's distribution. Such violations occur for the fastest half of response times for all four participants (significantly so for all participants except C.H.).

based trials will be faster than the analytic trials. That is, if participants successfully use a single unit to categorize ABCDE then they will tend to do so quickly. If they cannot use this route, their response time will tend to be slower. Thus, if the fast and slow response times tend to be based on single units and analytic integration, respectively, then we would predict violations of the analytic model to be limited to, or more pronounced for, the fast response times.

In light of these results, we concluded that category learning probably created new perceptual units. Large practice effects were found if and only if stimuli were unitizable (the first experiment), and responses after fourteen hours of training were faster for conjunctively defined categories than predicted by a charitably interpreted analytic model. The results shown in figure 9.6 only violate the analytic model if negative dependencies or independence is assumed between the five sampled response times that make up one

"All" judgment. Although it is beyond the scope of this chapter, we also have evidence
for violations of the analytic model for classes of positive dependencies, using Fourier
transformations to deconvolve shared input/output processes from the One task response-
time distribution (Goldstone 2000; Smith 1990).

There is still a remaining question: Exactly how do people become so fast at categorizing ABCDE in the "All" task? Two qualitatively different mechanisms could account for
the pronounced speed-up of the conjunctive categorization: a genuinely holistic match
process to a constructed unit, or an analytic model that incorporates interactive facilitation
among the component detectors. According to a holistic match process, a conjunctive
categorization is made by comparing the image of the presented item to an image that has
been stored over prolonged practice. The stored image may have parts, but either these
parts are arbitrarily small or they do not play a functional role in the recognition of the
image.

There is evidence supporting the gradual development of configural features. Neurophysiological findings suggest that some individual neurons represent familiar conjunctions of features (Perrett and Oram 1993; Perrett et al. 1984), and that prolonged training
can produce neurons that respond to configural patterns (Logothetis et al. 1995). However,
our results could also arise if detecting one component of "ABCDE" facilitates detection
of other components (Townsend and Wenger 2004). In either case, the process is appropriately labeled "unitization" in that the percepts associated with different components are
closely coupled. In fact, an interactive facilitation mechanism could be seen as the mechanism that implements holistic unit detection at a higher functional level of description.

Perceptual Learning via Differentiation

New perceptual representations can be created by chunking together elements that were
previously psychologically separated in a process of unitization, and the converse process
also occurs. This second process is dimension differentiation, according to which dimensions that are originally psychologically fused become separated and isolated. It is useful
to contrast dimension differentiation from the more basic learning process of learning to
selectively attend to one psychological dimension of stimulus. Selective attention assumes
that the different dimensions that make up a stimulus can actually be individually attended.
In his classic research on stimulus integrality and separability, Garner (1976, 1978) argues
that stimulus dimensions differ in how easily they can be isolated or extracted from each
other. Dimensions are said to be separable if it is possible to attend to one of the dimensions without attending to the other. Size and brightness are classic examples of separable
dimensions; making a categorization on the basis of size is not significantly slowed if there
is irrelevant variation on brightness. Dimensions are integral if variation along an irrelevant dimension cannot be ignored when trying to attend a relevant dimension. The classic
examples of integral dimensions are saturation and brightness, where saturation is related

to the amount of white mixed into a color, and brightness is related to the amount of light coming off of a color. For saturation and brightness, it is difficult to attend to only one of the dimensions (Burns and Shepp 1988; Melara et al. 1993).

From this work distinguishing integral from separate dimensions, one might conclude that selective attention can proceed with separable but not integral dimensions. However, one interesting possibility is that category learning can, to some extent, change the status of dimensions, transforming dimensions that were originally integral into more separable dimensions. Experience may change the underlying representation of a pair of dimensions such that they come to be treated as relatively independent and noninterfering sources of variation that compose an object. Seeing that stimuli in a set vary along two orthogonal dimensions may allow the dimensions to be teased apart and isolated, particularly if the two dimensions are differentially diagnostic for categorization. There is developmental evidence that dimensions that are easily isolated by adults, such as the brightness and size of a square, are treated as fused for four-year-old children (Kemler and Smith 1978; Smith and Kemler 1978). It is relatively difficult for children to decide whether two objects are identical on a particular dimension, but relatively easy for them to decide whether they are similar across many dimensions (Smith 1989). For example, children seem to be distracted by shape differences when they are instructed to make comparisons based on color. Adjectives that refer to single dimensions are learned by children relatively slowly compared to nouns (Smith et al. 1997).

The developmental trend toward increasingly differentiated dimensions is echoed by adult training studies. Under certain circumstances, color experts (art students and vision scientists) are better able to selectively attend to dimensions (e.g., hue, chroma, and value) that make up color than are nonexperts (Burns and Shepp 1988). Goldstone (1994) has shown that people who learn a categorization in which saturation is relevant and brightness is irrelevant (or vice versa) can learn to perform the categorization accurately, and as a result of category learning, they develop a selectively heightened sensitivity at making discriminations of saturation, relative to brightness. That is, categorization training that makes one dimension diagnostic and another dimension nondiagnostic can serve to split apart these dimensions, even if they are traditionally considered to be integral dimensions. These training studies show that in order to know how integral two dimensions are, one has to know something about the observer's history.

Goldstone and Steyvers (2001) used a category learning and transfer paradigm to explore whether genuinely arbitrary dimensions can become isolated from each other. Our subjects first learned to categorize a set of sixteen faces into two groups by receiving feedback from a computer, and then were transferred to a second categorization task. The stimuli varied along two arbitrary dimensions, A and B, that were created by morphing between randomly paired faces (Steyvers 1999). We created a set of stimuli with no preferred dimensional axes by assigning sixteen faces to coordinates that fall on a circle in the abstract space defined by dimensions A and B. To this end, a variable D was created that was assigned sixteen different values, from 0 to 360, in 22.5-degree steps. For each value assigned to D, the dimension A value for a face was equal to cosine (D) and the dimension B value was sine (D). The end result, shown in figure 9.7, is a set of faces that are organized on a circle with no privileged dimensional axes suggested by the set of faces.

With these faces, Goldstone and Steyvers asked whether the organization of the faces into dimensions could be influenced by the required categorization. Subjects were shown faces, asked to categorize them, and then received feedback on the correctness of their categorization. The categorization rules all involved splitting the sixteen faces into two

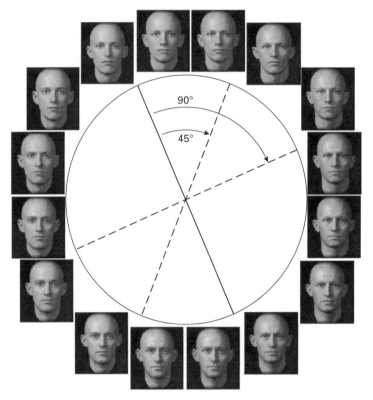

Figure 9.7
Stimuli from Goldstone and Steyvers (2001), experiment 3. The proportions of two randomly paired faces are negatively correlated such that the more of face 1 is present, the less of face 2 there will be. This negative correlation establishes the dimension on the X-axis, and a similar negative correlation between two other faces establishes the Y-axis dimension. A set of circularly arranged faces was created by varying degrees from 0 to 360, and assigning the face a value on the X-axis dimension based on the cosine of the degrees, and assigning the face's Y-axis value based on the sine of the degrees. Subjects learned two successive categorizations involving the faces. Each categorization split the faces into two equal groups with a straight line dividing them. The two category boundaries given to a subject were related to each other by either 45 or 90 degrees.

equal piles using straight lines such as those shown in figure 9.7. Each subject was given categorization training with one classification rule and then was transferred to a second categorization task governed by a different rule. The critical experimental manipulation was whether the final categorization rule involved a rotation of 45 or 90 degrees relative to the initial rule. Given that the initial categorization rules were randomly selected, the only difference in the 45- and 90-degree rotation conditions was whether the category boundary was shifted by two or four faces. When the category boundary was shifted by two faces in the 45-degree condition, the labels could either be preserved (six faces assigned to the same category) or reversed (two faces assigned to the same category), but the category boundary itself was the same for these two conditions. The results, shown in "Whole Face Dimensions" columns of figure 9.8, indicate that in the second phase of category learning, there was an advantage for the 90- over 45-degree rotation condition in these integral dimension conditions.

This is somewhat surprising, given that categorizations related by 90 degrees are completely incompatible in regard to their selective-attention demands. The dimension that was originally completely irrelevant becomes completely relevant. In the 45-degree condition, the originally relevant dimension is at least partially relevant later. However, categorizations related by 90 degrees do have an advantage as far as dimensional organization. The relevant dimensions for the two categorizations are compatible with each other in the

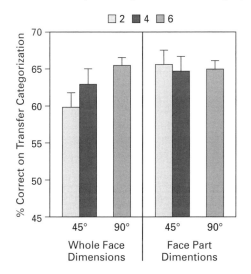

Figure 9.8
The 90-degree-rotation condition produced better transfer on the final categorization than the 45-degree condition, but only for overlapping face dimensions such as those in figure 9.7, and not spatially separated dimensions such as eyes and mouth.

sense of relying on independent sources of variation. For example, acquiring one dimension in figure 9.7 is compatible with later acquiring the 90-degree rotation of this dimension, because both are independent dimensions that can coexist without interference.

By analogy, categorizing rectangles on the basis of height is compatible with categorizing them on the basis of width because these two dimensions can each be separately registered and do not interfere with each other. Someone who thought about rectangles in terms of height would also be likely to think about them in terms of width. Organizing rectangles in terms of shape (ratio of width to height) and area is an alternative dimensional organization. A person who thinks in terms of rectangle shape might also be expected to think in terms of area because this is the remaining dimension along which rectangles vary once shape has been extracted. However, organizing rectangles in terms of height is incompatible with organizing them in terms of area because area is partially dependent on height. Thus, categorization rules separated by 90 degrees are inconsistent with respect to their selective attention demands because the dimension that was originally attended must be ignored and vice versa. However, the rules are consistent with respect to their dimensional organization of stimuli.

Our account for the advantage of a 90- over 45-degree rule rotation is that only the former rotation maintains a compatible dimensional interpretation of the stimuli across the two categorizations. If the relatively good transfer in the 90-degree rotation condition is because the two categorizations encourage the same differentiation of the faces into dimensions rather than crosscutting dimensions, then we should not expect the 90-degree rotation condition to produce better performance when dimension differentiation is not required— that is, with more separable stimuli. This is exactly what was found when we created dimensions by morphing select face parts rather than entire dimensions. One dimension morphed the eyes from one face to the eyes of another face, and the other dimension morphed mouths. These dimensions are more separable than those shown in figure 9.7 because people can attend to one dimension without showing much interference due to irrelevant variation on the other dimension (Garner 1976). With these more separable dimensions, participants should be able to selectively attend one dimension without as much need to differentiate fused dimensions. As shown by the right panel of figure 9.8, with these dimensions, the advantage for the 90-degree rotation was no longer found. This again suggests that the 90-degree advantage is due to participants' learning to isolate two originally fused dimensions from each other, and transferring this knowledge.

This conclusion is controversial. Op de Beeck and his colleagues (2003) created stimuli composed of novel, spatially overlapping dimensions. The shapes in figure 9.9 were created by combining seven sinusoidal functions (each with three parameters: frequency, phase, and amplitude), referred to individually as radial frequency components (RFCs), into a single, complex curve and then bending these to create closed contours.

While five of the seven RFCs remained fixed, two were chosen to have their amplitudes varied to define a two-dimensional space. Op de Beeck et al. (2003) showed that these

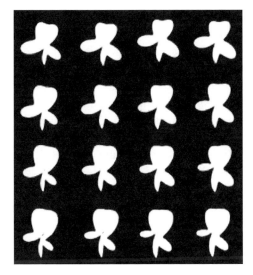

Figure 9.9
Stimuli used by Hockema et al. (2005), based on stimuli first developed by Op de Beeck et al. (2003), composed of two overlapping and integral dimensions. Looking from left to right, the amplitude of one radial frequency component (RFC) of the shapes is increased. Looking from top to bottom, a second RFC component is varied. These stimuli were purposefully blurred so that participants could not use local pixel features on the contour edges that might be correlated with the diagnostic dimensions. With these blurred stimuli participants needed to pay attention to relatively global aspects of the shape-based dimensions.

dimensions are relatively integral. With these stimuli there was no evidence that categorization via a horizontal or vertical boundary led to greater improvement in discriminability along the category-relevant dimension relative to the irrelevant dimension. On the basis of this result, they argued that category learning is only capable of altering weights to already separable dimensions, but not of making integral dimensions more separable.

Our dimension-differentiation account is not forced to predict that differentiation will occur for any set of dimensions within any set length of categorization training. Our account holds that some relatively integral dimensions can become differentiated, not that every arbitrary pair of indistinguishable dimensions can be well separated by categorization learning. Still, we found the RFC stimuli compelling, and were consequently interested in whether an improved training regime could lead to the differentiation of the RFC components (Hockema et al. 2005). In particular, we controlled the order of training trials to start with easy categorizations—shapes far from the category boundary—and gradually increase the difficulty to include shapes nearer to the boundary. Echoing classic results showing highly efficient learning with easy-to-hard training regimes (Mackintosh 1974), this training allowed our participants to eventually make categorizations that would have proved too difficult to learn in initial training. This training effectively challenged the perceptual system to adapt in order to support the categorization. After training, participants were better able to discriminate between stimuli near the categorization boundary that varied along the relevant, compared to irrelevant, dimension. This result indicates the kind of selective sensitization of a single dimension for which Op de Beeck and colleagues (2003) failed to find evidence. Further experiments showed that dynamic animations, varying on single dimensions, also successfully trained selective sensitization for an originally integral pair of dimensions. In light of these results, our current claim is that not all categorization training that would benefit from dimension differentiation will result in the desired differentiation. However, if care is taken to create training situations that push the perceptual system beyond its original capacity, then dimensions that were originally psychologically fused are not necessarily doomed to remain that way. Perceptual learning involves learning to selectively attend to relevant dimensions, but can also involve establishing what dimensions are available for selective attention in the first place. People not only learn appropriate weights for dimensions but also learn how to learn attentional weights for dimensions.

A Computational Reconciliation

Unitization involves the construction of a single functional unit out of component parts. Dimension differentiation divides wholes into separate component dimensions. There is an apparent contradiction between experience creating larger "chunks" via unitization and dividing an object into more clearly delineated components via differentiation. This incongruity can be transformed into a commonality at a more abstract level. Both mechanisms depend on the requirements established by tasks and stimuli. Objects will tend to be decomposed into their parts if the parts reflect independent sources of variation, or if the parts differ in their relevancy. Parts will tend to be unitized if they co-occur frequently, with all parts indicating a similar response. Thus, unitization and differentiation are both processes that build appropriately sized representations for the tasks at hand.

We have developed computational models to show how concept learning can lead to learning new perceptual organizations via unitization and differentiation (Gerganov et al. 2007; Goldstone 2003). In this pursuit, we have been drawn to neural networks that possess units that intervene between inputs and outputs and are capable of creating internal representations. For the current purposes, these intervening units can be interpreted as learned-feature detectors, and represent an organism's acquired perceptual vocabulary. Just as we perceive the world through the filter of our perceptual system, so the neural network does not have direct access to the input patterns, but rather only has access to the detectors that it develops.

The conceptual and perceptual learning by unitization and segmentation model, or CPLUS, is given a set of pictures as inputs and produces as output a categorization of each picture. Along the way to this categorization, the model comes up with a description of how the picture is segmented into pieces. The segmentation that CPLUS creates will tend to involve parts that (1) obey the Gestalt laws of perceptual organization by connecting object parts that have similar locations and orientations, (2) occur frequently in the set of presented pictures, and (3) are diagnostic for the categorization. For example, if the five input pictures of figure 9.10 are presented to the network and labeled as belonging to category A or category B, then originally random detectors typically become differentiated as shown.

This adaptation of the detectors reveals three important behavioral tendencies. First, detectors are created for parts that recur across the five objects, such as the lower square and upper rectangular antenna. Thus, the first input picture on the left will be represented by combining responses of the square and rectangular antenna detectors. Second, single, holistic detectors are created for objects such as the rightmost input picture that do not share any large pieces with other inputs. In this way, the model can explain how the same learning process unitizes complex configurations and differentiates other inputs into pieces. Third, the detectors act as filters that lie between the actual inputs and the categories. The

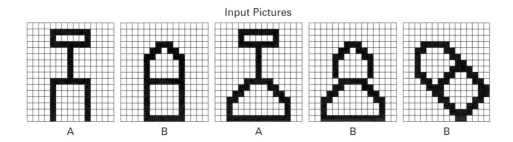

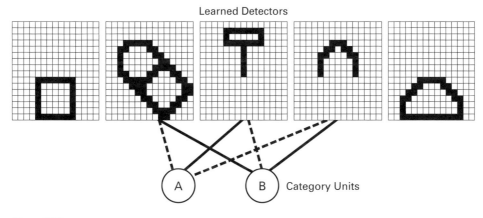

Figure 9.10
Sample output from the CPLUS (conceptual and perceptual learning by unitization and segmentation) model. After being exposed to the input pictures and their categorizations, the neural network creates detectors that can be assembled, like building blocks, to recreate the inputs. The detectors are learned at the same time that they are associated to categories. Solid lines represent excitatory connections; dashed lines represent inhibitory connections.

learned connections between the acquired detectors and the categories are shown by thick solid lines for positive connections and dashed lines for negative connections. The network learns to decompose the leftmost input picture into a square and rectangular antenna, but also learns that only the rectangular antenna is diagnostic for categorization, predicting that category A is present and that category B is not.

Although the mathematical details of the model are described elsewhere (Goldstone 2003), it is possible to give a functional description of the basic workings of the model that allow it to both separate stimuli into useful parts and create larger units. The heart of CPLUS is a competitive learning process (Rumelhart and Zipser 1985) in which detectors compete for the "right" to adapt toward randomly presented input patterns. In competitive learning algorithms, detectors start out as homogenous and undifferentiated. As inputs are presented, the detector that is most similar to a presented input adjusts its weights so that it is even more similar to the input, and inhibits the other detectors from learning to adapt toward the input. This leaves the other detectors available to become specialized for a different class of patterns. The originally homogenous detectors will be differentiated over time, and will split the input patterns into two categories. For another example of how small physical differences between detectors can developmentally snowball into substantially different modules, see Johnson (2000; see also chapter 15, this volume).

Competitive learning is typically applied to unsupervised categorization, in which case it takes entire patterns as input, and sorts these complete, whole input patterns into separate categories. However, CPLUS applies competitive learning to the problem of segmentation, by taking a single input pattern and sorting the pieces of the pattern into separate groups. Consistent with competitive learning, the pixel-to-detector weight that is closest to the pixel's actual value will adapt its weight toward the pixel's value, and inhibit other detectors from so adapting. This technique, by itself, segments a pattern into complementary parts. If one detector becomes specialized for a pixel, the other detector does not. Unfortunately, each detector can become specialized for a random set of pixels, rather than a coherent, psychologically plausible segmentation.

To create psychologically plausible segmentations, we modify the determination of winners. Topological constraints on detector creation are incorporated by two mechanisms: (1) input-to-detector weights "leak" to their neighbors by an amount proportional to their proximity in space, and (2) input-to-detector weights also spread to each other as a function of their orientation similarity, defined by the inner product of four orientation filters. The first mechanism produces detectors that tend to respond to cohesive, contiguous regions of an input. The second mechanism produces detectors that follow the principle of good continuation, dividing the figure X into two crossing lines rather than two kissing Vs, because the two halves of a diagonal line will be linked by their common orientation. Thus, if a detector wins for pixel Y (meaning that the detector receives more activation when pixel Y is on than any other detector), then the detector will also tend to handle pixels that are close to, and have similar orientations to, pixel Y. For an alternative approach to segmentation that uses synchronized oscillations rather than architecturally separated detectors to represent segmentations, see Mozer et al. (1992).

As described thus far, the algorithm is completely unsupervised, creating detectors as a function of statistical dependencies and bottom-up perceptual properties of the set of input images. However, much of the experimental evidence previously reviewed indicates a strong influence of learned categories on acquired perceptual encodings. This influence is incorporated into CPLUS by biasing diagnostic detectors to win the competition to learn the pattern. The diagnosticity of a detector is assumed to be directly proportional to the weight from the detector to the category label associated with an input pattern. The input-to-detector weights do not have to be set before the weights from detectors to categories are learned. In fact, in the actual operation of CPLUS, the detectors adapt at the same time that they become associated with categories to be learned. This core assumption of CPLUS allows it to create detectors only when they are useful for an important categorization rather than having to postulate a large initial set of detectors just in case one is needed for a future categorization task.

CPLUS differs from most other models of categorization in that it prominently features a perceptual segmentation process. Its ability to flexibly organize a pattern into learned parts is a large advantage to the extent that the world consists of objects that have parts that recur many times across many objects. CPLUS is inherently a componential model in which objects are broken down into parts during perception, and these parts are differentially associated with categories. Admittedly, there is little advantage to creating compositional representations for the five input pictures in figure 9.10. They can be represented by five holistic detectors just as effectively as by the shown componential representation. However, if we had a set of objects that each had five pieces, and each of those pieces had four variants, then the holistic strategy would require 1,024 (4^5) detectors whereas CPLUS requires only 20. In a world where objects are built from elementary blocks, a perceptual system that can take advantage of this fact stands to benefit considerably, both in terms of representational efficiency and generative flexibility (see also Griffiths and Ghahramani, 2006). A categorization advantage is also accrued when the building blocks are diagnostic for needed categories.

Recently we have incorporated even greater plasticity in the creation of feature detectors in CPLUS. The original version of CPLUS incorporated a hard-wired pressure to create detectors for stimulus elements that are close and create smoothly varying curves. Gerganov and colleagues (2007) have explored the possibility that these constraints themselves may be learned rather than hard-wired. If a set of input patterns mostly contains connected and smooth elements, then a neural network can internalize these regularities as it develops. Other researchers have proposed that visual detectors can be created by a system that simply internalizes statistical regularities extracted from a large set of natural photographic images (Olshausen and Field 1996); however, their detectors were assumed to adapt on evolutionary time scales, and hence be built in for any modern individual. In contrast, the newer version of CPLUS assumes that the process of learning constraints from an environment can take place in an individual's own lifetime. The empirical basis for this contention stems from developmental studies suggesting that some perceptual constraints appear to be learned rather than innate (Quinn and Bhatt 2006; Sheya and Smith 2006). Learning without constraints is impossible, but the exciting possibility still remains that constraints themselves can be learned.

Conclusion

The previously described neural network builds detectors at the same time that it builds connections between the detectors and categories. The psychological implication is that our perceptual systems do not have to be set in place before we start to use them. The concepts we need can and should influence the perceptual units we create. The influence of these concepts comes in at least two forms: unitizing originally individuated elements, and differentiating originally fused elements. Rather than viewing unitization and differentiation as contradictory, they are best viewed as aspects of the same process that bundles stimulus components if they diagnostically co-occur and separates these bundles from other statistically independent bundles. Under this conception, learning new features or detectors consists in learning how to carve a stimulus into useful components.

One of the most powerful ideas in cognitive science has been the notion that flexible cognition works by assembling a fixed set of building blocks into novel arrangements. Many of the most notable discoveries in cognitive science have involved finding these kinds of compositional encodings. In linguistics, phonemes have been represented by the presence or absence of fewer than twelve features such as *voiced, nasal,* and *strident* (Jakobson et al. 1963). Scenarios, such as ordering food in a restaurant, have been represented by Schank (1972) in terms of a set of twenty-three primitive concepts such as *physical-transfer, propel, grasp,* and *ingest.* In the field of object recognition, Biederman (1987) proposed a set of thirty-six geometric shapes such as *wedge* and *cylinder* to be used for representing objects such as telephones and flashlights. We are in complete agreement with these proposals in terms of the cognitive and computational advantage of creating representations by composing elements. The only difference, but a critical one, is that we believe these elements can be flexibly created during experience with an environment, rather than being fixed.

We have argued that the concepts we learn can reach down and influence the very perceptual descriptions that ground the concepts. This interactive cycle is figuratively shown in figure 9.11.

A person creates perceptual building blocks from his or her experiences in the world. Then, the person's subsequent experience of this same world is influenced by these learned building blocks. Naturally, cases of experience-induced hallucinations of figure 9.11's extremity are rare (but possible; Grossberg 2000), but this is a graphic, degenerate case

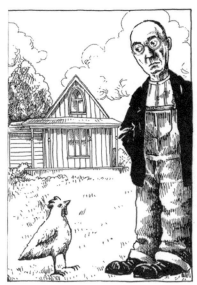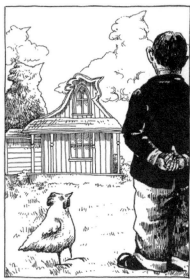

Figure 9.11
We learn about chickens from the world (left panel), and then turn around and interpret the world in terms of the chickens that we have learned (right panel). (Idea: Robert Goldstone; artwork: Joe Lee.)

of the everyday phenomenon in which our perceptions and conceptions are tightly coupled (Wisniewski and Medin 1994). Hopefully, the CPLUS model provides some reassurance that this interactive loop between perception and conception need not be viciously circular. In fact, it is because our experiences are necessarily based on our perceptual systems that these perceptual systems must be shaped so that our experiences are appropriate and useful for dealing with our world.

Acknowledgments

The research reported in this chapter has benefited greatly from comments and suggestions by Drew Hendrickson, Amy Needham, Mary Peterson, Paul Quinn, Richard Shiffrin, and Linda Smith. This research was funded by Department of Education, Institute of Education Sciences grant R305H050116, and National Science Foundation ROLE grant 0527920.

References

Behrmann M, Zemel RS, Mozer MC (1998) Object-based attention and occlusion: Evidence from normal participants and a computational model. J Exp Psychol Hum Percept Perform 24: 1011–1036.

Biederman I (1987) Recognition-by-components: A theory of human image understanding. Psychol Rev 94: 115–147.

Bukach CM, Gauthier I, Tarr MJ (2006) Beyond faces and modularity: The power of an expertise framework. Trends Cogn Sci 10: 159–166.

Burns B, Shepp BE (1988) Dimensional interactions and the structure of psychological space: The representation of hue, saturation, and brightness. Percept Psychophys 43: 494–507.

Busey TA, Vanderkolk JR (2005) Behavioral and electrophysiological evidence for configural processing in fingerprint experts. Vision Res 45: 431–448.

Cattell JM (1886) The time it takes to see and name objects. Mind 11: 63–65.

Elbert T, Pantev C, Wienbruch C, Rockstro, B, Taub E (1995) Increased cortical representation of the fingers of the left hand in string players. Science 270: 305–307.

Fahle M (1994) Human pattern recognition: Parallel processing and perceptual learning. Perception 23: 411–427.

Fahle M, Poggio T (2002) Perceptual learning. Cambridge, MA: MIT Press.

Garner WR (1976) Interaction of stimulus dimensions in concept and choice processes. Cognitive Psychol 8: 98–123.

Garner WR (1978) Selective attention to attributes and to stimuli. J Exp Psychology Gen 107: 287–308.

Gauthier I, Curran T, Curby KM, Collins D (2003) Perceptual interference evidence for a nonmodular account of face processing. Nat Neurosc 6: 428–432.

Gerganov A, Grinberg M, Quinn PC, Goldstone RL (2007) Simulating conceptually guided perceptual learning. In: Proceedings of the twenty-ninth Annual Conference of the Cognitive Science Society (McNamara DS, Trafton JG, eds), 287–292. Nashville, TN: Cognitive Science Society.

Gibson EJ (1991) An odyssey in learning and perception. Cambridge, MA: MIT Press.

Goldstone RL (1994) Influences of categorization on perceptual discrimination. J Exp Psychol Gen 123: 178–200.

Goldstone RL (2003) Learning to perceive while perceiving to learn. In: Perceptual organization in vision: Behavioral and neural perspectives (Kimchi R, Behrmann M, Olson C, eds), 233–278. Hillsdale, NJ: Lawrence Erlbaum.

Goldstone RL (1998) Perceptual learning. Annu Rev Psychol 49: 585–612.

Goldstone RL (2000) Unitization during category learning. J Exp Psychol Hum Percept Perform 26: 86–112.

Goldstone RL, Stevyers M (2001) The sensitization and differentiation of dimensions during category learning. J Exp Psychol Gen 130: 116–139.

Griffiths TL, Ghahramani Z (2006) Infinite latent feature models and the Indian buffet process. Adv Neural Info Proc Sys 18.

Grossberg S (2000) How hallucinations may arise from brain mechanisms of learning, attention, and volition. J Int Neuropsych Soc 6: 579–588.

Hockema SA, Blair MR, Goldstone RL (2005) Differentiation for novel dimensions. In: Proceedings of the twenty-seventh Annual Conference of the Cognitive Science Society (Bara BG, Barsalou L, Bucciarelli M, eds), 953–958. Hillsdale, NJ: Lawrence Erlbaum.

Hoffman DD, Richards WA (1984) Parts of recognition. Cognition 18: 65–96.

Jakobson R, Fant G, Halle M (1963) Preliminaries to speech analysis: The distinctive features and their correlates. Cambridge, MA: MIT Press.

Johnson MH (2000) Functional brain development in infants: Elements of an interactive specialization framework. Child Dev 71: 75–81.

Karni A, Sagi D (1993) The time course of learning a visual skill. Nature 365: 250–252.

Kemler DG, Smith LB (1978) Is there a developmental trend from integrality to separability in perception? J Exp Child Psychol 26: 498–507.

LaBerge D (1973) Attention and the measurement of perceptual learning. Mem Cognition 1: 268–276.

Logan GD, Taylor SE, Etherton JL (1996) Attention in the acquisition and expression of automaticity. J Exp Psychol Learn 22: 620–638.

Logothetis NK, Pauls J, Poggio T (1995) Shape representation in the inferior temporal cortex of monkeys. Curr Biol 5: 552–563.

Mackintosh NJ (1974) The psychology of animal learning. London: Academic Press.

Melara RD, Marks LE, Potts BC (1993) Primacy of dimensions in color perception. J Exp Psychol Hum Perc Perform 19: 1082–1104.

Mozer MC, Zemel RS, Behrmann M, Williams CKI (1992) Learning to segment images using dynamic feature binding. Neural Comput 4: 650–665.

Needham A (1999) The role of shape in 4-month-old infants' segregation of adjacent objects. Infant Behav Dev 22: 161–178.

Needham A, Baillargeon R (1998) Effects of prior experience in 4.5-month-old infants' object segregation. Infant Behav Dev 21: 1–24.

Needham A, Dueker G, Lockhead G (2005) Infants' formation and use of categories to segregate objects. Cognition 94: 215–240.

Notman LA, Sowden PT, Özgen E (2005) The nature of learned categorical perception effects: A psychophysical approach. Cognition 95: B1–B14.

Olshausen BA, Field DJ (1996) Emergence of simple cell receptive field properties by learning a sparse code for natural images. Nature 381: 607–609.

Op de Beeck H, Wagemans J, Vogels R (2003) The effect of category learning on the representation of shape: Dimensions can be biased but not differentiated. J Exp Psychol Gen 132: 491–511.

Perrett DI, Oram MW (1993) Neurophysiology of shape processing. Image Vision Comput 11: 317–333.

Perrett DI, Smith PAJ, Potter DD, Mistlin AJ, Head AD, Jeeves MA (1984) Neurones responsive to faces in the temporal cortex: Studies of functional organization, sensitivity to identity and relation to perception. Hum Neurobiol 3: 197–208.

Peterson MA (1994) Object recognition processes can and do operate before figure-ground organization. Curr Dir Psychol Sci 3: 105–111.

Peterson MA, Harvey EH, Weidenbacher HL (1991) Shape recognition inputs to figure-ground organization: Which route counts? J Exp Psychol Hum Perc Perform 17: 1075–1089.

Peterson MA, Gibson BS (1994) Must figure-ground organization precede object recognition? An assumption in peril. Psychol Sci 5: 253–259.

Peterson MA, Lampignano DW (2003) Implicit memory of novel figure-ground displays includes a history of cross-border competition. J Exp Psychol Hum Perc Perform 29: 808–822.

Puel JL, Bonfils P, Pujol R (1988) Selective attention modifies the active micromechanical properties of the cochlea. Brain Res 447: 380–383.

Quinn PC, Bhatt RS (2006) Are some Gestalt principles deployed more readily than others during early development? The case of lightness versus form similarity. J Exp Psychol Hum Perc Perform 32: 1221–1230.

Quinn PC, Schyns P (2003) What goes up may come down: Perceptual process and knowledge access in the organization of complex visual patterns by young infants. Cognitive Sci 27: 923–935.

Quinn PC, Schyns PG, Goldstone RL (2006) The interplay between perceptual organization and categorization in the representation of complex visual patterns by young infants. J Exp Child Psychol 95: 117–127.

Recanzone GH, Schreiner CE, Merzenich MM (1993) Plasticity in the frequency representation of primary auditory cortex following discrimination training in adult owl monkeys. J Neurosci 13: 87–103.

Recanzone GH, Merzenich MM, Jenkins WM (1992) Frequency discrimination training engaging a restricted skin surface results in an emergence of a cutaneous response zone in cortical area 3a. J Neurophysiol 67: 1057–1070.

Rumelhart DE, Zipser D (1985) Feature discovery by competitive learning. Cognitive Sci 9: 75–112.

Sagi D, Tanne D (1994) Perceptual learning: Learning to see. Curr Opin Neurobiol 4: 195–199.

Schank R (1972) Conceptual dependency: A theory of natural language understanding. Cognitive Psychol 3: 552–631.

Sheya A, Smith LB (2006) Perceptual features and the development of conceptual knowledge. Journal Cogn Dev 7: 455–476.

Shiffrin RM, Lightfoot N (1997) Perceptual learning of alphanumeric-like characters. In: The psychology of learning and motivation, volume 36 (Goldstone RL, Schyns PG, Medin DL, eds), 45–82. San Diego: Academic Press.

Shiu L, Pashler H (1992) Improvement in line orientation discrimination is retinally local but dependent on cognitive set. Percept Psychophys 52: 582–588.

Smith LB (1989) From global similarity to kinds of similarity: The construction of dimensions in development. In: Similarity and analogical reasoning (Vosniadou S, Ortony A, eds), 146–178. Cambridge: Cambridge University Press.

Smith LB, Gasser M, Sandhofer C (1997) Learning to talk about the properties of objects: A network model of the development of dimensions. In: The psychology of learning and motivation, volume 36 (Goldstone RL, Schyns PG, Medin DL, eds), 219–255. San Diego: Academic Press.

Smith LB, Kemler DG (1978) Levels of experienced dimensionality in children and adults. Cognitive Psychol 10: 502–532.

Smith PL (1990) Obtaining meaningful results from Fourier deconvolution of reaction time data. Psychol Bull 108: 533–550.

Sowden PT, Davies IRL, Roling P (2000) Perceptual learning of the detection of features in X-ray images: A functional role for improvements in adults' visual sensitivity? J Exp Psychol Hum Perc Perform 26: 379–390.

Steyvers M (1999) Morphing techniques for generating and manipulating face images. Behav Res Meth Ins C 31: 359–369.

Suga N, Ma X (2003) Multiparametric corticofugal modulation and plasticity of the auditory system. Nat Rev Neurosci 4: 783–794.

Tanaka JW, Curran T (2001) A neural basis for expert object recognition. Psychol Sci 12: 43–47.

Townsend JT, Wenger MJ (2004) A theory of interactive parallel processing: New capacity measures and predictions for a response time inequality series. Psychol Rev 111: 1003–1035.

Watanabe T, Náñez J, Sasaki Y (2001). Perceptual learning without perception. Nature 413: 844–848.

Wisniewski EJ, Medin DL (1994). On the interaction of theory and data in concept learning. Cognitive Sci 18: 221–281.

Zemel RS, Behrmann M, Mozer MC, Bavelier D (2002) Experience-dependent perceptual grouping and object-based attention. J Exp Psychol Hum Perc Perform 28: 202–217.

IV NUMBERS AND PROBABILITY

This section of the book covers the cognitive biology of quantities and values, which in the last decade has drawn considerable attention from researchers sensitive to the understanding of the origins of cognition. One product of that attention has been the development of sophisticated paradigms for both human and nonhuman species, providing evidence about the representation of magnitudes, numbers, and formal operations on these representations. This field has substantially benefited from comparing neuroscientific data with behavioral data obtained in nonhuman species and during human development.

Elizabeth Brannon and Jessica Cantlon review such data in their contribution (chapter 10), including applications of these parallel approaches instantiated in their own research. Indeed, the exploration of ontogenetic and phylogenetic paths is particularly fruitful in disentangling the ultimate nature of a concept, number, that for long has been presumed to be an abstraction deeply rooted in the possession of language. Data from other species (primates but also lower vertebrates) and from preverbal infants of course have the merit of eliminating the linguistic dimension and have already revealed aspects of the primitive conception of numerosity that preceded numerical cognition as we know it in human adults. The chapter is thus a mix of data from cognitive, developmental, and comparative psychology that culminates with a clear survey of the neural bases of numerical cognition.

In chapter 11, Edward Hubbard, Manuela Piazza, Philippe Pinel, and Stanislas Dehaene start with a heterogeneous set of data collected in human adults and infants, in other animals, and in other human cultures as well (taking into account the associated linguistic constraints), such as the Amazonian Munduruku. The main subject of their chapter is the neural localization of numerical competence. The empirical data, much of it stemming from the authors' own research, suggest a strong tie between numerical and spatial processing, such as in the SNARC (spatial-numerical association of response codes) effect or in the idea of the "number line." They identify the parietal cortex of the primate brain as the site where these interactions might give rise to number representations and operations.

Rochel Gelman, in chapter 12, takes the idea of natural number cognition as a case example for deepening the discussion on fundamental questions such as "What is a cognitive domain?" (distinguishing, more specifically, among core and noncore domains) and "How does learning enter a domain?"—the latter question very much related to the issue of the innate nature of domains. Empirical and theoretical experience in dealing with number understanding and arithmetic operations in infants (among other issues) lead her to establish a number of principles in the separation of core and noncore domains (based on criteria of structure, relevance, universality, explicitness, and so on). These she applies to the distinction among natural and rational numbers, offering insights into the organization of knowledge, its acquisition, and the nature of expertise.

In the last chapter of this section, Paul Glimcher (chapter 13) goes beyond the sheer concepts of number, magnitude, and their relative biological bases to delve further into a more applied domain, to which he has contributed as a leading thinker: neuroeconomics. This field has recently witnessed vast development, deriving its importance from interest among economists about behavior in situations of choice among alternatives associated with quantitatively differential outcomes, especially when numbers stand for monetary value. Whereas human studies are clearly important in psychology and economics for applied reasons, researchers in neuroeconomics have turned their attention to the biological bases of basic choice behavior, investigating the brain correlates of evaluation in situations where organisms (most usually, but not exclusively, primates) must choose among different amounts of physiological utility (such as fruit juice) trading them off with variable temporal delays or other input factors.

10 A Comparative Perspective on the Origin of Numerical Thinking

Elizabeth M. Brannon and Jessica F. Cantlon

The purpose of this book is to pinpoint how evolutionary and developmental studies can influence our understanding of the roots of human cognition. Numerical cognition is a domain in which considerable progress has been made toward discovering the underpinnings of adult cognition, and these advances have hinged upon studies of numerical cognition in human infants and nonhuman animals. The goal of this chapter is to highlight the main sources of evidence that lead to the conclusion that nonhuman animals, human infants, and adults share a nonverbal system for representing number as mental magnitudes.

To this end, we review experiments on the psychophysics of number discrimination in animals and human infants and explore the relationship between these data and studies of adult human numerical cognition. We also examine evidence that nonverbal representations of number are amenable to arithmetic operations, perceptual abstraction, and modality independence. Finally, we examine the extant data on the neural bases of numerical cognition in animals and early in human development as candidate precursors to the neural system underlying adult human numerical cognition.

The conclusion emerging from research in this domain is that animals, human infants, and adult humans share an evolutionarily and developmentally primitive system for basic numerical reasoning at both the cognitive and neural level. We believe that number representation is a quintessential example of continuity in cognitive processing throughout evolution and the lifespan.

Adult Humans Represent Number without Number Words

Numbers measure discrete quantity, yet number is universally represented in the mind as a continuous quantity. The main evidence for this idea is that Weber's Law of psychophysical judgment applies to nonverbal number discriminations just as it characterizes the discrimination of line length, brightness, or any other continuous dimension (Welford 1960; Stevens 1970). Weber's law states that successful detection of a change in stimulus intensity requires a proportional increment or decrement to a stimulus rather than an absolute change. For example, if an increment of 2 pounds is needed to detect a change in a 10-pound weight, then an increment of 4 pounds would be needed to detect a change in a 20-pound weight. When humans represent number nonverbally, discrimination is similarly controlled by the ratio between two values rather than their absolute difference. This suggests that number is represented as analog magnitudes.

In a classic demonstration of analog magnitude representation of symbolic number in adult humans, Moyer and Landauer (1967) presented two Arabic numerals to adult subjects and asked them to indicate which of the two digits was larger in numerical value. Figure 10.1 shows that reaction time (RT) was systematically influenced by both the linear distance between the values and the absolute magnitude of the values compared.

The greater the distance between the numerical values, the smaller the RT ; for example, participants were faster at deciding which was greater of 2 and 9 than of 2 and 5. When distance was held constant, RT became slower with numerical magnitude; for example, participants reacted faster when distinguishing between 2 and 3 than between 4 and 5. Thus, although number can be represented with arbitrary symbols—"2" or "two"—a continuous analog format underlies these symbols.

Numerical distance and magnitude effects have been replicated in many cultures with different symbolic number notation systems (on the Chinese system, see Campbell and

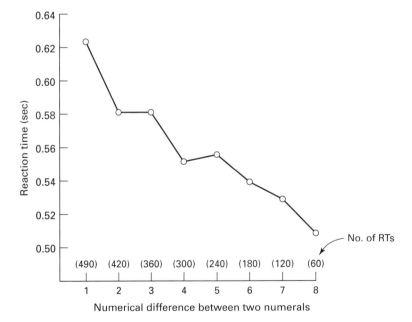

Figure 10.1
The time taken to choose the larger of two numerical symbols is a function of numerical distance. After Moyer and Landauer (1967).

Epp 2004; Iranian, see Dehaene et al. 1993; Kanji and Kana, see Takahashi and Green 1983). Such distance and magnitude effects are also found when humans compare the numerosity of dot arrays (Buckley and Gillman 1974; Cantlon and Brannon 2006). The universality of distance and magnitude effects in numerical performance highlights commonalities in the format of numerical representations, regardless of differences in cultural experience, language, and numerical notation.

Additional evidence that analog magnitude representations of number are language-independent and universal comes from recent studies of two indigenous Brazilian cultures, the Munduruku and the Piraha, both of which have languages that contain few number words. For example, the Munduruku language contains only number words for the values 1 to 5 and has no verbal algorithm for counting. Yet when Munduruku participants compared the relative magnitude of large numbers of dots (twenty vs. eighty) that were carefully controlled for surface area, perimeter, and density, their performance was quite similar to that of French-speaking control participants (Pica et al. 2004). In both groups, accuracy increased as the ratio between the two values (larger/smaller number) increased. Thus without numerical language, adult humans possess magnitude representations of number that obey Weber's Law.

Nonverbal Foundations of Numerical Thinking

Since the early twentieth century, a corpus of data has emerged that strongly supports the presence of a capacity for pure numerical representation in nonhuman animals. Many species of animals can represent number and ignore other variables that typically co-vary with number. Although this review focuses mainly on numerical competence in primates, many different animal species—fish (Agrillo et al. 2007), salamanders (Uller et al. 2003), pigeons (Roberts 1995), raccoons (Davis 1984), and rats (Meck and Church 1983)—have been shown to make quantity discriminations. Despite the fact that these studies vary in the tasks, stimuli, and even response formats they employed, their results converge on the conclusion that all species represent number in a common format that is ratio-dependent and obeys Weber's Law. For example, when chimpanzees (*Pan troglodytes*) or rhesus monkeys (*Macaca mulatta*) are given a choice between two food quantities they choose the option with the larger number of food morsels, but their ability to choose optimally is limited by the ratio between the two options (Beran and Beran 2004; Beran 2004).

Another recent study shows ratio dependence in nonverbal number discrimination even when continuous variables such as surface area and contour length are carefully controlled (Cantlon and Brannon 2006). Rhesus monkeys and adult college students were tested in a numerical ordering task; on each trial, two arrays of dots appeared and the subject was required to choose the smaller numerical value and ignore nonnumerical stimulus features such as the size or density of the elements. Figure 10.2 shows accuracy and RT in this task for the two species.

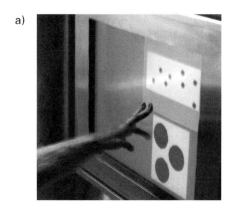

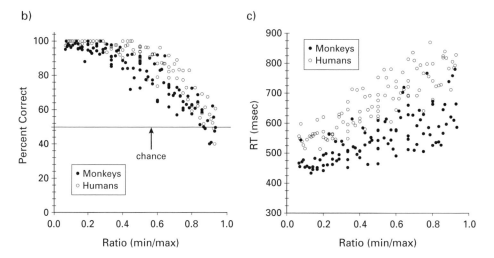

Figure 10.2
(a) A monkey choosing the numerically larger of two visual arrays. Accuracy (b) and RT (c) in a numerical comparison task as a function of the ratio between the two numerical values (smaller/larger) for monkeys (black circles) and college students (white circles). Data from Cantlon and Brannon (2006).

Accuracy and RT for both species were modulated by the ratio of the two values compared. These studies demonstrate that although no one would dispute the extraordinary mathematical capacity of the human mind, under some conditions we can observe continuity between the human mind and those of nonhuman animals.

Similarly, research undertaken over the last twenty-five years indicates that human infants in the first year of life represent number (see Feigenson et al. 2004 for review). The pattern of successful and unsuccessful numerical discriminations between groups of infants indicates that number discrimination is likely to be ratio-dependent even in the first year of life. For example, Xu and Spelke (2000) used a visual habituation paradigm in which six-month-old infants were repeatedly shown a series of images that contained a common number of elements, until infants' looking time substantially decreased. The babies were then tested with new images with either the same number or a new number of elements. When the displays were composed of eight or sixteen dots the infants spent more time looking at the test images with the new number of elements. When they had been habituated to eight or twelve dots—2:3 ratio—infants did not notice a change (see also Xu et al. 2005; Xu and Arriaga, 2007). Using a head-turn procedure Lipton and Spelke (2003) have shown a similar degree of ratio dependence in number discrimination when babies listen to sequences of sounds. Infants orient longer toward novel numbers of sounds and their ability to do so is dependent on the ratio between the familiar and the novel numbers of sounds. Finally, infants also show ratio dependence when discriminating changes in the number of times a puppet jumps (Wood and Spelke 2005).

Across these varying procedures and stimuli, six-month-old infants exhibit novelty effects when the discrimination involves a 1:2 ratio but fail to discriminate a 2:3 ratio (see table 10.1).

Sensitivity to numerical differences also increases with age such that by nine months of age infants can discriminate a 2:3 ratio in number (Lipton and Spelke 2003, 2004; Wood and Spelke 2005). An interesting twist to this pattern of ratio-dependent number discrimination and increasing precision over development is a recent study that indicates that when six-month-old infants are provided with redundant, and mutually reinforcing auditory and visual cues, they successfully discriminate a 2:3 ratio and overcome their inability to discriminate purely auditory or purely visual stimuli at this ratio (Jordan, Suanda and Brannon, in press). Thus, the ratio required for successful discrimination at a given age is not hard and fast but instead can be manipulated, and may be modulated by the salience of the numerical cue.

Table 10.1
Ratios of number, duration, and area for which six-month-old infants have succeeded or failed to discriminate

Dimension	Stimulus type	Success ratio	Failure ratio
Number (large sets > 4)	2-D shapes	1:2, 1:3	2:3
	Auditory tones	1:2	2:3
	Events	1:2	2:3
Duration	Audio and visual cues	1:2	2:3
Area of a single object	2-D cartoon face	1:2, 1:3, 1:4	2:3
Volume	Liquid in cylinder	1:3	Unknown
Length	Wooden dowel	1:2	Unknown
Summed area of multiple objects	Small sets (<4)	1:4	1:2, 1:3
	Large sets (>4)	1:4	1:2, 1:3

Adapted from Feigenson (2007)

A caveat to the general finding that nonverbal number discrimination is ratio-dependent is that human babies sometimes base their behavior on an entirely different cognitive system when they encounter small sets of objects. Convergent evidence from diverse methods suggests that infants are sometimes limited not by ratio but instead by absolute set size (Feigenson and Carey 2003, 2005; Feigenson et al. 2002; Xu 2003). For example, when infants watch graham crackers dropped into two buckets, they crawl to the bucket with the larger amount but only if each set is 3 or fewer (Feigenson et al. 2002). Similar results have been found with free-ranging rhesus monkeys given a similar choice (Hauser et al. 2000). One possibility is that babies and nonhuman animals rely on an object-tracking system when presented with small sets and that this system parallels the adult object-tracking system (Uller et al. 2001). Another possibility is that these findings account for the phenomenon known as *subitizing* whereby adults seem to rapidly and accurately recognize the number of elements in small sets without the need for counting. Further, there is a continuing debate over whether rapid appreciation of small values represents a distinct psychological process or is instead part of a continuum of Weber's Law that allows for almost no variability for small values (Balakrishnan and Ashby 1992; Gallistel and Gelman 1991).

The Relationship between Number and Continuous Variables

The research just described indicates that nonhuman animals and human infants are capable of representing number even when continuous variables such as time, area, and contour length do not co-vary with number. However, related questions are how the ability to discriminate number develops in relation to continuous variables and whether a common mechanism underlies discrimination of number and continuous variables. There is strong evidence from research with rats and pigeons that number and time may be represented similarly (Church and Meck 1984; Fetterman 1993; Meck and Church 1983; Meck et al. 1985; Roberts 1995; Roberts and Boisvert 1998; Roberts et al. 2000, 1995, 2002; Roberts and Mitchell 1994; Santi and Hope 2001). For example, Meck and Church (1983) found that when trained in a bisection procedure where number and time were confounded redundant cues, rats behaved as if they had encoded both time and number and showed similar sensitivity to changes in either. Moreover, methamphetamine affected number and time judgments to a similar degree in rats. These data formed the basis for an information-processing model of timing and counting that, twenty years later, continues to account for much data from nonverbal numerical reasoning tasks.

In the context of the development of number concepts in the human lifespan, Piaget's (1952) classic work on conservation has also suggested an important connection between how number concepts develop in relation to other quantitative dimensions such as area. Piaget argued that the number concept emerges out of comprehension of other quantitative dimensions and does not become independent of continuous variables until the child enters the concrete operational period. Although the development of looking-time procedures have revealed much earlier competencies in the numerical domain, recently some investigators have put forth a similar idea that numerical concepts emerge from the comprehension of continuous variables (see, e.g., Clearfield and Mix 1999, 2001; Mix et al. 2002; Newcombe 2002). In contrast with these ideas, research from our laboratory has suggested that number is often more salient for infants in the first year of life than continuous properties of sets. We have been comparing infants' sensitivity to changes in number, area, and time to determine the critical ratios needed for successful discrimination. Brannon and colleagues (2006) habituated babies to a single Elmo face and then tested them with a $2:3$, $1:2$, $1:3$, or $1:4$ ratio change (counterbalanced for change to smaller or larger Elmo). Infants succeeded at the $1:2$, $1:3$, and $1:4$ ratio changes and the difference in their looking-time scores increased with the ratio between familiar and novel areas. Infants were unable to discriminate the $2:3$ ratio change, demonstrating that at six months of age infants require a $1:2$ ratio change for successful discrimination of different areas. These data are also consistent with studies that have examined infants' ability to discriminate nonsolid substances (vanMarle, forthcoming; Gao et al. 2000; Huttenlocher et al. 2002)

A $1:2$ ratio is also needed for six-month-old infants to detect a change in a temporal interval. VanMarle and Wynn (2006) habituated babies to a puppet that danced and emitted a tone for a constant duration. Infants were then tested with the same puppet that danced and emitted a new tone whose duration differed from the first one by a $1:2$ or $2:3$ ratio. Infants successfully discriminated the $1:2$ but not the $2:3$ ratio change. Brannon and colleagues (2007) replicated the finding that six-month-old infants require a $1:2$ ratio duration change and further found that by ten months of age infants could discriminate a $2:3$ ratio change, which suggested that numerical and temporal discrimination may follow similar developmental trajectories.

Although infants are equally sensitive to numerical changes and changes in the area of a single element, research from our laboratory indicates that infants are far less sensitive to changes in the cumulative area of discrete elements. A recent series of studies from our lab suggests that six-month-old infants require a $1:4$ ratio to detect a change in the cumulative area of arrays of dots (Brannon et al. 2004; Cordes and Brannon 2008). These data are in marked conflict with recent claims that infants are more sensitive to continuous variables than to number (Clearfield and Mix 1999).

A common ratio of discrimination for number, area, and time suggests that there may be similarities in the way that these dimensions are represented or at least compared (Meck and Church 1983; Walsh 2003). For example, if there were a population of neurons whose firing rate was sensitive to numerosity, duration, and area, this would result in a common neural currency for these three dimensions akin to the Meck and Church proposal described earlier. Such a scenario would explain why infants are equally sensitive and show similar developmental trajectories for these three stimulus dimensions. However, it would be important to know whether there are any quantitative dimensions that follow different sensitivity or developmental trajectories (Feigenson 2007). For example, what ratio change is needed to detect changes in brightness or pitch? Understanding infants' sensitivity to dimensions that are and are not typically correlated with number would be informative as to the import of common ratios of discrimination for number, area, and duration.

Operations on Numerical Representations

A key advantage to representing number as analog magnitudes is that this allows addition and subtraction to work much like histogram arithmetic (Gallistel and Gelman 1992). Many models of foraging behavior assume that animals are calculating the rate of return and thus dividing the number of food items or the total amount of food they obtain by the time it took to procure the food (see Gallistel 1990 for a review). Thus, an important prediction is that animals, infants, and adults can not only represent number without language but also manipulate such representations arithmetically.

The simplest numerical operation is ordering: determining the numerically smallest or largest of two or more numerosities. As discussed earlier, monkeys and college students perform very similarly when given a numerical ordering task. There is also clear evidence from this study that when trained on one set of numerosities monkeys can transfer an ordinal rule (such as "Choose the smaller") to novel numerosities that are outside the training range. This suggests that number is a naturally ordered dimension for a monkey.

The behavioral signatures of the mental comparisons used to compare analog representations of numerical values are also common to humans and nonhuman animals. Semantic congruity systematically affects RT when humans make any type of ordinal comparison, such as which is smaller? Or which is farther? The semantic congruity effect refers to the finding that small values on a continuum, such as number, are more rapidly compared when participants are asked, "Which is smaller?" whereas large values are more rapidly compared when the question is "which is larger?" In other words, adults are faster to compare two numerical values when their overall magnitude is congruent with the verbal phrasing of the question.

Although it was originally thought that the semantic congruity effect was specific to comparisons that take place on discrete and symbolic representations (Banks and Flora 1977), a recent study illustrates that rhesus macaques also show a numerical semantic congruity effect (Cantlon and Brannon 2005). In that study a color cue served in lieu of the verbal questions "Which is smaller?" and "Which is larger?"

Monkeys were trained to choose the smaller of two dot arrays (see figure 10.3a) when the screen background was red and the larger of two dot arrays when the screen background was blue. As shown in figure 10.3b, monkeys, like humans, were much faster at choosing the smaller of two small values (red cue) than at choosing the larger of two small values (blue cue). Conversely, they were much faster at choosing the larger of two large

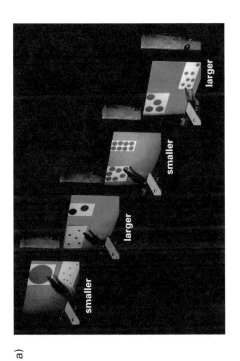

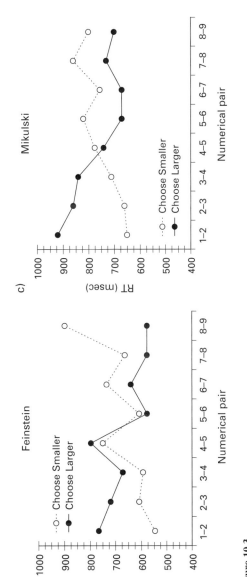

Figure 10.3

(a) Photograph of a monkey pressing the numerically smaller of two numerosities when the screen background was red and the numerically larger when the screen background was blue. (b) and (c) Reaction time was faster for small values when monkeys were given the red cue and required to choose the smaller of two numerosities and faster for the large values when given the blue cue and required to choose the larger of two numerosities. Data from Cantlon and Brannon (2005).

values than the smaller of two large values. Thus, the semantic congruity effect cannot be a byproduct of a language-specific comparative process but is instead, more generally, a hallmark of the psychological process for ordinally comparing analog representations of magnitude (Holyoak and Mah 1982; Petrusic et al. 1998).

Research on the development of ordinal number concepts indicates that by eleven months of age, infants detect reversals in the ordinal direction of a numerical sequence. In one set of studies infants were habituated to sequences of numerosity arrays where the sequence always progressed from smallest to largest or from largest to smallest. Infants were then tested with novel numerical values where the ordinal direction was maintained from that of habituation or reversed. Eleven-month-old babies looked longer when the ordinal direction was reversed, but nine-month-old infants showed no novelty preference, which suggests that sometime between nine and eleven months of age infants develop the ability to detect ordinal numerical relationships (Brannon 2002).

Analog magnitude representations of number are also amenable to arithmetic manipulation beyond ordinal comparison. Wynn (1992) first showed that infants' expectations are violated when an addition or subtraction event results in an arithmetically impossible outcome (figure 10.4). Five-month-old infants watched as a Mickey Mouse doll was occluded behind a screen and then observed a hand enter the stage and add a second doll behind the screen.

When the screen was lowered to reveal one doll, infants looked longer than when it was lowered to reveal two dolls. In contrast, when infants observed two dolls being occluded and a hand entered and removed one doll from behind the screen infants looked longer when the screen was lowered to reveal two dolls compared to when it was lowered to reveal one doll. McCrink and Wynn showed that nine-month-old infants showed a similar ability to notice violation of expectancy to arithmetically impossible events for large values (McCrink and Wynn 2004). These results suggest that infants make computations regarding analog magnitude representations of number. A recent study measured infants' brain waves from the surface of the scalp using the event-related potential method (ERP). ERPs were measured as infants watched impossible and possible arithmetic outcomes and reported a significant negative deflection in the ERP waveform between 330 and 530 ms during the arithmetically impossible condition (Berger et al. 2006).

Hauser and his colleagues adapted the Wynn paradigm for use with experimentally naïve monkeys free-ranging on an island in Puerto Rico (Flombaum et al. 2005; Hauser, MacNeilage, and Ware, 1996). For example, in one study monkeys viewed a stage with four lemons and then watched as an experimenter first raised an occluder in front of the stage that blocked the lemons from view and then added four more lemons to the stage behind the occluder. The occluder was then removed to reveal a possible outcome of eight lemons or an impossible outcome of four lemons. Monkeys looked significantly longer at the four-lemon outcome, which suggests that their expectation was violated. No difference in looking time were found when the monkeys were shown a 2 + 2 operation and tested

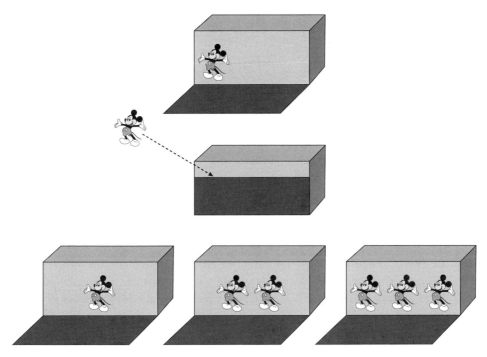

Figure 10.4
Example of an addition problem presented to preverbal infants. Infants watch as a Mickey Mouse doll is placed on a stage and then occluded by a screen. A hand then enters the stage and places a second Mickey Mouse doll behind the screen. When the screen is lowered, on some trials two dolls are visible (possible) and on other trials one or three dolls are visible (impossible). Infants look longer at the arithmetically impossible outcomes than at the possible outcome.

with an outcome of 4 or 6. Thus, monkeys appear to track addition operations with large sets but only detect violations in the outcome of addition operations when the ratio between the observed and expected outcome is favorable.

One chimpanzee (Sheba) has even been shown to add using symbols. Sheba was first trained to match numerosities with the Arabic numerals 0 to 4 (Boysen and Berntson 1989) and was then trained to associate the Arabic numeral 4 with four food items, the Arabic numeral 3 with three food items, and so on. Once the chimpanzee was proficient at associating the Arabic numerals 0 to 4 with their respective quantities, she was tested on her ability to spontaneously add the Arabic numerals. Sheba was given a choice among three occluded food caches that were each labeled with a pair of Arabic numerals. The sum of the two Arabic numerals reflected the total number of food items in the occluded cache. When given a choice among these caches, Sheba chose the cache that was labeled with the greatest sum on a significant proportion of trials. These data showed that a symbol-trained chimpanzee can choose an amount that corresponds to the sum of two Arabic numerals, at least for sets totaling less than four items. However, less clear from these results is whether the mental arithmetic performed by the chimpanzee in this study is comparable to nonverbal arithmetic in humans.

We recently tested macaque monkeys on a nonverbal addition task with a large range of addition problems and numerical values (Cantlon and Brannon 2007a).

Monkeys were presented with two sets of dots on a touchscreen monitor separated by a delay (see figure 10.5a). The numerical value of each set varied randomly from one to sixteen items. Following the presentation of these two sets, monkeys were required to choose between two arrays: one with a number of dots equal to the sum of the two sets and a second, distractor, array that contained a different number of dots. Monkeys' accuracy on each of the addition problems was modulated by the numerical ratio between the correct sum and the distractor choice (see figure 10.5b). The qualitative similarity between the addition performance of monkeys in this study and that of humans in prior studies (Barth et al. 2006; Pica et al. 2004) is striking; when humans nonverbally add two sets of objects together to represent their sum, their performance is similarly modulated by the ratio between the numerical values of choice stimuli. Humans and nonhuman primates thus appear to share a system for basic arithmetic that is part of a broader set of skills for reasoning about number.

a)

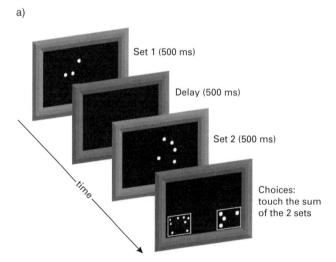

Figure 10.5
(a) Monkeys were presented with one array followed by a second array of elements and then given a choice between two arrays where only one was equal to the numerical sum of the addends. Monkeys were rewarded for choosing the numerical sum. (b) Accuracy was a function of the ratio between the correct sum and the incorrect choice.

b)

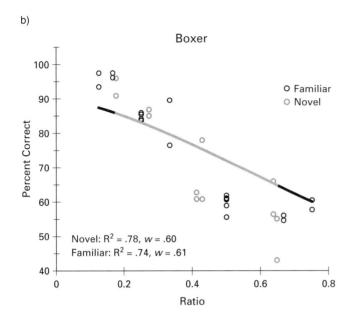

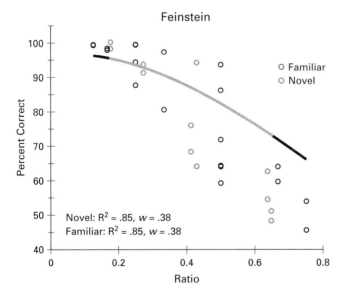

Figure 10.5
(continued)

An Adaptive Strategy vs. a Last Resort

Early views on animal numerical ability focused on the idea that number is an unnatural artificial dimension that can be represented by animals only under conditions of extensive training (Davis and Perusse 1988; Davis and Memmott 1982). More recent research, however, suggests that many animals attend to the numerical attributes of their world spontaneously and automatically (see Hauser et al. 2003; Flombaum et al. 2005; Lewis et al. 2005; Santos et al. 2005). This is nicely illustrated by demonstrations that ratio-dependent number discrimination can be found in tamarin monkeys (*Saguinus oedipus*) without training in numerical tasks (Hauser et al. 2003). Hauser and colleagues presented cotton-top tamarins with auditory sequences of speech syllables in a familiarization-discrimination paradigm. They tested whether tamarins would look longer at a speech stream consisting of a novel number of speech syllables following familiarization with a standard number of syllables. They controlled for the nonnumerical variables of sequence duration, item duration, interstimulus interval, and intensity to ensure that tamarins discriminated the number of syllables as opposed to these other dimensions.

Tamarins' ability to discriminate the speech streams was dependent on the ratio between the number of syllables in the familiar and novel streams. Tamarins discriminated sequences of four versus eight, four versus six, and eight versus twelve syllables but not four versus five and eight versus ten syllables. Thus, tamarins' sensitivity for numerical discrimination did not exceed a 2:3 ratio for the values tested in this experiment. The fact that untrained monkeys spontaneously represented the numerical values of the sets suggests that number is a salient attribute of a set of items for monkeys in their natural environments. Further, the mechanism of representation that was spontaneously employed by these animals appears to be an analog magnitude enumeration system, since numerical discrimination was constrained by the ratio between the familiar and novel numerical values.

However, despite the fact that monkeys exhibit looking preferences that demonstrate a spontaneous capacity for number discrimination, laboratory studies have often found that animals require long training periods before they reliably attend to the numerical attribute of a stimulus (Davis and Memmott 1982). This has led some researchers to propose that nonhuman animals only attend to numerical value as a last resort, when there are no other salient dimensions on which they could base their decisions. An implication of the last-resort hypothesis is that any other stimulus attribute should be more salient to an animal than number.

We recently explored this idea by testing number-experienced and number-naïve monkeys on a matching task in which they were allowed to freely choose the basis for matching during nondifferentially reinforced probe trials from two dimensions: number and either color, shape, or cumulative surface area (Cantlon and Brannon 2007b). Monkeys were initially trained on a matching task in which number was initially confounded with one of these alternative dimensions. Then, probe trials were introduced in which number was pitted against the alternative dimension (color, shape, or surface area). During these probe trials, monkeys were rewarded no matter which dimension they selected as the match. The last-resort hypothesis predicts that both number-experienced and number-naïve monkeys would prefer to match stimuli on the basis of nonnumerical dimensions such as color, shape, and surface area over number. Further, the last-resort hypothesis predicts that monkeys without previous laboratory experience of discriminating numerical values would be especially prone to match stimuli according to nonnumerical properties rather than matching on the basis of number.

Contrary to the last-resort hypothesis, we found that both number-experienced and number-naïve monkeys represented the numerical values of the stimuli even though this was not required by our task; when number was easy to discriminate, both groups of monkeys preferred number as the basis for matching over color, shape, and cumulative surface area. Monkeys spontaneously represented the numerical values of the stimuli when they could have easily solved the task by representing only the color, shape, or cumulative surface area of the stimuli. These data demonstrate that numerical value is a salient feature of the environment for monkeys, and their proclivity for representing numerical values depends on the difficulty of the numerical discrimination.

Similar to the debates in the animal literature, there have been claims that infants only track area when number and area are both available as cues (Clearfield and Mix 1999; Mix et al. 2002; Newcombe 2002). However, the review provided earlier of the comparative psychophysics of number and area are not consistent with this interpretation. Instead, human infants show similar sensitivity to number and area and are in fact much less sensitive to the cumulative area of a discrete array than they are to number. Thus our review demonstrates that neither human infants nor monkeys are biased to attend to area over number.

Apples and Oranges, Sounds and Sights: How Abstract Are Nonverbal Number Representations?

An important aspect of number representations is that they do not take into account the features of the sets they represent. Thus, three telephones, three ice cubes, and three vultures are all equally good examples of "three-ness." Heterogeneous collections provide a good test of this abstraction principle. Can animals and young children represent number with equal ease when sets are homogeneous as when they are heterogeneous? A recent pair of studies from our laboratory explored this question. Monkeys were required to choose the numerically smaller of two arrays across conditions where the degree of perceptual variability in the arrays was systematically varied. Monkeys show no difference in accuracy on sets with high perceptual variability (where elements vary in size, shape, and color) as opposed to sets with low perceptual variability (with homogeneous elements). Similarly, four-to-five-year-old children tested in the same task showed no impairment on heterogeneous stimuli on this numerical ordering task (Cantlon et al. 2007). Thus, under some circumstances monkeys and children ignore the identity of elements and instead represent only the abstract number in an array.

A critical property of abstract conceptual numerical representation is that it is supramodal. Although it is quite obvious that number words and Arabic numerals allow us to use language to numerically equate sets experienced in different modalities (for example, three sights, three sounds, three touches), a study by Barth and colleagues (2003) demonstrated that the nonverbal representations of number held by adults are also independent of the sensory modality in which they are originally perceived. In their study, adults were just as accurate at making relative numerosity judgments for two sequences presented in different sensory modalities as for two sequences presented in a single modality.

The question of cross-modal number matching in animals and human infants has, however, been a bit contentious. Starkey et al. (1983, 1990) first employed a preferential looking method to test whether infants would spontaneously look at a visual array that numerically matched a sequence of drumbeats. Many previous studies in domains other than number had already shown that infants look preferentially toward visual stimuli that correspond to a sound track (Spelke 1976; Kuhl and Meltzoff 1982; Patterson and Werker 2002); for example, when infants hear a specific speech sound, they look preferentially at a face that articulates that speech sound compared with a face that articulates a different speech sound (Kuhl and Meltzoff 1982). Starkey and colleagues (1983, 1990) presented infants with side-by-side slides of two or three household objects while an experimenter who was out of the infants' view hit a drum two or three times. Infants preferentially looked toward the visual display that numerically matched the number of drumbeats they heard. Unfortunately, when other researchers varied parameters (such as the rate and duration of the tones) that often co-vary with number—or even the identity of the visual objects displayed—they had difficulty replicating these results (Mix et al. 1997; Moore et al. 1987). In some cases infants had no preference for the matching visual array, whereas in other cases they preferred to look at the nonmatching array.

Using a similar preferential looking-time method with infants and monkeys, Jordan and colleagues (Jordan et al. 2005; Jordan and Brannon 2006) demonstrated that monkeys and infants make spontaneous numerical correspondences across modalities for small sets of objects. Monkeys and infants were seated in front of two monitors, one of which displayed two conspecifics vocalizing and the other of which contained three conspecifics vocalizing (see figure 10.6a). All participants heard one chorus of two or three conspecifics vocalizing synchronously with the videos.

This paradigm differed from past tests in that it used nonarbitrarily related stimuli and avoided temporal confounds by presenting the sounds as a chorus rather than a sequence. Monkeys and infants looked longer at a video of three conspecific faces when they heard a soundtrack of three conspecifics vocalizing compared to when they heard two conspeci-

a)   b)

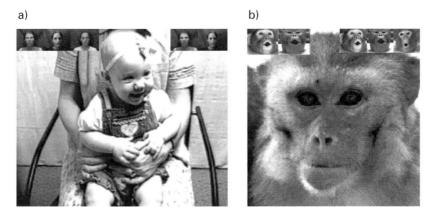

Figure 10.6
(a) A seven-month-old infant and video images with which infants were tested. (b) A rhesus macaque and video images with which monkeys were tested. In both experiments individual human infants and monkeys heard a chorus of two or three conspecifics vocalizing. Stimuli from Jordan et al. (2005) and Jordan and Brannon (2006).

fics vocalizing, whereas monkeys and infants who heard a soundtrack of only two conspecifics vocalizing showed the opposite looking preference (see figure 10.6b). Importantly, the actors in the videos were unfamiliar to the participants and the onset and offset of voices and mouth movements were equated to prevent synchrony cues.

Although this pair of studies suggested that monkeys and human babies can represent number independently of the sensory modality in which a number representation is formed, important questions remained. Are infants and monkeys accessing analog magnitude representations of number when matching across sensory modalities as would be indicated if performance was ratio-dependent? And is cross-modal matching limited to socially relevant contexts such as perceiving conspecifics? A recent study from our lab examined these questions. Monkeys were trained to match the number of tones in a one-to-nine-tone sequence with the numerical value of a visual array of dots (figure 10.7a; Jordan, Maclean and Brannon, in press).

Monkeys' performance on this task was significantly above chance and exhibited the characteristics of ratio dependence (figure 10.7b). Monkeys matched the numerical values of the stimuli across sensory modalities, indicating that the capacity for analog numerical representation is abstracted from its input channel.

Taken together with studies from adult humans, these studies demonstrate that the cognitive mechanisms underlying nonverbal numerical representation in monkeys and humans are cut to the same pattern: monkeys and humans represent numerical values as amodal approximate mental magnitudes; consequently, their performance obeys Weber's Law, no matter what numerical task is tested or how the stimuli are presented.

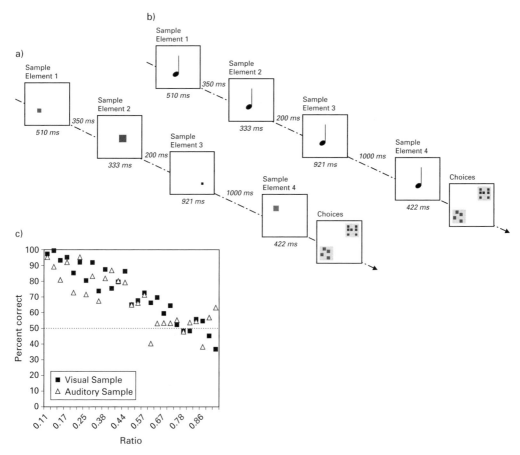

Figure 10.7
(a) Example of a successive visual array sample in a delayed numerical match-to-sample trial. (b) Example of a successive auditory array sample in a delayed numerical match-to-sample trial. (c) Accuracy was dependent on the ratio between the correct numerical match and the incorrect alternative and was similar for trials with auditory and visual samples.

How Does the Brain Represent Number?

As reviewed by Edward M. Hubbard and colleagues (see chapter 11 of this volume), the intraparietal sulcus (IPS) has been implicated as critically important for representing the meaning of number. Patient studies have revealed that damage to the parietal cortex typically results in a form of acalculia that disrupts understanding of the meaning of numbers (see Lemer et al. 2003; Cohen and Dehaene 2000). In contrast, damage to other brain areas can disrupt memorized arithmetic facts but leaves an understanding of number intact (Varley et al. 2005; Cohen and Dehaene 2000). Functional imaging of the normal brain demonstrates that the IPS is activated by numerical stimuli, regardless of their notation (that is, "3," "three," ". . . ," or "♪♪♪") and irrespective of whether stimuli are presented in the visual or auditory modality (Eger et al. 2003).

Research by Piazza and colleagues (2004, 2007) suggests that the IPS also responds to nonsymbolic numerical stimuli. Using an event-related adaptation paradigm they found that the BOLD signal (blood-oxygen-level dependent changes) decreased to repeated presentations of a standard numerosity but that recovery of the BOLD signal was systematically related to the degree to which a deviant value differed from the standard value (figure 10.8a and 10.8b; but see Shuman and Kanwisher 2004).

This region did not, however, respond to stimuli that deviated from the standard stimuli in element shape but not number. This event-related adaptation paradigm has recently produced evidence that four-year-old children and adults show overlapping activation in the IPS in response to number and not shape changes (Cantlon et al. 2006). At four years of age, children have limited experience with numerical symbols such as number words and written numerals. Thus, if the IPS plays a causal role in numerical thinking, it should respond during numerical judgments regardless of an individual's experience with numbers. Our finding that four-year-old children evoke activity in the IPS in response to numerical deviants but not shape deviants provides empirical support for this prediction.

Convergent evidence for the role of the parietal cortex in number representations comes from a handful of recent studies demonstrating that single cells in the parietal cortex encode number. In a series of studies, Nieder and Miller (Nieder et al. 2002; Nieder and Miller 2004; Nieder et al. 2006) identified cells in the prefrontal cortex and the fundus of the intraparietal sulcus of rhesus monkeys that are selective for a given numerosity (see figure 10.9). Monkeys viewed arrays that contained one to five elements and were required to indicate whether a second, nonidentical, array matched the sample numerosity.

Individual neurons showed a maximal firing rate to one numerosity and decreased firing rate as a function of distance from the preferred number. These neurons responded to specific numerical values regardless of nonnumerical stimulus attributes such as cumulative circumference, surface area, or density. The tuning curves for number-selective neurons increased in their bandwidth with increasing number leading to increasing representational overlap with magnitude. This extraordinary discovery of number cells in the monkey brain provides a compelling physiological correlate of the behavioral magnitude and distance effects.

Recently, Roitman and colleagues (2007) found another type of numerical neuronal coding in the macaque monkey. The purpose of this study was to measure numerical sensitivity in the brains of monkeys without any number discrimination training and to examine the neuronal response to large numerical values. In addition, since the dominant models of nonverbal numerical processing include a stage at which total numerical

a)

Stream of habituation stimuli
(16 dots)

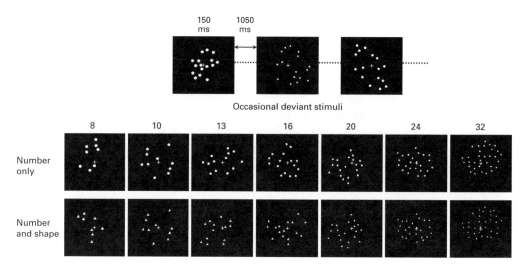

Occasional deviant stimuli

b)

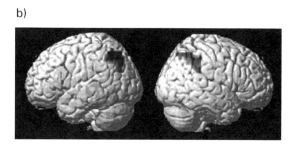

c)

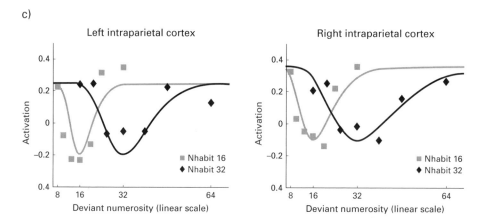

Figure 10.8
(a) Stimuli used in a passive viewing event–related fMRI adaptation experiment with number and shape deviants.
(b) Brain region in human adults that responded more to a number change than a shape change. (c) Brain activation (percentage change in BOLD signal relative to habituation stimuli) elicited to numerical values is systematically related to degree to which novel value deviates from habituation value. Data from Piazza et al. (2004).

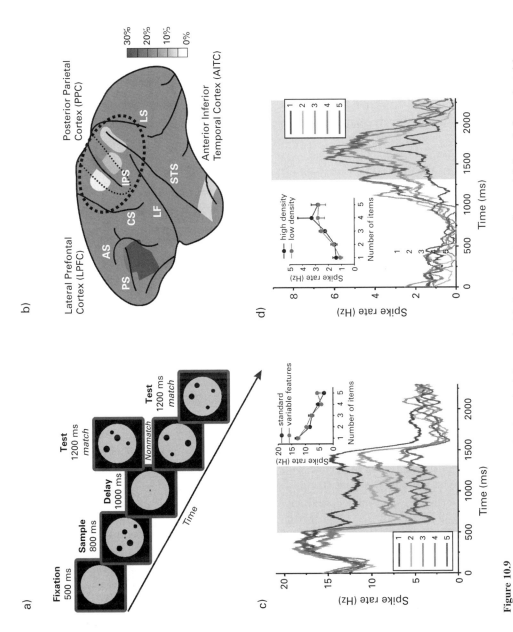

Figure 10.9

(a) Task structure for monkeys tested in electrophysiology study. Monkeys viewed sample array briefly and after a short delay were required to indicate whether a second array matched or did not match the numerosity of the sample. (b) Lateral view of a monkey brain that illustrates recording sites and is color coded to reflect relative proportion of number selective cells. (c) and (d) Firing rate as a function of sample numerosity during sample or delay interval for two distinct neurons selective for the numerosities 1 and 4, respectively. Data from Nieder and Miller (2004).

magnitude is represented, one goal was to identify summation or accumulation neurons rather than neurons that show sensitivity to particular cardinal values.

Recordings were made from LIP neurons while monkeys performed a delayed saccade task that had an incidental numerical component. Once the response field of a given neuron was well-identified, monkeys performed a delayed saccade task where they were required to fixate a central cue as a target, a single red circle, which was presented in the periphery away from the response field (see figure 10.10a).

An array of dots was briefly presented in the mapped response field of the neuron. In standard trials the stimuli contained the same number of dots on every trial, but on some trials a deviant number of dots was presented that differed from the standard by at least a 2:1 ratio. When the fixation stimulus extinguished this was the cue for the monkey to make a saccade to the target. Accurate saccadic eye movements on these deviant trials was rewarded with three times as much juice as the standard trials.

The numerical stimulus in this task was totally irrelevant to the monkeys' successful performance of the delayed saccade-to-target task. Nonetheless, behavioral evidence indicated that monkeys were sensitive to the numerical deviants: RT was significantly faster to the target on trials in which a deviant numerical array was presented. Despite the fact that numerical discrimination was not required by the task, monkeys did it anyway, presumably because numerical deviants signified a greater expected reward.

Another important aspect of the design was that each neuron was tested with two or more different standard values so that any given value that served as a standard also served as a deviant. This feature of the experimental design allowed a test of whether the neurons were driven by the reward properties or the numerical value.

LIP neurons showed a very different profile of number selectivity than the cardinal-number cells found by Nieder and colleagues (Nieder et al. 2002; Nieder and Miller 2004; Nieder et al. 2006). Sixty-five percent of the neurons were number selective; however, all of these cells preferred either the largest numerosity tested or the smallest numerosity tested and no intermediate number cells were found. That is, about half of all number-selective neurons increased firing rate with magnitude whereas the other half decreased firing rate with magnitude. Figure 10.10b shows an example of a single LIP neuron whose firing rate increased with number and another neuron whose firing rate decreased with number. Importantly, reward value had no influence on firing rate for neurons in this task.

Collectively, these data suggest that there may be at least two populations of neurons in the parietal cortex that together allow for the complex behavioral discriminations reviewed earlier in the chapter. The Nieder and Miller (Nieder et al. 2002; Nieder and Miller 2004; Nieder et al. 2006) cells from the fundus of the IPS are cardinal in that they prefer a specific numerical value, in contrast, the cells described by Roitman and colleagues (2007) respond monotonically to number.

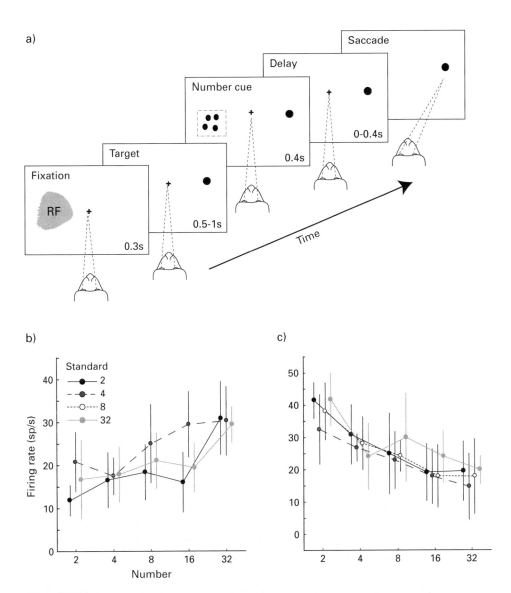

Figure 10.10
(a) Task structure for monkeys tested in an implicit number electrophysiology study. Monkeys participated in a delayed saccade task while numerosity images were briefly presented in the receptive field of an LIP neuron. (b) A single neuron for which firing rate increased with number. (c) A single neuron for which firing rate decreased with number (data from Roitman et al. 2007).

Conclusions

Numerical cognition is a conceptual domain that affords tractable conclusions about the principles and origins of thought. Adult humans possess a symbolic and linguistically mediated system for representing number that allows precise computations such as $749 \times 253 = 189,497$, but alongside this system, and perhaps even grounding that system, is a primitive, language-independent, analog representational system. This system represents number as analog magnitudes that are proportional to the numerosities to which they correspond. It likely evolved before humans diverged from other nonhuman primates, and perhaps substantially earlier, since many nonprimate species also represent number. This nonverbal number system is also rooted early in human development, suggesting that representing the numerical attributes of the world around us is a core computational mechanism that likely bestows adaptive advantages (Spelke 2000).

Recent studies have made important advances in determining which tools are included in this evolutionarily primitive system for mathematical thinking. Nonhuman primates, human adults, and developing humans in the first year of life all share an ability to roughly equate, compare, and perform basic arithmetic on numerical values independent of variability in other quantitative dimensions such as surface area, density, and perimeter. These numerical representations are abstract and independent of the sensory and perceptual features of the input. Furthermore, the ability to form pure numerical representations is not a laborious process compared with other domains of representation; rather, humans and monkeys form numerical representations spontaneously, without extensive training or experience. Since all of these capacities share the behavioral signatures of ratio dependence, a reasonable proposal is that they belong to a common psychological system for representing and mentally manipulating numerical quantity.

Current data indicate that the brain systems underlying numerical thinking appear to be shared by monkeys and humans. Neural activity in homologous regions of the parietal cortex has been shown to underlie nonsymbolic numerical representation in children and nonhuman primates as well as both symbolic and nonsymbolic numerical processing in adult humans. A current controversy in this area of research concerns the specificity of this brain region for numerical processing (Hubbard et al. 2005; see also chapter 11, this volume; Pinel et al. 2001; Shuman and Kanwisher 2004). In particular, the intraparietal sulcus has been identified as a region important in a variety of cognitive tasks, including spatial processing, attention, and decision making in adult humans. The links between numerical cognition and any or all of these other domains in the brain may shed light on the cognitive antecedents of pure numerical representation in humans.

We believe that the progress that has been made thus far in researching the nonverbal underpinnings of numerical cognition is testament to the value of numerical cognition as an ideal case study of human cognitive evolution and development. Yet the psychological and neural properties of this domain require further elaboration. How do cardinal and ordinal number cells together yield the complex nonverbal numerical computations described here? Do numerical representations transcend all sensory modalities or are vision and audition privileged? Are modality-specific representations converted into modality-independent representations? What is the relationship between the representation of number, time, and area? Is the common ratio of discriminability seen for number, time, and area in infancy meaningful or coincidental? As we find answers to these questions we will come to understand how abstract information is organized in the mind and brain, in the absence of language.

Acknowledgments

Elizabeth M. Brannon is supported by NIMH RO1 MH066154, NICHD RO1 HD49912, an NSF CAREER award, and a Merck Scholars award. Jessica F. Cantlon is supported by an NSF graduate fellowship and an APA Elizabeth Munsterberg Koppitz dissertation award.

References

Agrillo C, Dadda M, Bisazza A (2007) Quantity discrimination in a female mosquitofish. Anim Cogn 10: 63–70.

Balakrishnan JD, Ashby FG (1992) Subitizing: Magical numbers or mere superstition. Psychol Res 54: 80–90.

Banks WP, Flora J (1977) Semantic and perceptual processes in symbolic comparisons. J Exp Psychol Hum Percept Perform 3: 278–290.

Barth H, Kanwisher N, Spelke E (2003) The construction of large number representations in adults. Cognition 86: 201–221.

Barth H, La Mont K, Lipton J, Dehaene S, Kanwisher N, Spelke E (2006) Nonsymbolic arithmetic in adults and young children. Cognition 98: 199–222.

Beran MJ (2004) Chimpanzees (*Pan troglodytes*) respond to nonvisible sets after one-by-one addition and removal of items. J Comp Psychol 118: 25–36.

Beran MJ, Beran MM (2004) Chimpanzees remember the results of one-by-one addition of food items to sets over extended time periods. Psychol Sci 15: 94–99.

Berger A, Tzur G, Posner MI (2006) Infant brains detect arithmetic errors. P Natl Acad Sci USA 103: 12649–12653.

Boysen ST, Berntson GG (1989) Numerical competence in a chimpanzee (*Pan troglodytes*). J Comp Psychol 103: 23–31.

Brannon EM (2002) The development of ordinal numerical knowledge in infancy. Cognition 83: 223–240.

Brannon EM, Abbott S, Lutz D (2004) Number bias for the discrimination of large visual sets in infancy. Cognition 93: B59–B68.

Brannon EM, Lutz D, Cordes S (2006) The development of area discrimination and its implications for number representation in infancy. Developmental Sci 9: F59–F64.

Brannon EM, Suanda SH, Libertus K (2007) Increasing precision in temporal discriminations over development parallels the development of number discrimination. Developmental Sci 10: 770–777.

Buckley PB, Gillman CB (1974) Comparisons of digit and dot patterns. J Exp Psychol 103: 1131–1136.

Campbell JID, Epp LJ (2004) An encoding-complex approach to numerical cognition in Chinese-English bilinguals. Can J Exp Psychol 58: 229–244.

Cantlon JF, Brannon EM (2005) Semantic congruity affects numerical judgments similarly in monkeys and humans. P Natl Acad Sci USA 102: 16507–16511.

Cantlon JF, Brannon EM (2006) Shared system for ordering small and large numbers in monkeys and humans. Psychol Sci 17: 402–407.

Cantlon JF, Brannon EM (2007a). Basic math in monkeys and college students PLoS Biol 5: e328.

Cantlon JF, Brannon EM (2007b) How much does number matter to a monkey (*Macaca mulatta*)? J Exp Psychol Anim B 33: 32–41.

Cantlon JF, Brannon EM, Carter EJ, Pelphrey KA (2006) Functional imaging of numerical processing in adults and 4-y-old children. PLoS Biol 4: 844–854.

Cantlon J, Fink R, Safford KE, Brannon EM (2007) Heterogeneity differentially affects children's performance in a matching and ordinal numerical task. Developmental Sci 10: 431–440.

Church RM, Meck WH (1984) The numerical attribute of stimuli. In: Animal cognition (Roitblat HL, Bever TG, Terrace HS, eds), 445–464. Hillsdale, NJ: Lawrence Erlbaum.

Clearfield MW, Mix KS (1999) Number versus contour length in infants' discrimination of small visual sets. Psychol Sci 10: 408–411.

Clearfield MW, Mix KS (2001) Infant use continuous quantity—not number—to discriminate small visual sets. J Cogn Dev 2: 243–260.

Cohen L, Dehaene S (2000) Calculating without reading: Unsuspected residual abilities in pure alexia. Cogn Neuropsychol 17: 563–583.

Cordes S, Brannon EM (2008) The difficulties of representing continuous extent in infancy: Using number is just easier. Child Dev 79: 476–489.

Davis H (1984) Discrimination of the number three by a raccoon (*Procyon lotor*). Anim Learn Behav 12: 409–413.

Davis H, Memmott J (1982) Counting behavior in animals: A critical evaluation. Psychol Bull 92: 547–571.

Davis H, Perusse R (1988) Numerical competence in animals: Definitional issues, current evidence and a new research agenda. Behav Brain Sci 11: 561–579.

Dehaene S, Bossini S, Giraux P (1993) The mental representation of parity and number magnitude. J Exp Psychol Gen 122: 371–396.

Eger E, Sterzer P, Russ MO, Giraud AL, Kleinschmidt A (2003) A supramodal number representation in human intraparietal cortex. Neuron 37: 719–725.

Feigenson LR (2007) The equality of quantity. Trends Cogn Sci 11: 185–187.

Feigenson L, Carey S (2003) Tracking individuals via object-files: evidence from infants' manual search. Developmental Sci 6: 568–584.

Feigenson L, Carey S (2005) On the limits of infants' quantification of small object arrays. Cognition 97: 295–313.

Feigenson L, Carey S, Hauser M (2002) The representations underlying infants' choice of more: Object files versus analog magnitudes. Psychol Sci 13: 150–156.

Feigenson L, Dehaene S, Spelke E (2004) Core systems of number. Trends Cogn Sci 8: 307–314.

Fetterman JG (1993) Numerosity discrimination: Both time and number matter. J Exp Psychol Anim B 19: 149–164.

Flombaum JI, Junge JA, Hauser MD (2005) Rhesus monkeys (*Macaca mulatta*) spontaneously compute addition operations over large numbers. Cognition 97: 315–325.

Gallistel CR (1990) The organization of learning. Cambridge, MA: MIT Press.

Gallistel CR, Gelman R (1991) Subitizing: The preverbal counting process. In: Memories, thoughts and emotions: Essays in honor of George Mandler (Kessen W, Ortony A, Craik F, eds), 65–81. Hillsdale, NJ: Lawrence Erlbaum.

Gallistel CR, Gelman R (1992) Preverbal and verbal counting and computation. Cognition 44: 43–74.

Gao F, Levine SC, Huttenlocher J (2000) What do infants know about continuous quantity? J Exp Child Psychol 77: 20–29.

Hauser MD, Carey S, Hauser LB (2000) Spontaneous number representation in semi–free ranging rhesus monkeys. P Roy Soc Lond B Bio 267: 829–833.

Hauser MD, MacNeilage P, Ware M (1996) Numerical representations in primates. Proc Natl Acad Sci USA 93: 1514–1517.

Hauser MD, Tsao F, Garcia P, Spelke ES (2003) Evolutionary foundations of number: Spontaneous representation of numerical magnitudes by cotton-top tamarins. P Roy Soc Lond B Bio 270: 1441–1446.

Holyoak KJ, Mah WA (1982) Cognitive reference points in judgments of symbolic magnitude. Cognitive Psychol 14: 328–352.

Hubbard EM, Piazza M, Pinel P, Dehaene S (2005) Interaction between number and space in parietal cortex. Nat Rev Neurosci 6: 435–448.

Huttenlocher J, Duffy S, Levine S (2002) Infants and toddlers discriminate amount: Are they measuring? Psychol Sci 13: 244–249.

Jordan KE, Brannon EM (2006) The multisensory representation of number in infancy. P Natl Acad Sci USA 103: 3486–3489.

Jordan KE, Brannon EM, Logothetis NK, Ghazanfar AA (2005) Monkeys match the number of voices they hear to the number of faces they see. Curr Biol 15: 1–5.

Jordan KE, Maclean EL, Brannon EM (in press). Monkeys abstract number across sounds and sights. Cognition.

Jordan KE, Suanda SH, Brannon EM (in press) Intersensory redundancy accelerates preverbal numerical competence. Cognition.

Kuhl PK, Meltzoff, AN (1982) The bimodal perception of speech in infancy. Science 218: 1138–1141.

Lemer C, Dehaene S, Spelke E, Cohen L (2003) Approximate quantities and exact number words: dissociable systems. Neuropsychologia 41: 1942–1958.

Lewis KP, Jaffe S, Brannon EM (2005) Analog number representations in mongoose lemurs (*Eulemur mongoz*): Evidence from a search task. Anim Cogn 8: 247–252.

Lipton J, Spelke E (2003) Origins of number sense: Large-number discrimination in human infants. Psychol Sci 14: 396–401.

Lipton J, Spelke E (2004) Discrimination of large and small numerosities by human infants. Infancy 5: 271–290.

McCrink K, Wynn K (2004) Large-number addition and subtraction by 9-month-old infants. Psychol Sci 15: 776–781.

Meck WH, Church RM (1983) A mode control model of counting and timing processes. J Exp Psychol Anim B 9: 320–334.

Meck WH, Church RM, Gibbon J (1985) Temporal integration in duration and number discrimination. J Exp Psychol Anim B 11: 591–597.

Mix KS, Levine SC, Huttenlocher J (1997) Numerical abstraction in infants: Another look. Dev Psychol 33: 423–428.

Mix KS, Huttenlocher J, Levine SC (2002) Multiple cues for quantification in infancy: Is number one of them? Psychol Bull 128: 278–294.

Moore D, Benenson J, Reznick JS, Peterson M, Kagan J (1987) Effect of auditory numerical information on infants' looking behavior: Contradictory evidence. Dev Psychol 23: 665–670.

Moyer RS, Landauer TK (1967) Time required for judgements of numerical inequality. Nature 215: 1519–1520.

Newcombe N (2002) The nativist-empiricist controversy in the context of recent research on spatial and quantitative development. Psychol Sci 13: 395–401.

Nieder A, Freedman DJ, Miller EK (2002) Representation of the quantity of visual items in the primate prefrontal cortex. Science 297: 1708–1711.

Nieder A, Miller EK (2004) A parieto-frontal network for visual numerical information in the monkey. P Natl Acad Sci USA 101: 7457–7462.

Nieder A, Diester I, Tudusciuc O (2006) Temporal and spatial enumeration processes in the primate parietal cortex. Science 313: 1431–1435.

Patterson ML, Werker JF (2002) Infants' ability to match dynamic phonetic and gender, information in the face and voice. J Exp Child Psychol 81: 93–115.

Petrusic WM, Baranski JV, Kennedy R (1998) Similarity comparisons with remembered and perceived magnitudes: Memory psychophysics and fundamental measurement. Mem Cognition 26: 1041–1055.

Piaget J (1952) The child's conception of number. New York: Norton.

Piazza M, Izard V, Pinel P, Le Bihan D, Dehaene S (2004) Tuning curves for approximate numerosity in the human intraparietal sulcus. Neuron 44: 547–555.

Piazza M, Pinel P, Le Bihan D, Dehaene S (2007) A magnitude code common to numerosities and number symbols in human intraparietal cortex. Neuron 53: 293–305.

Pica P, Lemer C, Izard W, Dehaene S (2004) Exact and approximate arithmetic in an Amazonian indigene group. Science 306: 499–503.

Pinel P, Dehaene S, Riviere D, Le Bihan D (2001) Modulation of parietal activation by semantic distance in a number comparison task. Neuroimage 14: 1013–1026.

Roberts WA (1995) Simultaneous numerical and temporal processing in the pigeon. Curr Dir Psychol Sci 4: 47–51.

Roberts WA, Mitchell S (1994) Can a pigeon simultaneously process temporal and numerical information. J Exp Psychol Anim B 20: 66–78.

Roberts WA, Macuda T, Brodbeck DR (1995) Memory for number of light-flashes in the pigeon. Anim Learn Behav 23: 182–188.

Roberts WA, Boisvert MJ (1998) Using the peak procedure to measure timing and counting processes in pigeons. J Exp Psychol Anim B 24: 416–430.

Roberts WA, Coughlin R, Roberts S (2000) Pigeons flexibly time or count on cue. Psychol Sci 11: 218–222.

Roberts WA, Roberts S, Kit KA (2002) Pigeons presented with sequences of light flashes use behavior to count but not to time. J Exp Psychol Anim B 28: 137–150.

Roitman J, Brannon EM, Platt ML (2007) Monotonic coding of numerosity in macaque lateral intraparietal area. PLoS Biol 5(8): e208; doi:10.1371/journal.pbio.0050208.

Santi A, Hope C (2001) Errors in pigeons' memory for number of events. Anim Learn Behav 29: 208–220.

Santos LR, Barnes JL, Mahajan N (2005) Expectations about numerical events in four lemur species: *Eulemur fulvus, Eulemur mongoz, Lemur catta* and *Varecia rubra*). Anim Cogn 8: 253–262.

Shuman M, Kanwisher N (2004) Numerical magnitude in the human parietal lobe; tests of representational generality and domain specificity. Neuron 44: 557–569.

Spelke E (1976) Infants' intermodal perception of events. Cognitive Psychol 8: 533–560.

Spelke ES (2000) Core knowledge. Am Psychol 55: 1233–1243.

Starkey P, Spelke ES, Gelman R (1983) Detection of intermodal numerical correspondences by human infants. Science 222: 179–181.

Starkey P, Spelke ES, Gelman R (1990) Numerical abstraction by human infants. Cognition 36: 97–127.

Stevens SS (1970) Neural events and the psychophysical law. Science 170: 1043–1050.

Takahashi A, Green D (1983) Numerical judgments with Kanji and Kana. Neuropsychologia 21: 259–263.

Uller C, Hauser M, Carey S (2001) Spontaneous representation of number in cotton-top tamarins (*Saguinus oedipus*). J Comp Psychol 115: 248–257.

Uller C, Jaeger R, Guidry G, Martin C (2003) Salamanders (*Plethodon cinereus*) go for more: Rudiments of number in an amphibian. Anim Cogn 6: 105–112.

vanMarle K, Wynn K (2006) Six-month-old infants use analog magnitudes to represent duration. Developmental Sci 9: F41–F49.

vanMarle K (forthcoming). Infants' sensitivity to continuous quantity: The relationship between discrete and continuous quantification.

Varley RA, Klessinger NJC, Romanowski CAJ, Siegal M (2005). Agrammatic but numerate. P Natl Acad Sci USA 102: 3519–3524.

Walsh V (2003) A theory of magnitude: Common cortical metrics of time, space and quantity. Trends Cogn Sci 7: 483–488.

Welford AT (1960) The measurement of sensory-motor performance: Survey and reappraisal of twelve years' progress. Ergonomics 3: 189–230.

Wood J, Spelke ES (2005) Chronometric studies of numerical cognition in 5-month-old infants. Cognition 97: 23–29.

Wynn K (1992). Addition and subtraction by human infants. Nature 358: 749–750.

Xu F (2003) Numerosity discrimination in infants: Evidence for two systems of representations. Cognition 89: B15–B25.

Xu F, Spelke ES (2000) Large number discrimination in 6-month-old infants. Cognition 74: B1–B11.

Xu F, Spelke E, Goddard S (2005) Number sense in human infants. Developmental Sci 8: 88–101.

Xu F, Arriaga R (2007) Number discrimination in 10-month-old infants. Brit J Dev Psychol 25: 103–108.

11 Numerical and Spatial Intuitions: A Role for Posterior Parietal Cortex?

Edward M. Hubbard, Manuela Piazza, Philippe Pinel, and Stanislas Dehaene

Historically, many mathematical advances have been developed through the use of conceptual mappings between numbers and space. From the most elementary aspects of mathematics, such as the notion of measurement, all the way up to the concepts of the real number line, Cartesian coordinates, the complex plane, and even the proof of Fermat's Last Theorem, metaphors by which numbers are made to correspond to spatial positions permeate mathematical thinking (Dehaene 1997; Singh 1997). The evolution of these culturally defined representations of number has been critical to the development of mathematics. In this chapter, we review and update our previous models (Dehaene et al. 2003; Hubbard et al. 2005) discussing the neural mechanisms that might underpin these cultural achievements. We begin by reviewing recent behavioral, patient, and transcranial magnetic stimulation (TMS) data showing that certain aspects of numerical understanding depend on spatial representations (for reviews of the behavioral literature, see also Fias and Fischer 2005; Gevers and Lammertyn 2005). We then turn to neuroimaging data in humans that suggest how the deep connection between numbers and space may be mediated by circuitry in the parietal lobe. Drawing on recent work in monkey physiology and human neuroimaging studies establishing tentative homologies, we then present a refined hypothesis concerning specific neural regions in the intraparietal sulcus (IPS) involved in these numerical and spatial processes, including the human homologues of the lateral intraparietal (hLIP) and ventral intraparietal (hVIP) regions. To date, these two lines of research have been largely independent, as most studies of numerical cognition have been conducted in humans using functional imaging, while the most detailed studies of spatial processing have been conducted in monkeys, using single-unit electrophysiology. However, this division is breaking down, as single-unit data have revealed "number neurons" in the macaque IPS, while many recent human neuroimaging studies have focused on establishing human-monkey homologies in the parietal lobe. We conclude by discussing the development of numerical-spatial interactions within the context of the "neuronal recycling" hypothesis (Dehaene 2005; Dehaene and Cohen 2007).

Behavioral Studies of Numerical Spatial Interactions

Numerous behavioral paradigms have demonstrated a close connection between numbers and space, in which smaller numbers are represented on the left side of space, and larger numbers on the right. In this section, we will examine three important questions that have guided research in this area. First, how automatic is this association between numbers and space? Second, what level of spatial representation is involved? And third, what role do cultural factors play in the orientation of these numerical-spatial associations?

Automaticity of Numerical-Spatial Interactions

The simplest demonstration of a connection between numbers and space is the spatial-numerical association of response codes (SNARC) effect (Dehaene et al. 1993). When subjects are asked to classify numbers as even or odd (parity judgment), smaller numbers are responded to more quickly when responses are made on the left side of space, while larger numbers are responded to more quickly when responses are made on the right (figure 11.1a).

This association of numbers and space occurs despite the fact that the task itself has nothing to do with numerical magnitude. Indeed, the SNARC effect can occur with non-numerical tasks such as judging phonemic content of number words (Fias et al. 1996) or even in tasks where the digit itself is completely irrelevant to the task. In one series of experiments, subjects were asked to perform an orientation discrimination task on a triangle or line superimposed on a digit, and to respond with the left or right hand. In this task, a SNARC effect was observed, suggesting that numerical magnitude was processed automatically (Fias et al. 2001; Lammertyn et al. 2002). However, this effect was reduced or absent when subjects were asked to report the colors of the digit, or when asked to identify a shape (circle or square) superimposed on the digits.

Even simply presenting a digit automatically draws attention to either the left or right visual field based on the relative size of the number (Fischer et al. 2003). Fisher and colleagues presented single-digit numbers (1, 2, 8, or 9) at fixation, followed by a target in either the left or right visual field that participants responded to as quickly as they could (detection reaction time [RT]). The magnitude of the number influenced the direction of the allocation of attention, and thus the detection RT (figure 11.1b). Digits 1 and 2 automatically directed attention to the left visual field and thus facilitated the response to left-sided targets, whereas the opposite was true for 8 and 9, even though the digit was noninformative and completely irrelevant. In a recent follow-up it has been shown that these shifts of attention can have perceptual consequences. For instance, numerical cues induced the phenomenon of prior entry, in which objects at attended locations are perceived as appearing earlier than objects at nonattended locations (Casarotti et al. 2007). Similarly, in a backward priming experiment, Stoianov and colleagues (2007) found that

a. SNARC Effect

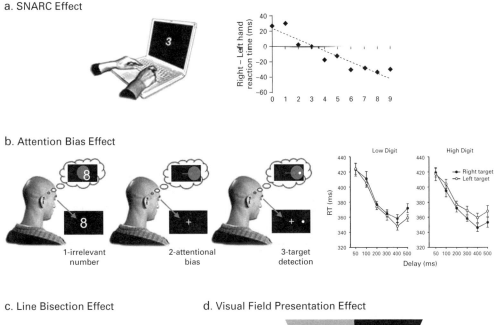

b. Attention Bias Effect

c. Line Bisection Effect

d. Visual Field Presentation Effect

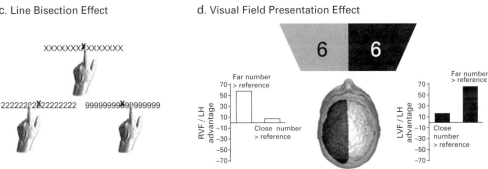

Figure 11.1
Behavioral studies demonstrating numerical-spatial interactions. (a) SNARC effect. Subjects respond whether a number is even or odd. Right-minus left-hand reaction time differences are plotted, with values greater than 0 indicating a left-hand advantage. Adapted from Dehaene et al. (1993). (b) Attention bias effect. Presentation of a noninformative digit at fixation leads to an automatic shift of attention to the left or right, and subsequently faster responses to visual targets. Graphs indicate reaction times to detect a visual target on the left or right side of space after presentation of a "low" or "high" digit. Open symbols indicate left-sided targets and filled symbols, right-sided targets. Adapted from Fischer et al. (2003). (c) Line bisection effect. When asked to point toward the midpoint of a line, subjects are accurate when the line is composed of x's (center indicated by bold x). However, when the line is composed of 2's or 9's, pointing deviates from the midpoint. (d) Visual field presentation effect. When a number is presented in one visual field, an interaction between numerical distance and visual field is observed. Numbers that are smaller than the standard show an advantage for LVF/RH presentation, while numbers that are larger than the standard show an advantage for RVF/LH presentation. Adapted from Lavidor et al. (2004).

responses for smaller numbers were faster when they were followed by a cue on the left side of the screen than when they were followed by a cue on the right side of the screen; the converse was true for larger numbers. This backward priming effect suggests that it takes a brief amount of time for the processing of numerical magnitude to evoke a spatial location. However, other recent studies have demonstrated that the presence of such orienting of attention is not entirely automatic, but rather is sensitive to top-down control and task set (Galfano et al. 2006; Ristic et al. 2006).

In a third demonstration of automatic numerical-spatial interactions, line bisection can be biased when the lines are composed of numbers (Calabria and Rossetti 2005; Fischer 2001). When asked to indicate the midpoint of a line composed of x's, subjects were accurate. However, when asked to indicate the midpoint of a line composed of either the digit 9 or the French word *neuf* (nine) subjects deviated to the right. When the line is composed of 2's or the French word *deux* (two) subjects deviated to the left (figure 11.1c). The suggestion is that the numbers automatically bias attention to the left or the right, and that the bisection of the lines therefore deviates in the same direction.

Spatial Reference Frames

A second question relevant to our purposes here is to determine the coordinate frame in which the SNARC effect arises. Several findings have suggested that an abstract, effector-independent cross-modal representation of space is involved. For example, it is known that the SNARC effect occurs even when the hands are crossed: large numbers continue to be associated with the right-hand side of space, even when responses on that side are made with the left hand (Dehaene et al. 1993). This observation suggests that the effect depends on eye- or world-centered coordinates, rather than hand-centered coordinates (although hand also makes an independent contribution; see Wood et al. 2006). Similar data from cross-modal visual-tactile attentional studies have shown that noninformative tactile stimuli to either hand improved detection thresholds on the same side of space even when the hands are crossed (Spence et al. 2000), suggesting that similar mechanisms may underlie both the spatial representation in the SNARC effect and in cross-modal spatial cuing. Neuroimaging studies of these cross-modal cuing effects consistently find parietal lobe activation (Kennett et al. 2001; Macaluso and Driver 2005; Macaluso et al. 2003), a point we will return to.

Additionally, the SNARC effect arises when subjects are asked to perform the parity judgment by pointing (Fischer 2003) or by moving their eyes, instead of a manual response (Fischer et al. 2004; Schwarz and Keus 2004). Finally, it has recently been shown that it is possible to obtain a SNARC effect with foot-pedal responses, demonstrating that the effect is not merely linked to effectors involved with writing but is a more general stimulus-response compatibility effect (Schwarz and Müller 2006). Bearing in mind that a noninformative digit automatically biases attention toward the left or right (Fischer et al. 2003), even though the response has nothing to do with the digit, these results suggest that numerical-spatial interactions occur in effector-independent, stable spatial coordinate frames.

A related question is the relation between the SNARC effect and the Simon effect, in which responses are faster when the stimulus and response occur at corresponding spatial locations. In the case of the SNARC, relative numerical magnitude may evoke corresponding spatial locations in representational space rather than physical space. Using the additive-factors method (AFM), two studies have yielded contradictory results. Mapelli and colleagues (2003) found that the SNARC effect, unlike the Simon effect, did not decay with time, and that it did not interact with the Simon effect. On this basis, they argued that the two effects were distinct. However, Keus and colleagues (2005), using the same AFM logic, found that the two effects did interact, suggesting that they share a common stage. More recently, Gevers and colleagues (2005) noted that both the SNARC and the Simon effect violate one of the assumptions of the AFM, namely, stage robustness, and as such the AFM logic is not appropriate for these questions. Rather, they showed that whether the SNARC and Simon interacted depended on the task relevance of the magnitude code (parity judgment vs. magnitude comparison), thereby demonstrating that the two effects do not conform to the AFM logic. To account for their results, Gevers and colleagues proposed a "dual-route" model of the SNARC, which involves activation of spatial codes indirectly via numerical codes, and which predicts a slight delay between stimulus onset and the elicitation of the spatial code, as seen in the Stoianov et al. (2007) study mentioned earlier. This account also suggests a partially shared architecture for the SNARC and Simon effects (see also Rusconi et al. 2006).

Another related question is when do these numerical-spatial interactions arise in the processing chain leading from stimulus to response? A recent study using a dual-task paradigm demonstrated a backward compatibility effect by showing that when subjects were asked to verbally respond "one" or "two" for different stimuli, even though digits were not presented, the automatic activation of numerical information interfered with responding to the orientation of an arrow (Caessens et al. 2004). This study indicates that SNARC-like influences occur at a task- and modality-independent level. Other studies have suggested that the SNARC effect best correlates with the response-locked (as opposed to stimulus-locked) event-related potentials (ERPs) and begins to emerge at a response selection stage (Gevers et al. 2006; Keus et al. 2005). However, given the delay in the elicitation of the spatial code seen in previous studies, and the relatively short response times in a traditional parity judgment task (400 to 500 ms), this temporal overlap may obscure other ERP components, such as those linked with shifts of attention, that may also play an important role in the genesis of the SNARC effect. These methodological considerations suggest that it may be premature to conclude that the SNARC effect is elicited only after substantial processing.

Indeed, interference between numerical and spatial information can arise even from spatial congruity of the stimulus, rather than the response (figure 11.1d; see Lavidor et al.

2004). The classic "numerical distance effect" is the finding that responses are increasingly faster as the numerical distance between the compared numbers increases (Dehaene et al. 1990; Moyer and Landauer 1967). However, when numbers were presented to the left (LVF) or right (RVF) of fixation, the magnitude of the distance effect was modulated, such that numbers smaller than the standard showed an advantage for LVF presentation, and numbers that are larger than the standard showed an advantage for RVF presentation. This effect is highly reminiscent of the SNARC effect (compare figures 11.1a and 11.1d). Taken together, these results suggest that numerical-spatial interactions arise at a central level, independent of input-modality or output-effector, and that they depend on spatial compatibility in both the input and output processes.

Cultural Factors

Even though these associations are automatic and depend on abstract representations of number and space, the *direction* of the effect—smaller numbers left, larger numbers right—might be determined by cultural factors such as the direction of writing or the conventional orientation of mathematical graph axes. For example, American children do not show a SNARC effect until age nine, showing that substantial education is required before these links become automatic (Berch et al. 1999). Indeed, the SNARC effect tends to reverse in Iranian subjects who write from right to left (Dehaene et al. 1993; Zebian 2005). As Fias and Fischer (2005) note, the direction of reading influences a whole host of ordering behaviors, and its influence is probably not limited to the SNARC effect.

Interestingly, when children are asked to map numbers onto a spatially oriented line, their responses change with age from a logarithmic to a linear encoding (Siegler and Opfer 2003) between the ages of seven and nine. However, this change seems to occur in stages, as seven-year-old children are likely to map the range 0 to 100 in a linear fashion but map the range 0 to 1000 in a logarithmic fashion. That is, they dedicate more space to small numbers than to large numbers, placing 10 near the middle of the 0 to 100 segment, rather spacing the numbers equally across the entire range. More recently, Opfer and Siegler (2007) replicated this developmental trend, and have shown that training on just one number (5, 150, or 750) can lead to rapid recalibration from logarithmic to linear representations in eight-year-old children who demonstrated logarithmic scaling of the mental number line on a pretest. This feedback was most effective where the discrepancy between the linear and logarithmic representations was greatest (at 150) and generalized across the entire mental number line in an all-or-none fashion, even though only one value was trained.

In the Amazon, Australia, and Africa, one can still find some cultures with a drastically reduced verbal lexicon for numbers. These cultures provide a more extreme situation for studying cultural universals and cultural differences in the number domain. Gordon (2004) studied the Piraha, who only have names for one and two, while Pica and colleagues (2004) studied the Munduruku, who have names for numbers about up to five. In both cases, a competence for approximate numerosity was demonstrated, suggesting that this intuition arises in a strictly nonverbal form even in remote cultures without formal education. For instance, adult and children Munduruku could perform an approximate addition task where one set of dots was added to another set of dots in a can, and the task was to decide if the total was larger or smaller than a third number. Even with very small numbers, in a subtraction condition where Western control subjects could perform with exact precision (e. g., 6-4), the Munduruku performance remained approximate and could be modeled mathematically by Weber's Law, suggesting that their spontaneous representation of number is an approximate logarithmic number line. Recently, we were able to show that uneducated Munduruku adults also have intuitions of number-space mappings (Dehaene et al. 2008). When presented with a nonsymbolic version of the Opfer-Siegler task (Siegler and Opfer 2003), with a horizontal line labeled with one dot at left and ten dots at right, they spontaneously understood that other numbers go to specific places on this physical number line. Furthermore, like young children with larger numbers, they spontaneously adopted a logarithmic spacing: for them the middle of the interval 1-10 was closer to the geometric mean (3 or 4) than to the arithmetic mean (5.5). It is likely that experience with counting, arithmetic, measurement, or other aspects modifies this internal representation by giving us access to a linear coordinate scheme, but exactly which cultural factors are involved and whether they also affect the direction of the SNARC effect remains unknown.

Studies of cultural influences on the SNARC effect are made more difficult because mathematical conventions are now essentially universal and often conflict with other cultural conventions. For instance, Japanese subjects were faster to respond to small numbers with the lower response button and large numbers with the upper response button (Ito and Hatta 2004), despite the fact that Japanese subjects use both left-to-right (like Western subjects) and top-to-bottom (which would have predicted the opposite pattern of SNARC effects) writing systems. It is possible that this discrepancy is due to graphing conventions (where small = bottom left). In another recent study, Chinese speakers in Taiwan were tested with three different writing systems, which are used in different writing situations. Arabic numerals appear in horizontal text, whereas simple Chinese characters appear in vertical text. Complex Chinese characters are used only in formal situations, such as check writing, and are not associated with a particular writing direction. A horizontal, left-to-right SNARC effect was found for the Arabic numerals, but not for either of the other two systems, while a vertical top-to-bottom SNARC was found for the simple Chinese characters, but not for the other two systems (Hung et al. 2008). These data add weight to the idea that the orientation of the SNARC effect is influenced by the direction of writing and demonstrates that the mappings are flexible, depending on numerical context.

Additionally, priming different types of spatial representation affects the orientation of the SNARC effect (Bachtold et al. 1998). Subjects were presented with a magnitude task (greater or less than 6) after being primed with either an image of a ruler or an image of a clock. After being primed with a ruler, the standard SNARC effect was observed (small-left, large-right). However, after being primed with a clock face, subjects showed a reverse SNARC effect (small-right, large-left) consistent with the representation of time on the clock face.

In sum, various paradigms suggest that numbers automatically elicit task-, modality-, and effector-independent spatial representations, even when these spatial representations are not strictly relevant to the task. Although cognitive and cultural factors clearly play some role in the orientation of these effects, the existence of spatial-numerical interference is robust. In the next section we relate these effects to monkey physiology and human neuroimaging studies of parietal regions involved in the appropriate representations of numbers and space.

Patient and TMS Studies Examining Numerical-Spatial Interactions

Joint deficits of space and number are frequently observed in patients with lesions of the parietal lobes. Classic evidence for this comes from studies of patients with Gerstmann's syndrome, which often involves dyscalculia, and spatial problems such as left-right confusion and finger agnosia (Benton 1992; Gerstmann 1940; Mayer et al. 1999; Roux et al. 2003). Recently, a case of pure Gerstmann's syndrome due to a subangular lesion has been identified (Mayer et al. 1999). After substantial testing of all the elements of Gerstmann's syndrome, the authors suggested that the common deficit linking the symptoms in this patient was a deficit in visuospatial manipulations, consistent with our hypothesis of numerical-spatial interaction in the parietal lobe. Interpretation of such symptom-association data remains complicated, however, because it could be due to the mere anatomical proximity of functionally distinct systems. Indeed, numerous studies have questioned the unity of Gerstmann's syndrome by showing that its defining features can be dissociated in both patient (Benton 1992) and intracranial stimulation studies (Roux et al. 2003).

Recent studies support a role for the right parietal lobe in the connection between numbers and space by demonstrating distortions in number processing in patients with hemi-spatial neglect (Vuilleumier et al. 2004; Zorzi et al. 2002). Patients with neglect ignore the contralesional (usually left) portion of space, including internal representational space in mental images, a condition known as "representational neglect" (Bisiach and Luzzatti 1978; see figure 11.2a).

In a classic test of neglect, patients, when asked to bisect a line, neglect the left half of the line, and therefore place the perceived midpoint of the line to the right of center (Driver and Vuilleumier 2001). In one recent study Zorzi and colleagues (2002) demonstrated that neglect patients have deficits in numerical tasks that closely correspond to those seen in physical line bisection tasks. When patients with neglect were asked to state the midpoint number of various numerical intervals—say, to give the numerical midpoint of 3 and 15—they deviated "to the right" (toward larger values), and for the smallest interval (3) they deviated "to the left" (toward smaller values), consistent with the "cross-over" effect

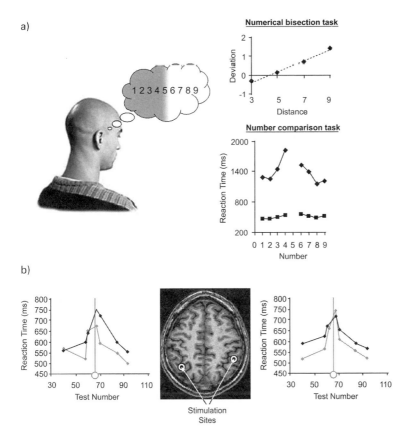

Figure 11.2
Hemispheric effects in numerical-spatial interactions. (a) Neglect patients demonstrate severe deficits in numerical distance and number bisection tasks. The upper graph shows the deviation on a number-interval bisection task, as a function of interval size (adapted from Zorzi et al. 2002), while the lower graph shows reaction times on a magnitude judgment task with 5 as the standard (adapted from Vuilleumier et al. 2004). (b) When rTMS is applied to the angular gyrus, responding to a number greater than the standard takes longer than in the no-stimulation condition. Adapted from Göbel et al. (2001).

observed in patients with spatial neglect. This was despite the fact that both the problem input and the response were given in a nonspatial spoken form. This numerical bias reflects a purely representational form of neglect (Bisiach and Luzzatti 1978), and suggests that numerical bisection involves an internal stage of representation on a spatially oriented "number line." Patients with right parietal lobe damage but no neglect do not show this pattern (Zorzi et al. 2002; for data suggesting that line and number bisection are doubly dissociable, see Doricchi et al. 2005). Additional follow-up studies have shown that the effect of neglect differs across tasks, such that the SNARC effect remains unaffected, despite impaired bisection performance, suggesting that the effect of neglect may vary depending on whether the task requires implicit or explicit access to the mental number line (Priftis et al. 2006). A second study showed that these representational deficits extend to the clock and ruler tasks described above (Vuilleumier et al. 2004; figure 11.2b). Wearing leftward adapting prisms tends to improve both spatial (Frassinetti et al. 2002; Rossetti et al. 1998) and representational neglect (Rode et al. 2001), including numerical neglect (Rossetti et al. 2004), further suggesting that the neural mechanisms that underlie spatial abilities are critical for certain numerical tasks.

Joint deficits of space and number can also be induced by TMS in normal subjects. TMS over the left angular gyrus, but not the left supramarginal gyrus or corresponding sites in the right hemisphere, both disrupted performance on a visuospatial search task and caused a deficit in numerical processing when subjects performed a magnitude judgment, but only for numbers greater than the midpoint of the interval (Göbel et al. 2001; figure 11.2c). In a follow-up study, Göbel and colleagues (2006) compared right parietal TMS with occipital stimulation while subjects were asked to report the midpoint of a verbally presented numerical interval. Parietal stimulation led to neglect-like responses, replicating the results found in patients with neglect, whereas occipital stimulation had no effect.

In the first study to directly examine the effects of TMS on the SNARC effect, Rusconi and colleagues (2008) tested both the SNARC and the Simon effect while they administered TMS over one of four different sites: anterior or posterior portions of the posterior parietal lobule (PPL) in either the left or right hemisphere. They found that stimulation over anterior PPL sites interfered with the Simon, but not SNARC, effect, whereas stimulation of posterior PPL sites interfered with both the Simon and the SNARC effect, consistent with the behavioral evidence reviewed earlier, which suggests that the two effects depend on partially shared neural circuits. Note that this localization is consistent with the role we had previously proposed for posterior parietal regions, such as the human homologue of lateral intraparietal (hLIP; see more in the next section), in the generation of the SNARC effect (Hubbard et al. 2005).

In general, these results suggest that numerical manipulations are critically dependent on intact spatial representations, and that the neural mechanisms of numerical-spatial interactions might be the same ones that subserve spatial cognition in the intact brain. One caveat is that both lesion and TMS effects probably encompass large amounts of cortex and thus may cause multiple independent impairments, suggesting the need for more fine-grained analysis of the neural substrates of these functions.

The Parietal Basis of Number Processing

The past ten years has seen an explosion of interest in the neural basis of basic mathematical processes such as subitizing, numerosity estimation, addition, subtraction, and multiplication (Dehaene 1997; Dehaene et al. 2004). One of the main findings from this line of research is that the neural circuitry critical for abstract representations of quantity is housed in the parietal lobe, in regions overlapping with neural circuitry involved in spatial representations.

The triple-code model of number processing (Dehaene 1992) proposes that numbers can be mentally represented in a nonverbal *quantity* representation (a semantic representation of the size and distance relations between numbers, which may be category-specific), a *verbal* system (where numerals are represented lexically, phonologically, and syntactically, much like any other type of word), and a *visual* system (in which numbers can be encoded as strings of Arabic numerals). The quantity system is thought to be located in the parietal cortex, and this system may be critical for mediating the observed interactions between numerical and spatial representations.

Functional magnetic resonance imaging (fMRI) has been used to test this model and to localize the nonverbal quantity system. Numerous results indicate that number comparison typically involves the left and right parietal lobes. In some experiments, for instance, subjects were asked to compare two numbers and decide which one was larger (Pinel et al. 2001, 2004). Irrespective of whether the numbers were presented as digits or as words, an identical behavioral distance effect was observed. FMRI indicated that the activation of the left and right intraparietal sulci (IPS) showed a tight correlation with the behavioral distance effect: the activation signal in this region also showed an inverse relation to the distance between the numbers to be compared. On the basis of this and other fMRI experiments of arithmetic tasks such as calculation (Chochon et al. 1999), approximation (Dehaene et al. 1999), or even the mere detection of digits (Eger et al. 2003), a meta-analysis has suggested that the bilateral horizontal segment of the IPS (HIPS) may play a particular role in quantity representation (Dehaene et al. 2003). In some cases, the activation also extended to dorsal parietal sites thought to be involved in orienting spatial attention.

Crucially, the quantity system in the parietal lobe might be part of a broader network of areas involved in nonnumerical magnitude representation (Fias et al. 2003; Pinel et al. 2004). Pinel and colleagues (2004) measured fMRI responses during three tasks: luminance comparison, size comparison, and numerical magnitude comparison. Because all three tasks demonstrate a distance effect, it was possible to match task difficultly by varying the discriminability of the stimuli for each subject. FMRI revealed a network of areas that were activated during each of the three tasks. An anterior region of the IPS was activated by all three tasks, but other mid-IPS regions were activated only by numerical comparison, suggesting a distributed, partially overlapping network of regions.

To further examine the neural basis of this quantity system, Simon and colleagues (2002) used fMRI to examine the topographical relation of calculation-related activation to other spatial and language areas in the human parietal lobe. They found that manual tasks (grasping and pointing) activated a large overlapping region in the anterior parietal cortex, with the greatest extent of activation for grasping, which recruited an additional anterior intraparietal region bilaterally (possibly coinciding with area hAIP [human anterior intraparietal area]; see the next section). Posterior to this was a region selectively activated by calculation alone, specifically in the horizontal segment of the intraparietal sulcus (HIPS). The posterior parietal cortex was activated by all visuospatial tasks (grasping, pointing, saccades, and spatial attention), consistent with previous data (Corbetta and Shulman 2002). Finally, calculation and phoneme detection jointly activated a portion of the IPS lying underneath the left angular gyrus. Overall, these results suggest that calculation activates the fundus of the IPS in a region close to, or within, hVIP surrounded by a network of areas involved in manual, visuospatial, and verbal tasks.

Neurons Sensitive to Number

Several animal species spontaneously keep track of number (Dehaene et al. 1998; Hauser et al. 2000; Hauser et al. 2002) and can be trained to use symbolic representations of number in a variety of tasks (Boysen and Berntson 1989; Harris and Washburn 2005; Matsuzawa 1985). Additionally, it has been shown that many of the signatures of semantic numerosity processing, such as the distance effect, are present in macaque monkeys, suggesting a shared evolutionary basis for such effects (Cantlon and Brannon 2005, 2006). Physiological recordings have demonstrated that there are neurons in the parietal cortex of cats (Thompson et al. 1970) and macaques (Nieder and Miller 2004; Sawamura et al. 2002) that respond selectively to number (for a recent review, see Nieder 2005). These results suggest that there may be an evolutionary necessity to keep track of the number of objects and events in the environment, and that, at least at a rudimentary level, the ability to estimate numerosity may be present in many nonhuman animals.

Recently, Andreas Nieder and Earl Miller (Nieder et al. 2002; Nieder and Miller 2003, 2004) recorded from single neurons in awake monkeys trained to perform a visual number match-to-sample task. Many neurons were selectively tuned to a preferred numerosity; some responded preferentially to sets of one object, others to two objects, and so on up to five objects. The tuning was coarse, and became increasingly imprecise as numerosity increased. Importantly, a large proportion of these number-selective neurons were originally observed in the dorsolateral prefrontal cortex, but more recently another population of neurons with a shorter latency has been found in the parietal lobe (Nieder and Miller 2004). In a more recent study, Nieder and colleagues (2006) showed that some number-selective neurons also demonstrated motion selectivity, consistent with their localization to VIP, a plausible homolog of the human HIPS area active during many number tasks.

Piazza and colleagues (2004) used an adaptation method to investigate whether such numerosity tuning exists in humans, and thus to link human fMRI responses to those obtained with monkeys. During fMRI, they repeatedly presented participants with sets of dots with a fixed number, say, sixteen. The purpose was to "adapt" the neural population coding for this value, thus leading putative human number neurons to progressively reduce their firing rate, as observed in macaque electrophysiological experiments (Miller et al.

1991). They then presented occasional deviant numbers, which ranged from half to twice the adapted number. FMRI revealed that only two regions, the left and right IPS, responded to the change in numerosity by increasing their activation in relation to the distance between the adapted number and the deviant one, regardless of the direction of the change (more or less dots). In a follow-up study, Cantlon and colleagues (2006) replicated these findings and showed that four-year-old children demonstrated similar adaptation in the IPS, which overlapped with the regions showing adaptation in the adults. Interestingly, these effects were stronger in the right hemisphere than in the left, suggesting a potential developmental difference between the two hemispheres for the representation of numerosity. Piazza and colleagues (2007) have recently extended this adaptation effect to a cross-notation paradigm, where it was shown that digits lead to adaptation for similar quantities of dots, and vice versa, but not when the numerosities are less similar, thereby showing that digits and numerosity converge on the same neural populations in adult subjects.

These human fMRI and monkey electrophysiological data yielded similar tuning profiles, suggesting that humans and macaque monkeys possess similar populations of intraparietal number-sensitive neurons. In both the single-unit recording studies and the human fMRI studies, responses closely matched predicted responses from computational models (Dehaene and Changeux 1993; Verguts and Fias 2004). Specifically, the firing rates assumed a Gaussian distribution only if plotted on a logarithmic scale. This logarithmic compression is commonly seen in human numerical tasks (Dehaene 2002), and is reflected in decreased word-frequency with numerical magnitude, and local increases for reference numerals such as 10, 20, 50, or 100 in many of the world's languages (Dehaene and Mehler 1992). Thus, even the fine-grained properties of adult numerical abilities can be predicted from the responses of neurons in the parietal cortex.

The Parietal Basis of Spatial Cognition

Recent work in both electrophysiology (Cohen and Andersen 2002; Colby and Goldberg 1999) and neuroimaging (Orban et al. 2004) has begun to converge on specific regions of the parietal lobe as the possible neural bases for the spatial representations that we discuss here. On the basis of architectonic (Lewis and Van Essen 2000a), connectivity (Felleman and Van Essen 1991; Lewis and Van Essen 2000b), and physiological criteria, the intraparietal sulcus has been divided into numerous subregions that represent space in a variety of different frames of reference. Identification of putative human homologs of macaque IPS regions is tentative, both because the parietal and frontal cortex is differentially expanded in humans compared with similar regions in macaques (Van Essen et al. 2001) and because direct comparisons between monkey and human fMRI responses to the same stimuli have revealed important differences (Orban et al. 2006; Orban et al. 2003). Nevertheless, the overall pattern of posterior-to-anterior organization, with a systematic transformation from sensory to effector-specific properties, presents striking parallels with that observed in previous studies of monkey physiology (Culham and Valyear 2006; Simon et al. 2002). We will focus on three of these putative homologies, areas hLIP, hVIP and hAIP, where *h* identifies these as putative human homologs of the aforementioned monkey areas.

Area LIP and hLIP

Many neurons in macaque area LIP are organized into a retinotopic map (Ben Hamed et al. 2001), represent target position in an eye-centered frame of reference (Colby et al. 1995; but see Mullette-Gillman et al. 2005), and are highly active during memory-guided saccades (Colby et al. 1993; Colby et al. 1996; Snyder et al. 2000). Additionally, these neurons are involved in spatial updating, even before an eye movement is made (Colby et al. 1995; Duhamel et al. 1992). Reversible inactivation of this region leads to deficits in saccade execution, demonstrating its causal role in eye movements (Li and Andersen 2001; Wardak et al. 2002).

Recent neuroimaging studies have demonstrated as many as four retinotopic maps within the posterior portion of the human intraparietal sulcus, and there is still debate as to which of these maps constitutes hLIP, and whether the additional maps are evolution-arily new (Schluppeck et al. 2005; Sereno et al. 2001; Silver et al. 2005; Swisher et al. 2007). Despite this ambiguity, recent studies have shown that posterior IPS responds in an effector-independent manner (Astafiev et al. 2003; Medendorp et al. 2005) and is jointly active for attending, pointing, and making saccades to peripheral targets (see also Simon et al. 2002). In addition, this region demonstrates delay-period activity (Schluppeck et al. 2006) and is involved in spatial updating (Medendorp et al. 2003; Merriam et al. 2003), as is macaque LIP. More recently, Morris and colleagues (2007) have used TMS to show that inactivation of this region leads to deficits in a double-step saccade paradigm. Taken together, these results suggest that at least one of the maps identified in the posterior parietal cortex is the human homolog of macaque LIP.

Area VIP and hVIP

Macaque area VIP contains populations of neurons that represent targets in either a head-centered or eye-centered frame of reference (Duhamel et al. 1997, 1998), although some receptive fields (RFs) are partially shifting or gain-modulated by eye position (Avillac et al. 2005). That is, when the eyes are moved around in the visual field, the best stimulus location either remains fixed relative to the position of the head (head-centered) or shifts partway between the position relative to the eyes and that relative to the head (partially shifting receptive fields). Additionally, many VIP neurons have joint tactile and visual motion-determined receptive fields (Duhamel et al. 1998), and are strongly driven by optic flow fields (Bremmer et al. 2002; Zhang et al. 2004). To date, two fMRI studies have attempted to identify hVIP. Bremmer and colleagues (2001) tested for regions that were conjointly activated by visual, tactile, and auditory motion. Only one such region was identified in the fundus of the IPS, anterior to hLIP, and consistent with the known organization in the monkey. In another study, Sereno and Huang (2006) mapped visual and tactile responsiveness, and demonstrated the presence of visual and tactile maps in the mid-IPS near to, but slightly mesial and superior to, the peaks of the Bremmer et al. study. They found that these maps were spatially aligned, so that voxels showing responses to a specific location in the visual field also responded to tactile stimulation on corresponding portions of the face, further suggesting that this is the human homolog of macaque VIP.

Area AIP and hAIP

Macaque area AIP represents space in hand-centered coordinates, and is crucial for fine grasping (Iwamura et al. 1994; Taira et al. 1990). Neurons in this area are bimodal (visual-tactile; see Murata et al. 2000; Saito et al. 2003; Taira et al. 1990), so that when the hand moves, the visual receptive field remains in a fixed position relative to the hand. Neurons in this area, in combination with neurons in the caudal intraparietal area (CIP), which extracts 3-D shape, are critical for correctly reaching to and grasping 3-D objects (Sakata et al. 1999; Shikata et al. 2001) and tools (Hihara et al. 2003; Iriki et al. 1996; Obayashi et al. 2001). Neurons in monkey area AIP respond in a hand-centered manner and are involved in fine grasping, but not necessarily in the transport phase of the action. Several studies have used these properties to identify hAIP (for a review see Culham et al. 2006). In the first study of this kind, regions of the IPS that responded when subjects grasped objects were identified (Binkofski et al. 1998). Interestingly, the region identified by fMRI overlapped nearly completely with a region that was damaged in a patient who demonstrated a selective impairment in fine grasping behavior (Binkofski et al. 1998). Other studies identified a region of the anterior IPS that responded more strongly to grasping than to reaching (Culham et al. 2003) or to finger pointing (Simon et al. 2002). As expected from monkey maps, activations in these regions putatively homologous to area AIP consistently lie anterior to the activations identified with the putative hLIP and hVIP.

Overlap with Numerical Activations

Crucially, the regions that have been consistently activated in arithmetic tasks overlap with, or are intermingled with, putative area hVIP, consistent with the localization derived from anatomical criteria in the monkey (see figure 11.3).

It is possible that this overlap accounts for the interaction between representations of number and space. At present, however, this co-localization remains only tentative, given that these regions have commonly been defined on the basis of average foci of brain activation in a normalized template space. Future studies should concentrate on higher-resolution studies in which hLIP, hVIP, and hAIP are identified in individual subjects. Once these regions have been identified on an individual-subject basis, activation related to number processing can be compared to these predefined regions of interest.

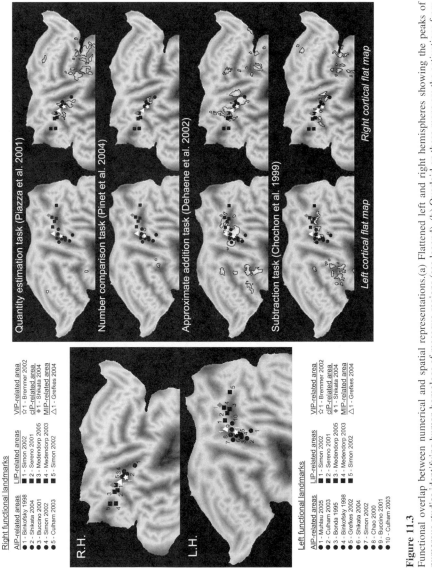

Figure 11.3

Functional overlap between numerical and spatial representations. (a) Flattened left and right hemispheres showing the peaks of numerous studies identifying human homologs of macaque regions (see legend). (b) Overlaid on these maps are the activations from four different types of numerical studies: addition, subtraction, estimation, and comparison (outlined in black). Estimation and comparison activated circumscribed regions overlapping hVIP consistent with macaque physiology data. Addition and subtraction activated larger networks, including hLIP, consistent with our hypothesis that numerical operations may also depend on hVIP-hLIP circuitry and interactions.

A Possible Role for hLIP in Shifts of Attention Along the Mental Number Line

These considerations lead us to speculate that shifts of attention along the mental number line may be mediated by shifts of attention in hLIP in the same manner that shifts of attention in the external world are mediated by hLIP. This hypothesis may explain many of the behavioral and patient data reviewed. First, the finding that the SNARC effect is present even when the hands are crossed (Dehaene et al. 1993) is consistent with the stable, eye-centered spatial representation in hLIP, and with data suggesting that multisensory (tactile-visual) attentional effects show similar remapping in space, including the activation of posterior IPS regions. Second, this hypothesis would explain why the SNARC effect is effector-independent (Dehaene et al. 1993; Fischer 2003; Schwarz and Keus 2004), given that area hLIP contains an effector-independent representation of space. Finally, this hypothesis can explain the results of the Fischer studies (Fischer 2001; Fischer et al. 2003), in which presentation of numbers leads to automatic shifts of attention to the left or to the right. We suggest that all of these effects arise from a common neural mechanism, namely, the flow of some activation from a quantity representation in area hVIP to interconnected hLIP neurons involved in programming overt and covert shifts to the contralateral side of space (Corbetta and Shulman 2002).

Similarly, in patients with neglect, we suggest that area hLIP is damaged or functionally disconnected, leading to the failure to attend to both the left side of space and the left side of the number line. It is clear that neglect is not a unitary syndrome (Halligan and Marshall 1998): some authors pin its neural substrate to the superior temporal lobe (Karnath et al. 2004), but most others place it in the parietal lobe (Mort et al. 2003). One recent proposal suggests that neglect is composed of two deficits, a spatial one, dependent on posterior superior parietal structures (including the IPS) and a memory one, dependent on the superior temporal sulcus (Malhotra et al. 2004). In light of this debate, it is interesting that transient inactivation of monkey LIP leads to neglect-like phenomena (Wardak et al. 2002; 2004). We suggest that damage to this region is responsible for not only the observed deficits in shifts of attention to external space, but also for shifts of attention along internal representations of the mental number line.

We have begun to test this idea, using fMRI, by using the classical SNARC task during whole-brain fMRI scanning (Hubbard et al. forthcoming). Subjects classified Arabic numerals as odd or even by making bimanual responses with normal or crossed hands. Four parietal regions of interest were studied, three showing lateralized activations for hands (putative hAIP), space (dorsal IPS), and saccades (putative hLIP), and a fourth active during mental arithmetic (putative hVIP). During parity judgment, number size elicited a systematic pattern of lateralized activation, which was found only in the saccade region (hLIP). In this region, a significant interaction between hemisphere and numerical size indicated that large numbers tended to cause more activation in the left hLIP, preferentially coding for the rightward side of space, while small numbers tended to cause more activation of the right hLIP, suggesting a biased attention toward the left side of space. This is the first positive evidence that this posterior parietal region, a putative homolog of macaque area LIP, may be the site of number-space interactions exemplified by the SNARC effect.

Predictions and Conclusions

Our view of the links between number and space in the parietal cortex leads to several testable predictions. First, we predict that shifts of attention along the number line make use of the same hLIP-hVIP circuitry that is involved in the development of multisensory, world-centered representations of space (Deneve and Pouget 2004; Pouget et al. 2002). This implies that the same computational transformations that support spatial updating would be critical for arithmetic operations that create shifts of the locus of activation along an internal number line (see figure 11.3). Indeed, the problem of computing a world-centered spatial representation by combining two separate population codes for eye and retinal location is formally identical to that of computing an approximate addition or subtraction by combining two population codes for numerosity (Deneve and Pouget 2004; Pouget et al. 2002). Thus, the parietal mechanisms that are thought to support spatial transformation might be ideally suited to support arithmetic transformations as well.

Future studies can test this prediction by comparing patterns of fMRI activation during spatial updating and numerical tasks. We would predict that when subjects compute additions or subtractions on numerical symbols, they will shift their attention to the left for subtraction problems, and to the right for addition problems, leading to increased activation of contralateral hLIP. Second, we predict that behavioral paradigms in which attention is shifted to the left should interfere with addition, while rightward attentional shifts should interfere with subtraction. Third, once number neurons can be recorded in animals during performance of simple addition and subtraction tasks, we predict that one should observe numerical equivalents of the partially shifting receptive fields and gain fields observed in the spatial domain.

Each of these examples might be thought of as examples of "neuronal recycling" in which preexisting neural circuits, evolved for more basic functions (in this case visuospatial processing, multisensory integration, and numerosity processing), are modified by education to perform more advanced functions (Dehaene 2005; Dehaene and Cohen 2007). Although number and space are already tightly linked by functional and anatomical links that probably exist in other animals, these links are expanded upon, within the mathematical domain, by the human-specific ability to draw metaphors between distinct domains, thus creating a cultural expanded concept of the "number line."

According to the neuronal recycling model, the very possibility of retraining these circuits to perform more advanced functions, such as the mental number line, may be dependent on the distance between the function that these circuits originally evolved to serve, and their use in abstract reasoning, such as in the case of mathematics. Thus, certain mathematical concepts such as the concept of zero, of negative numbers, or of complex numbers may be difficult to grasp because they require an important reorganization of the internal representation of numbers, associated with a considerable amount of neuronal recycling. To take a more advanced mathematical example, fractal objects such as Cantor dust, the Koch snowflake, and the Sierpinski gasket may be difficult to understand because they violate the normal connection between area and perimeter that may constitute a strong evolutionary expectation built into the very structure of our parietal circuitry for object properties in space. By better understanding the neural foundations that make such abstractions possible, we may come to a deeper appreciation of the drastic reorganization necessary to attain such mathematical insights and may be able to develop better methods for explaining and teaching such profound mathematical ideas to children.

Acknowledgments

The authors thank Mariano Sigman, Lisa E. Williams, and Anna J. Wilson for valuable comments on earlier versions of this chapter. This research is supported by the Institute National de la Santé et de la Recherche Médicale (S.D. and P.P.), Collège de France (S.D.), a James S. McDonnell Centennial Fellowship (S.D.), a NUMBRA postdoctoral fellowship (E.M.H.), and a Marie-Curie individual fellowship (M.P.).

References

Astafiev SV, Shulman GL, Stanley CM, Snyder AZ, Van Essen DC, Corbetta M (2003) Functional organization of human intraparietal and frontal cortex for attending, looking, and pointing. J Neurosci 23: 4689–4699.

Avillac M, Deneve S, Olivier E, Pouget A, Duhamel JR (2005) Reference frames for representing visual and tactile locations in parietal cortex. Nat Neurosci 8: 941–949.

Bachtold D, Baumuller M, Brugger P (1998) Stimulus-response compatibility in representational space. Neuropsychologia 36: 731–735.

Ben Hamed S, Duhamel JR, Bremmer F, Graf W (2001) Representation of the visual field in the lateral intraparietal area of macaque monkeys: A quantitative receptive field analysis. Exp Brain Res 140: 127–144.

Benton AL (1992) Gerstmann's syndrome. Arch Neurol 49: 445–447.

Berch DB, Foley EJ, Hill RJ, Ryan PM (1999) Extracting parity and magnitude from Arabic numerals: Developmental changes in number processing and mental representation. J Exp Child Psychol 74: 286–308.

Binkofski R, Dohle C, Posse S, Stephan KM, Hefter H, Seitz RJ, Freund H-J (1998) Human anterior intraparietal area subserves prehension. Neurology 50: 1253–1259.

Bisiach E, Luzzatti C (1978) Unilateral neglect of representational space. Cortex 14: 129–133.

Boysen ST, Berntson GG (1989) Numerical competence in a chimpanzee (Pan troglodytes). J Comp Psychol 103: 23–31.

Bonda E, Petrides M, Frey S, Evans A (1995) Neural correlates of mental transformations of the body-in-space. Proc Natl Acad Sci USA 92: 11180–11184.

Bremmer F, Duhamel JR, Ben Hamed S, Graf W (2002) Heading encoding in the macaque ventral intraparietal area (VIP). Eur J Neurosci 16: 1554–1568.

Bremmer F, Schlack A, Shah NJ, Zafiris O, Kubischik M, Hoffmann K-P, Zilles K, Fink GR (2001) Polymodal motion processing in posterior parietal and premotor cortex: A human fMRI study strongly implies equivalencies between humans and monkeys. Neuron 29: 287–296.

Buccino G, Binkofski R, Fink GR, Fadiga L, Fogassi L, Gallese V, Seitz RJ, Zilles K, Rizzolatti G, Freund H-J (2001) Action observation activates premotor and parietal areas in a somatotopic manner: An fMRI study. Eur J Neurosci 13: 400–404.

Caessens B, Hommel B, Reynvoet B, van der Goten K (2004) Backward-compatibility effects with irrelevant stimulus-response overlap: The case of the SNARC effect. J Gen Psychol 131: 411–425.

Calabria M, Rossetti Y (2005) Interference between number processing and line bisection: A methodology. Neuropsychologia 43: 779–783.

Cantlon JF, Brannon EM (2005) Semantic congruity affects numerical judgments similarly in monkeys and humans. P Natl Acad Sci USA 102: 16507–16511.

Cantlon JF, Brannon EM (2006) Shared system for ordering small and large numbers in monkeys and humans. Psychol Sci 17: 401–406.

Cantlon JF, Brannon EM, Carter EJ, Pelphrey KA (2006) Functional imaging of numerical processing in adults and 4-y-old children. PLoS Biol 4: e125.

Casarotti M, Michielin M, Zorzi M, Umilta C (2007) Temporal order judgment reveals how number magnitude affects visuospatial attention. Cognition 102: 101–117.

Chao LL, Martin A (2000) Represntation of manipulable man-made objects in the dorsal stream. Neuroimage 12: 478–484.

Chochon F, Cohen L, van de Moortele PF, Dehaene S (1999) Differential contributions of the left and right inferior parietal lobules to number processing. J Cognitive Neurosci 11: 617–630.

Cohen YE, Andersen RA (2002) A common reference frame for movement plans in the posterior parietal cortex. Nat Rev Neurosci 3: 553–562.

Colby CL, Duhamel JR, Goldberg ME (1993) The analysis of visual space by the lateral intraparietal area of the monkey: the role of extraretinal signals. Prog Brain Res 95: 307–316.

Colby CL, Duhamel JR, Goldberg ME (1995) Oculocentric spatial representation in parietal cortex. Cereb Cortex 5: 470–481.

Colby CL, Duhamel JR, Goldberg ME (1996) Visual, presaccadic, and cognitive activation of single neurons in monkey lateral intraparietal area. J Neurophysiol 76: 2841–2852.

Colby CL, Goldberg ME (1999) Space and attention in parietal cortex. Annu Rev Neurosci 22: 319–349.

Corbetta M, Shulman GL (2002) Control of goal-directed and stimulus-driven attention in the brain. Nat Rev Neurosci 3: 201–215.

Culham JC, Cavina-Pratesi C, Singhal A (2006) The role of parietal cortex in visuomotor control: What have we learned from neuroimaging? Neuropsychologia 44: 2668–2684.

Culham JC, Danckert SL, DeSouza JF, Gati JS, Menon RS, Goodale MA (2003) Visually guided grasping produces fMRI activation in dorsal but not ventral stream brain areas. Exp Brain Res 153: 180–189.

Culham JC, Valyear KF (2006) Human parietal cortex in action. Curr Opin Neurobiol 16: 205–212.

Dehaene S (1992) Varieties of numerical abilities. Cognition 44: 1–42.

Dehaene S (1997) The number sense: How the mind creates mathematics. New York: Oxford University Press.

Dehaene S (2002) Neuroscience. Single-neuron arithmetic. Science 297: 1652–1653.

Dehaene S (2005) Evolution of human cortical circuits for reading and arithmetic: The "neuronal recycling" hypothesis. In: From monkey brain to human brain (Dehaene S, Duhamel JR, Hauser MD, Rizzolatti G, eds), 133–158. Cambridge, MA: MIT Press.

Dehaene S, Bossini S, Giraux P (1993) The mental representation of parity and numerical magnitude. J Exp Psych Gen 122: 371–396.

Dehaene S, Changeux J-P (1993) Development of elementary numerical abilities: A neuronal model. J Cognitive Neurosci 5: 390–407.

Dehaene S, Cohen L (2007) Cultural recycling of cortical maps. Neuron 56: 384–398.

Dehaene S, Dehaene-Lambertz G, Cohen L (1998) Abstract representations of numbers in the animal and human brain. Trends Neurosci 21: 355–361.

Dehaene S, Dupoux E, Mehler J (1990) Is numerical comparison digital? Analogical and symbolic effects in two-digit number comparison. J Exp Psych Human 16: 626–641.

Dehaene S, Izard V, Spelke E, Pica P (2008) Log or linear? Distinct intuitions of the number scale in Western and Amazonian indigene cultures. Science 320: 1217–1220.

Dehaene S, Mehler J (1992) Cross-linguistic regularities in the frequency of number words. Cognition 43: 1–29.

Dehaene S, Molko N, Cohen L, Wilson AJ (2004) Arithmetic and the brain. Curr Opin Neurobiol 14: 218–224.

Dehaene S, Piazza M, Pinel P, Cohen L (2003) Three parietal circuits for number processing. Cognitive Neuropsychol 20: 487–506.

Dehaene S, Spelke E, Pinel P, Stanescu R, Tsivkin S (1999) Sources of mathematical thinking: Behavioral and brain-imaging evidence. Science 284: 970–974.

Deneve S, Pouget A (2004) Bayesian multisensory integration and cross-modal spatial links. J Physiol 98: 249–258.

Doricchi F, Guariglia P, Gasparini M, Tomaiuolo F (2005) Dissociation between physical and mental number line bisection in right hemisphere brain damage. Nat Neurosci 8: 1663–1665.

Driver J, Vuilleumier P (2001) Perceptual awareness and its loss in unilateral neglect and extinction. Cognition 79: 39–88.

Duhamel JR, Bremmer F, Ben Hamed S, Graf W (1997) Spatial invariance of visual receptive fields in parietal cortex neurons. Nature 389: 845–858.

Duhamel JR, Colby CL, Goldberg ME (1992) The updating of the representation of visual space in parietal cortex by intended eye movements. Science 255: 90–92.

Duhamel JR, Colby CL, Goldberg ME (1998) Ventral intraparietal area of the macaque: Congruent visual and somatic response properties. J Neurophysiol 79: 126–136.

Eger E, Sterzer P, Russ MO, Giraud A-L, Kleinschmidt A (2003) A supramodal number representation in human intraparietal cortex. Neuron 37: 719–725.

Felleman DJ, Van Essen DC (1991) Distributed hierarchical processing in the primate cerebral cortex. Cereb Cortex 1: 1–47.

Fias W, Brysbaert M, Geypens F, d'Ydewalle G (1996) The importance of magnitude information in numerical processing: Evidence from the SNARC effect. Mathematical Cogn 2: 95–110.

Fias W, Fischer MH (2005) Spatial representation of Numbers. In: Handbook of mathematical cognition (Campbell JID, ed). 43–54. New York: Psychology Press.

Fias W, Lammertyn J, Reynvoet B, Dupont P, Orban GA (2003) Parietal representation of symbolic and non-symbolic magnitude. J Cognitive Neurosci 15: 47–56.

Fias W, Lauwereyns J, Lammertyn J (2001) Irrelevant digits affect feature-based attention depending on the overlap of neural circuits. Cogn Brain Res 12: 415–423.

Fischer MH (2001) Number processing induces spatial performance biases. Neurology 57: 822–826.

Fischer MH (2003) Spatial representations in number processing-evidence from a pointing task. Vis Cogn 10: 493–508.

Fischer MH, Castel AD, Dodd MD, Pratt J (2003) Perceiving numbers causes spatial shifts of attention. Nat Neurosci 6: 555–556.

Fischer MH, Warlop N, Hill RL, Fias W (2004) Oculomotor bias induced by number perception. Exp Psychol 51: 91–97.

Frassinetti F, Angeli V, Meneghello F, Avanzi S, Ladavas E (2002) Long-lasting amelioration of visuospatial neglect by prism adaptation. Brain 125: 608–623.

Galfano G, Rusconi E, Umilta C (2006) Number magnitude orients attention, but not against one's will. Psychon B Rev 13: 869–874.

Gerstmann J (1940) Syndrome of finger agnosia, disorientation for right and left, agraphia, acalculia. Arch Neurolog Psych 44: 398–408.

Gevers W, Caessens B, Fias W (2005) Towards a common processing architecture underlying Simon and SNARC effects. Eur J Cogn Psychol 17: 659–673.

Gevers W, Lammertyn J (2005) The hunt for SNARC. Psychol Sci 47: 10–21.

Gevers W, Ratinckx E, De Baene W, Fias W (2006) Further evidence that the SNARC effect is processed along a dual-route architecture: Evidence from the Lateralized Readiness Potential. Exp Psychol 53: 58–68.

Göbel SM, Calabria M, Farne A, Rossetti Y (2006) Parietal rTMS distorts the mental number line: simulating "spatial" neglect in healthy subjects. Neuropsychologia 44: 860–868.

Göbel SM, Walsh V, Rushworth MFS (2001) The mental number line and the human angular gyrus. Neuroimage 14: 1278–1289.

Gordon P (2004) Numerical cognition without words: Evidence from Amazonia. Science 306: 496–499.

Grefkes C, Weiss PH, Zilles K, Fink GR (2002) Crossmodal processing of object features in human anterior intraparietal cortex: An fMRI study implies equivalencies between humans and monkeys. Neuron 35: 173–184.

Grefkes C, Ritzl A, Zilles K, Fink GR (2004) Human medial intraparietal cortex subserves visuomotor coordinate transformation. Neuroimage 23: 1494–1506.

Halligan PW, Marshall JC (1998) Visuospatial neglect: The ultimate deconstruction? Brain Cogn 37: 419–438.

Harris EH, Washburn DA (2005) Macaques' (Macaca mulatta) use of numerical cues in maze trials. Anim Cogn 8: 190–199.

Hauser MD, Carey S, Hauser LB (2000) Spontaneous number representation in semi-free-ranging rhesus monkeys. P Roy Soc Lond B Bio 267: 829–833.

Hauser MD, Dehaene S, Dehaene-Lambertz G, Patalano AL (2002) Spontaneous number discrimination of multi-format auditory stimuli in cotton-top tamarins (Saguinus oedipus). Cognition 86: B23–B32.

Hihara S, Obayashi S, Tanaka M, Iriki A (2003) Rapid learning of sequential tool use by macaque monkeys. Physiol Behav 78: 427–434.

Hubbard EM, Piazza M, Pinel P, Dehaene S (2005) Interactions between number and space in parietal cortex. Nat Rev Neurosci 6: 435–448.

Hubbard EM, Pinel P, Jobert A, Le Bihan D, Dehaene S (forthcoming) The place for the SNARC: Interactions between numerical and spatial representations in parietal cortex.

Hung Y-h, Hung DL, Tzeng OJ-L, Wu DH (2008) Flexible spatial mapping of different notations of numbers in Chinese readers. Cognition 106: 1441–1450.

Iriki A, Tanaka M, Iwamura Y (1996) Coding of modified body schema during tool use by macaque postcentral neurones. NeuroReport 7: 2325–2330.

Ito Y, Hatta T (2004) Spatial structure of quantitative representation of numbers: Evidence from the SNARC effect. Mem Cognition 32: 662–673.

Iwamura Y, Iriki A, Tanaka M (1994) Bilateral hand representation in the postcentral somatosensory cortex. Nature 369: 554–556.

Karnath HO, Fruhmann Berger M, Kuker W, Rorden C (2004) The anatomy of spatial neglect based on voxelwise statistical analysis: A study of 140 patients. Cereb Cortex 14: 1164–1172.

Kennett S, Eimer M, Spence C, Driver J (2001) Tactile-visual links in exogenous spatial attention under different postures: Convergent evidence from psychophysics and ERPs. J Cognitive Neurosci 13: 462–478.

Keus IM, Jenks KM, Schwarz W (2005) Psychophysiological evidence that the SNARC effect has its functional locus in a response selection stage. Cogn Brain Res 24: 48–56.

Keus IM, Schwarz W (2005) Searching for the functional locus of the SNARC effect: Evidence for a response-related origin. Mem Cognition 33: 681–695.

Lammertyn J, Fias W, Lauwereyns J (2002) Semantic influences on feature-based attention due to overlap of neural circuits. Cortex 38: 878–882.

Lavidor M, Brinksman V, Göbel SM (2004) Hemispheric asymmetry and the mental number line: Comparison of double-digit numbers. Neuropsychologia 42: 1927–1933.

Lewis JW, Van Essen DC (2000a) Mapping of architectonic subdivisions in the macaque monkey, with emphasis on parieto-occipital cortex. J Comp Neurol 428: 79–111.

Lewis JW, Van Essen DC (2000b) Corticocortical connections of visual, sensorimotor, and multimodal processing areas in the parietal lobe of the macaque monkey. J Comp Neurol 428: 112–137.

Li CS, Andersen RA (2001) Inactivation of macaque lateral intraparietal area delays initiation of the second saccade predominantly from contralesional eye positions in a double-saccade task. Exp Brain Res 137: 45–57.

Macaluso E, Driver J (2005) Multisensory spatial interactions: A window onto functional integration in the human brain. Trends Neurosci 28: 264–271.

Macaluso E, Driver J, Frith CD (2003) Multimodal spatial representations engaged in human parietal cortex during both saccadic and manual spatial orienting. Curr Biol 13: 990–999.

Malhotra P, Mannan S, Driver J, Husain M (2004) Impaired spatial working memory: One component of the visual neglect syndrome? Cortex 40: 667–676.

Mapelli D, Rusconi E, Umilta C (2003) The SNARC effect: An instance of the Simon effect? Cognition 88: B1–B10.

Matsuzawa T (1985) Use of numbers by a chimpanzee. Nature 315: 57–59.

Mayer E, Martory M-D, Pegna AJ, Landis T, Delavelle J, Annoni J-M (1999) A pure case of Gerstmann syndrome with a subangular lesion. Brain 122: 1107–1120.

Medendorp WP, Goltz HC, Crawford JD, Villis T (2005) Integration of target and effector information in human posterior parietal cortex for the planning of action. J Neurophys 93: 954–962.

Medendorp WP, Goltz HC, Villis T, Crawford JD (2003) Gaze-centered updating of visual space in human parietal cortex. J Neurosci 23: 6209–6214.

Merriam EP, Genovese GR, Colby CL (2003) Spatial updating in human parietal cortex. Neuron 39: 361–373.

Miller EK, Li L, Desimone R (1991) A neural mechanism for working and recognition memory in inferior temporal cortex. Science 254: 1377–1379.

Morris AP, Chambers CD, Mattingley JB (2007) Parietal stimulation destabilizes spatial updating across saccadic eye movements. P Natl Acad Sci USA 104: 9069–9074.

Mort DJ, Malhotra P, Mannan SK, Rorden C, Pambakian A, Kennard C, Husain M (2003) The anatomy of visual neglect. Brain 126: 1986–1997.

Moyer RS, Landauer TK (1967) Time required for judgments of numerical inequality. Nature 215: 1519–1520.

Muhlau M, Hermsdorfer J, Goldenberg G, Wohlschlager AM, Castrop F, Stahl R, Rottinger M, Erhard P, Haslinger B, Ceballos-Baumann AO, Conrad B, Boecker H (2005) Left inferior parietal dominance in gesture imitation: an fMRI study. Neuropsychologia 43: 1086–1098.

Mullette-Gillman OA, Cohen YE, Groh JM (2005) Eye-centered, head-centered, and complex coding of visual and auditory targets in the intraparietal sulcus. J Neurophysiol 94: 2331–2352.

Murata A, Gallese V, Luppino G, Kaseda M, Sakata H (2000) Selectivity for the shape, size, and orientation of objects for grasping in neurons of monkey parietal area AIP. J Neurophysiol 83: 2580–2601.

Nieder A (2005) Counting on neurons: the neurobiology of numerical competence. Nat Rev Neurosci 6: 177–190.

Nieder A, Diester I, Tudusciuc O (2006) Temporal and spatial enumeration processes in the primate parietal cortex. Science 313: 1431–1435.

Nieder A, Freedman DJ, Miller EK (2002) Representation of the quantity of visual items in the primate prefrontal cortex. Science 297: 1708–1711.

Nieder A, Miller EK (2003) Coding of cognitive magnitude: compressed scaling of numerical information in the primate prefrontal cortex. Neuron 37: 149–157.

Nieder A, Miller EK (2004) A parieto-frontal network for visual numerical information in the monkey. P Natl Acad Sci USA 101: 7457–7462.

Obayashi S, Suhara T, Kawabe K, Okauchi T, Maeda J, Akine Y, Onoe H, Iriki A (2001) Functional brain mapping of monkey tool use. Neuroimage 14: 853–861.

Opfer JE, Siegler RS (2007) Representational change and children's numerical estimation. Cognitive Psychol 55: 169–195.

Orban GA, Claeys K, Nelissen K, Smans R, Sunaert S, Todd JT, Wardak C, Durand JB, Vanduffel W (2006) Mapping the parietal cortex of human and non-human primates. Neuropsychologia 44: 2647–2667.

Orban GA, Fize D, Peuskens H, Denys K, Nelissen K, Sunaert S, Todd J, Vanduffel W (2003) Similarities and differences in motion processing between the human and macaque brain: Evidence from fMRI. Neuropsychologia 41: 1757–1768.

Orban GA, Van Essen D, Vanduffel W (2004) Comparative mapping of higher visual areas in monkeys and humans. Trends Cogn Sci 8: 315–324.

Piazza M, Giacomini E, Le Bihan D, Dehaene S (2003) Single-trial classification of parallel pre-attentive and serial attentive processes using functional magnetic resonance imaging. Proc Roy Soc Lond B 270: 1237–1245.

Piazza M, Izard V, Pinel P, Le Bihan D, Dehaene S (2004) Tuning curves for approximate numerosity in the human intraparietal sulcus. Neuron 44: 547–555.

Piazza M, Pinel P, Le Bihan D, Dehaene S (2007) A magnitude code common to numerosities and number symbols in human intraparietal cortex. Neuron 53: 293–305.

Pica P, Lemer C, Izard V, Dehaene S (2004) Exact and approximate arithmetic in an Amazonian indigene group. Science 306: 499–503.

Pinel P, Dehaene S, Riviere D, Le Bihan D (2001) Modulation of parietal activation by semantic distance in a number comparison task. Neuroimage 14: 1013–1026.

Pinel P, Piazza M, Le Bihan D, Dehaene S (2004) Distributed and overlapping cerebral representations of number, size, and luminance during comparative judgments. Neuron 41: 983–993.

Pouget A, Deneve S, Duhamel JR (2002) A computational perspective on the neural basis of multisensory spatial representations. Nat Rev Neurosci 3: 741–747.

Priftis K, Zorzi M, Meneghello F, Marenzi R, Umilta C (2006) Explicit vs. implicit processing of representational space in neglect: Dissociations in accessing the mental number line. J Cognitive Neurosci 18: 680–688.

Ristic J, Wright A, Kingstone A (2006) The number line effect reflects top-down control. Psychon Bull Rev 13: 862–868.

Rode G, Rossetti Y, Boisson D (2001) Prism adaptation improves representational neglect. Neuropsychologia 39: 1250–1254.

Rossetti Y, Jacquin-Courtois S, Rode G, Ota H, Michel C, Boisson D (2004) Does action make the link between number and space representation? Visuo-manual adaptation improves number bisection in unilateral neglect. Psychol Sci 15: 426–430.

Rossetti Y, Rode G, Pisella L, Farne A, Li L, Boisson D, Perenin MT (1998) Prism adaptation to a rightward optical deviation rehabilitates left hemispatial neglect. Nature 395: 166–169.

Roux F-E, Boetto S, Sacko O, Chollet F, Trémoulet M (2003) Writing, calculating, and finger recognition in the region of the angular gyrus: a cortical stimulation study of Gerstmann syndrome. J Neurosurg 99: 716–727.

Rusconi E, Turatto M, Umiltà C (2008) Two orienting mechanisms in posterior parietal lobule: An rTMS study of the Simon and SNARC effects. Cognitive Neuropsychol, in press.

Rusconi E, Umilta C, Galfano G (2006) Breaking ranks: Space and number may march to the beat of a different drum. Cortex 42: 1124–1127.

Saito DN, Okada T, Morita Y, Yonekura Y, Sadato N (2003) Tactile-visual cross-modal shape matching: A functional MRI study. Cogn Brain Res 17: 14–25.

Sakata H, Taira M, Kusunoki M, Murata A, Tsutsui K, Tanaka Y, Shein WN, Miyashita Y (1999) Neural representation of three-dimensional features of manipulation objects with stereopsis. Exp Brain Res 128: 160–169.

Sawamura H, Shima K, Tanji J (2002) Numerical representation for action in the parietal cortex of the monkey. Nature 415: 918–922.

Schluppeck D, Curtis CE, Glimcher PW, Heeger DJ (2006) Sustained activity in topographic areas of human posterior parietal cortex during memory-guided saccades. J Neurosci 26: 5098–5108.

Schluppeck D, Glimcher PW, Heeger DJ (2005) Topographic organization for delayed saccades in human posterior parietal cortex. J Neurophysiol 94: 1372–1384.

Schwarz W, Keus IM (2004) Moving the eyes along the mental number line: Comparing SNARC effects with saccadic and manual responses. Percept Psychophys 66: 651–664.

Schwarz W, Müller D (2006) Spatial associations in number-related tasks: A Comparison of manual and pedal responses. Exp Psychol 53: 4–15.

Sereno MI, Huang RS (2006) A human parietal face area contains aligned head-centered visual and tactile maps. Nat Neurosci 9: 1337–1343.

Sereno MI, Pitzalis S, Martinez A (2001) Mapping of contralateral space in retinotopic coordinates by a parietal cortical area in humans. Science 294: 1350–1354.

Shikata E, Hamzei F, Glauche V, Knab R, Dettmers C, Weiller C, Buchel C (2001) Surface orientation discrimination activates caudal and anterior intraparietal sulcus in humans: An event-related fMRI study. J Neurophysiol 5: 1309–1314.

Shikata E, Hamzei F, Glauche V, Koch M, Weiller C, Binkofski F, Buchel C (2003) Functional properties and interaction of the anterior and posterior intraparietal areas in humans. Eur J Neurosci 17: 1105–1110.

Siegler RS, Opfer JE (2003) The development of numerical estimation: Evidence for multiple representations of numerical quantity. Psychol Sci 14: 237–243.

Silver MA, Ress D, Heeger DJ (2005) Topographic maps of visual spatial attention in human parietal cortex. J Neurophysiol 94: 1358–1371.

Simon O, Mangin JF, Cohen L, Le Bihan D, Dehaene S (2002) Topographical layout of hand, eye, calculation, and language-related areas in the human parietal lobe. Neuron 33: 475–487.

Singh S (1997) Fermat's Last Theorem. London: Fourth Estate.

Snyder LH, Batista AP, Andersen RA (2000) Intention-related activity in the posterior parietal cortex: A review. Vision Res 40: 1433–1441.

Spence C, Pavani F, Driver J (2000) Crossmodal links between vision and touch in covert endogenous spatial attention. J Exp Psychol Hum Percept Perform 26: 1298–1319.

Stanescu-Cosson R, Pinel P, van De Moortele PF, Le Bihan D, Cohen L, Dehaene S (2000) Understanding dissociations in dyscalculia: A brain imaging study of the impact of number size on the cerebral networks for exact and approximate calculation. Brain 123: 2240–2255.

Stoianov I, Kramer P, Umilta C, Zorzi M (2008) Visuospatial priming of the mental number line. Cognition 106: 770–779.

Swisher JD, Halko MA, Merabet LB, McMains SA, Somers DC (2007) Visual topography of human intraparietal sulcus. J Neurosci 27: 5326–5337.

Taira M, Georgopolous AP, Murata A, Sakata H (1990) Parietal cortex neurons of the monkey related to the visual guidance of hand movement. Exp Brain Res 79: 155–166.

Thompson RF, Mayers KS, Robertson RT, Patterson CJ (1970) Number coding in association cortex of the cat. Science 168: 271–273.

Van Essen DC, Lewis JW, Drury HA, Hadjikhani N, Tootell RBH, Bakircioglu M, Miller MI (2001) Mapping visual cortex in monkeys and humans using surface-based atlases. Vision Res 41: 1359–1378.

Verguts T, Fias W (2004) Representation of number in animals and humans: A neural model. J Cognitive Neurosci 16: 1493–1504.

Vuilleumier P, Ortigue S, Brugger P (2004) The number space and neglect. Cortex 40: 399–410.

Wardak C, Olivier E, Duhamel JR (2002) Saccadic target selection deficits after lateral intraparietal area inactivation in monkeys. J Neurosci 22: 9877–9884.

Wardak C, Olivier E, Duhamel JR (2004) A deficit in covert attention after parietal cortex inactivation in the monkey. Neuron 42: 501–508.

Wood G, Nuerk HC, Willmes K (2006) Crossed hands and the SNARC effect: A failure to replicate Dehaene, Bossini and Giraux (1993). Cortex 42: 1069–1079.

Zebian S (2005) Linkages between number concepts, spatial thinking, and directionality of writing: The SNARC effect and the reverse SNARC effect in English and Arabic monoliterates, biliterates, and illiterate Arabic speakers. J Cogn Culture 5: 165–190.

Zhang T, Heuer HW, Britten KH (2004) Parietal area VIP neuronal responses to heading stimuli are encoded in head-centered coordinates. Neuron 42: 993–1001.

Zorzi M, Priftis K, Umiltà C (2002) Neglect disrupts the mental number line. Nature 417: 138–139.

12 Learning in Core and Noncore Domains

Rochel Gelman

Different researchers have different ideas regarding the domain-specific approach to learning and its implications for an account of early cognitive development and learning. This leads me to focus on the oft-repeated question: What is a domain? I start with this question, then I discuss the difference between core and noncore domains, and follow with the respective distinctions between domains that have an innate basis and those that do not. The distinction between core and noncore domains dispels the widespread interpretation that all domain-specific theoretical accounts imply a commitment to a new form of nativism.

The Notion of a Domain

I and other developmentalists hold that an area of knowledge constitutes a domain if it has a set of coherent principles that form a structure and contains domain-specific entities that are domain-specific and that can combine to form other entities within the domain (Gelman 1990; Spelke 2000). The domain of causality is about the kinds of conditions that lead objects to move and transform as well as how they move or change. It dominates several classes of items, including those that are separably movable and those that are not. Regarding the former, we can distinguish between those that move by themselves and those that do not.[1] These are of course the classes of animate and inanimate objects. Different considerations apply regarding both the nature of the object and its sources of energy. Setting aside machines, the energy for separably movable animate objects is from within or inside the organism, whereas that for inanimates is external. Importantly, the kind of material the object is made of and the material's composition and are yoked to these causal distinctions. As predicted, even preschoolers treat machines as a separate default category from either the animate or inanimate ones, given the ambiguity between machines' inanimate material and their seemingly self-generated motion (Gelman 2002).

The distinction between the classes of animate and inanimate objects that are separably movable goes hand in hand with the fact that animate objects are composed of biological matter and honor biomechanical principles as well as principles of mechanics, whereas inanimate objects are composed of nonbiological material and honor only principles of mechanics. Further, animate motions have a quality of purpose or function. This is a direct consequence of their governance by control mechanisms that make it possible for animates to respond (adjust) to environments—be these social or nonsocial—and adapt to unforeseeable changes in circumstances. Such considerations mean that the priors for learning about animates include principles that are social, including collaboration, reciprocity, and the capacity to perceive and communicate (Gelman et al. 1995; Gelman and Lucariello 2002).

The present definition of domain implies that different domains are organized according to different principles and include only those entities that are constrained by the given principles. So the entities of the causality domain are qualitatively different from those for the domain of language. The causality domain does not contain any basic linguistic elements that are combined to make a sentence. The principles for generating phonemes, morphemes, and sentences are organized by principles that constitute linguistic structures. It makes no sense to ask whether the "movement" of the word *how* in sentences (1) and (2) is due to internal biological energy or forces of nature.

1.   He knows *how* to go there.

2.   *How* does he know to go there?

For yet another domain, that of arithmetic and the subordinate principles that govern counting, still different entities and structures are involved. It does not matter how large an entity is when one engages counting principles to generate a cardinal value to add to or subtract from another quantity. Indeed, the to-be-counted entities need not even be objects. They can be imaginary playmates, good ideas at a conference, or cracks in the sidewalk. The entities generated by the counting principles are such that they can be combined to produce yet further examples of quantities within the domain.

To repeat: Whenever we can state that a unique set of principles serves to capture the structure of a domain of knowledge and the entities within it, either by themselves or ones generated according to the combination rules of the structure, it is appropriate to postulate a kind of domain-specific knowledge.

Core and Noncore Domains

Domains can either be based on innate skeletal structures or acquired later on in development. This is a crucial point. It is a mistake to assume that all domains of knowledge are based on innate skeletal structures. Indeed, thus far the discussion of what counts as a domain is neutral as to whether a given domain is innate or not. I call domains that benefit from biological underpinnings *core* domains (Gelman and Williams 1998), in way that is similar to Spelke (2000). Domains of organized knowledge that are acquired later are called *noncore* domains. Thus, I reserve the phrase *core domain* for domains that have an innate origin and noncore domain for those that require the acquisition of both the structure and related content. Examples of noncore domains include chess, sushi making, and all kinds of advanced fields in physics, mathematics, movie making, computer science, and so on. Importantly, it is a mistake to label information-processing operations—such as discrimination, attention, or classification—as domains. These are processes that are orthogonal to the distinction between core and noncore domains. They may or may not be variables that differ across domains. But, this is a theoretical position that remains to be tested.

We know from the literature on adult cognitive psychology that it is always much easier to learn more about a content domain if we already possess a coherent understanding of that domain. We also know that it is difficult to acquire new conceptual structures. One has to work at the goal of building a new domain of knowledge for many years, and it helps to have formal tutoring about what to learn and what to practice (Bransford et al. 1999). Often when one is exposed to a new domain it seems incomprehensible. For example, beginning chemistry undergraduates in their first class might think that the words "bond," "attraction," "model," and so forth are related to business and cannot imagine why these terms are being used in chemistry. These students surely are not in a position to understand the technical meaning of these terms as they are used in chemistry and therefore are at risk for misunderstanding them or even of dropping the course. We know from research that such knowledge is the kind attributed to experts and we know that it takes a great deal of work over many, many years to acquire expertise for any noncore domain (Ericsson 2006). A characterization of noncore domains is presented in a later section.

For young children, having some nascent mental structures for various domains means that they have a leg up when it comes to learning about the data that can put flesh on these early structures. A core domain's principles serve to outline the equivalence class of inputs that are relevant, that can nurture the acquisition of the domain-relevant body of knowledge. Of course the notion of "skeletal" is a metaphor meant to capture the idea that core domains do not start out being knowledge-rich or even complete. Nevertheless, no matter how nascent these mental structures may be, they are mental structures. And, like all bodily structures, they are actively used to engage with relevant environments—those that have the potential to nourish their growth. They accomplish this by directing attention and permitting the uptake into memory of relevant data in the environment. In this way, they provide a way to gather together domain-relevant memories within a common structure. This line of reasoning highlights the role of structure mapping as a fundamental learning mechanism.

More on Core Domains

Natural number arithmetic is an example of a core domain. Importantly, the principles of arithmetic (addition, subtraction, and ordering) and their entities (numerons and separate, orderable discrete and continuous quantities) do not overlap with those involved in the causal principles and their link to separably movable animate and inanimate objects. As a result, examples of relevant entities and their properties are distinctly different. For no matter what the conceptual or perceptual entities are, if you think they constitute a to-be-counted collection of separate entities, you can count them. It even is permissible to decide to count the spaces between telephone poles (a favorite game of many young American children) or collect for counting the temporary set of every person and writing utensil in a particular room. This is because there is no principled restriction on the kinds of items that can be counted. The only requirement is that the items be taken to be perceptually or conceptually separable. I later develop the evidence and argument that skeletal structures in the domain of positive natural number arithmetic benefit from nonverbal structures that define relevance regarding the verbal instantiation of counting and its related principles of arithmetic.

Now consider the domains of animate and inanimate causality. There is no question that the nature and characteristics of the entities really do matter. The way one plans to interact with an object is constrained by the kind of entity it is and its environment. If the entity is an animate object, when deciding whether to pet it or run away as fast possible I will take into account the object's size, how it moves, how fast it can move, whether it has teeth, and so on. If I want to move two desks, I have to take into account their size and likely weight as well as my own limits. I will do the same should I be asked to also lift the two men sitting in chairs. I know that I do not have the kind of strength it takes to lift and move the men, whereas I might be able to push the desks. So objects' material, weight, and size definitely do matter when I consider the conditions under which they move. This contrast accomplishes what we want–an a priori account of psychological relevance. If the learner's goal is to engage in counting, then attention has to be paid to identifying and keeping as separate the to-be-counted entities but not their particular attributes, let alone their weight.

Similarly, if the learner's goal is to think about animate or inanimate objects, then attention has to be given to the information that provides clues about animacy or inanimacy, for example, whether the object communicates with and responds in kind to like objects, moves by itself, and is made up of what we consider biological material. Food surely is another core domain. We care about the color of a kind of food, whereas we rarely care about the color of an artifact or countable entity. It is noteworthy that children as young as two years of age also take the color of food into account (Macario 1991).

Defining Core Domains

So how should we think about core domains? I offer the following of criteria.

1. Core domains are *mental structures*. To start, they are far from fully developed, which is why I use the metaphor of "skeletal." Despite their incompleteness, they are structures

that actively engage the environment from the start. This a consequence of their being biological, mental organizations that function to collect domain-relevant data and hence provide the needed "memory drawer" for the buildup of knowledge that is organized in a way that is consistent with the principles of the domain.

2. Core domains help us solve the problem of *selective attention*. They provide a way for us to avoid the common circular argument that selective attention is due to salience and salience directs attention. Potential relevant candidate data are those that that fit the equivalence class outlined by the principles of the domain, which define the relevance dimensions.

3. They are *universal*. One reason to say that core domains are universal is that they can support learning about any data sets that cohere as domain-relevant examples of the structure of the core domain. The particular set of examples of inputs can vary across cultures. There are no known restrictions of the possibility of adopting any healthy infant into any language culture. Children in different language communities all learn to speak in sentences that share the organization of Noun Phrase and Verb Phrase as well as key combination rules. In a similar way, children everywhere think about instances of animate and inanimate objects as belonging to separate categories, even though the particular examples vary from culture to culture. For these reasons, we can expect variability across cultures as far as the particular language that is spoken, the different instances of animals that will be known, and so on. Since the kind of data a given culture offers young children varies as a function of geography, urbanization, and other factors, it follows that the range of knowledge about the animate-inanimate domain will vary. Still, the organizing principles will be the same during early acquisition (Waxman et al. 2007).

Linguists who posit that there are universal principles supporting language acquisition do not expect children to learn their language in two days. The main idea is that the learning occurs on the fly and without formal instruction. The same considerations hold for other domains. We now know that even infants abstract and process numerical displays and reason about the effects of numerical operations (Cordes and Brannon 2006). They also make inferences about unseen causes (Saxe et al. 2006).

When we posit that young learners use universal innate principles to find relevant inputs, we end up with a challenge. Given that the learner's self-generated attention is a key contributor to what counts as relevant data, we no longer can assume that we know what inputs will or will not foster such active learning. Nor do we know how many examples or how much of each example is necessary. The challenge to is find the kind of theory of learning that accounts for early learnings that occur on the fly, without formal instruction and the extent to which these early acquisitions serve as bridges or barriers to later learnings. We also need to study the nature of relevant environments so as to develop a theory of supporting inputs for learning. At present, many assume that learning takes place whenever an organism is presented with sufficient examples of any kind of inputs.

Ethologists constitute a notable exception to this generalization. They take it granted that innate learning dispositions have to encounter environments that are examples of existing predilections. A given biological predisposition must encounter particular inputs for the behavior in question to develop. The terms "innate" and "learned" are not opposite nor mutually exclusive. (See Gelman and Williams 1998, for further discussion.)

4. Core domains are akin to *labeled and structured memory drawers* where data acceptable to the domain are incorporated. This provides an account of how it is possible to build up a coherent knowledge domain.

5. Core domains support *learning on the fly*. They support this type of learning because of the child's active tendencies to search for supporting environments in the physical, social, or communicative worlds offered by the environment. The fact that learning occurs on the fly and is a function of what the child attends to is why many students of young children's early cognitive development have moved in to postulate core domains. It also is related to efforts to enrich early learning with core domain examples of domain-relevant learning environments such as preschools and daycare centers (Gelman et al., forthcoming).

6. The principles of the structure and entities within a domain are *implicit*. They cannot be stated by an adult (not to mention an infant), any more than a nonexpert adult can state linguistic principles.

7. Children are highly *motivated to learn* in these domains. They ask relevant questions, including how a remote control works, why a parent says the car battery is dead, what number comes after 100, 1000, and so forth. I well remember a little girl in a schoolyard telling me she was too busy to talk. She had set herself to count to "a million." I asked when she thought she would get there. Her reply was, "A very, very, very long time." She pointed out that she needed to eat, sleep, and probably would be very old.

Many young children's inclinations to self-correct and rehearse are part of their overall tendencies to put into place the competencies that are within their purview. Examples of young children self-correcting their efforts or even rehearsing what they have just learned are ubiquitous in the developmental literature. A common report from parents has to do with their children asking, "What's that?" after the parents have answered the question many, many times. Such rituals can go on for days and, then, for no obvious reason, drop off the radar screen. In a related way, we are finding that the children from right across the socioeconomic spectrum in the preschools where we work are eager to have us ask more questions about unfamiliar animate and inanimate objects (Gelman and Brenneman 2004).

8. The number of core domains is probably *relatively small*. A core domain is only going to be as large as is necessary for each individual to possess universal shared knowledge without formal instruction. Just as the core domain of language supports the acquisition

of different languages in different language communities, different language-cultural communities favor differential uptake of the relevant data that they offer. Nevertheless, the underlying structure of the core domain should be common—at least to start.

On Early Learning

The Role of Structure Mapping

For me, the most important learning mechanism is *structure mapping*. Possessing an existing structure, the human mind will run it roughshod over the environment, finding those data that are isomorphic to what it already has stored in a structured way. It could be that an infant first identifies the examples of the relevant patterned inputs and then maps to the relevant structure. Subsequently further sections of the pattern are put in place. In any case, the details that are assimilated fit into a growing set of the class of relevant data that fill in the basic structure.

Importantly, input data may vary considerably in terms of surface characteristics as long as they are in the class of data that are recognizable by the domain's principles. This carries with it the implication that the input stimuli do not have to be identical; in fact, they are most likely to be variants of the same underlying structure. Multiple examples offer a number of advantages: They provide different ways of doing the same thing, opportunities to compare and contrast items to zero in on whether they are in the same domain. Given an existing structure, a child can self-monitor and self-correct, saying, "That's not right; try again." In fact, in our counting protocols, we have examples of children saying, "One, two, three, five—no, try dat again!" for five trials, then getting it right and saying, "Whew!" Nobody tells children to do this; they just do it. We see a lot of this kind spontaneous correction or rehearsal of learning that is related to the available structure.

Natural Number

There is a very large literature now on whether babies and young preschoolers count, can order displays representing different numerical values, and process the effect of addition and subtraction on an expected value. For a number of years the evidence did not favor this position. Instead it was held that infants respond to overall quantity variables that are confounds on numerosity, as might be the overall length or area of a display (see Mix et al. 1997). The tide has once again turned to favoring the view that infants do abstract number from dot displays (Cordes et al. 2007; see also Brannon and Cantlon, chapter 10, this volume).

The various studies that report the use of nonverbal counting as well as addition, subtraction, and ordering lend credence to our account of how these operations benefit beginning learners' acquisition of the language of counting and simple arithmetic.

It is crucial to keep in mind my view that counting principles are embedded in the domain of positive natural number under addition and subtraction. If so, the meaning of a count word does not stand alone. Given the fact that available structures can pick out isomorphs, the use rules for verbal counting can be mapped to the underlying nonverbal counting principles that young children bring to their verbal environment. Since people use their mental structures to find data that feed these structures, this means that beginning language learners are likely to attend to and start to learn the nonsense string of sounds that constitutes the verbal counting list ("one-two-three" etc.). Keep in mind that there is nothing about the sound "won" that dictates it will be followed by the sound "too" and so on.

The principled requirements for verbal counting lists are that the words follow some basic rules: (1) The *one-to-one* principle. If you are going to count, you have to have available a set of tags that can be placed one for one, for each of the items, without skipping, jumping, or using the same tag more than once. (2) The *stable order* principle. Whatever the mental tags are, they have to be used in a stable order over trials. If they were not, you would not know how to treat the last tag—the total amount. This relates to (3) the *cardinal value*, which is conserved over irrelevant changes. The relevant arithmetic principles are ordering, adding, and subtracting. Counting itself is constrained by three principles. If you want to know whether the last tag used in a tagging list is *understood as a cardinal number*, it is important to consider whether a child relates these to arithmetic principles; it helps also to determine how the child treats the effects of adding and subtracting.

Count words behave differently than adjectives, even when they are in the same position in a sentence. It is acceptable to say of a set of four round circles that "a circle is round" or to speak of "a round circle," but one cannot say "a circle is four" or speak of "a four circle."

What about addition and subtraction? A rather long time ago, I started studying whether very young children two and a half to five years keep track of the number-specific effects of addition and subtraction. In one series of experiments, I used a magic show that was modeled after discussions with people in Philadelphia who specialized in doing magic with children (Gelman 1972). The procedure is a modification of a shell game. It starts with an adult showing a child two small toys on one plate and three on another plate (see figure 12.1). One plate is randomly dubbed the winner, the other the loser. The adult does not mention number but does say several times which is the winner plate and which is the loser plate. Henceforth both plates are covered by cans and the child is to guess where the winner is. The child picks up a can, and if it hides the winner plate the child gets a prize to immediately to put in an envelope. If the child does not see a winner, he or she is asked where it is, at which point the child picks up the other one and then gets a prize. The use of a correction procedure is deliberate: it helps children realize that we are not doing anything unusual, at least from their point of view. This set-up continues for ten or eleven trials, at which point the children encounter a surreptitiously altered display either because items were rearranged or because they changed in color, kind, or number).

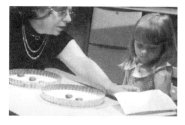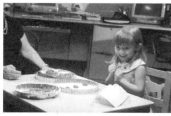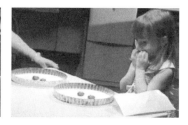

Figure 12.1
The three phases of the Gelman (1972) "magic game," shown from left to right. In phase 1, the child is shown uncovered displays and told that one is the winner, the other the loser. She is asked to identify each and told about winning prizes that will be stored in the envelope. To start phase 2, the displays are covered and shuffled for ten or eleven trials. When she picks up a winner, she gets a prize. In phase 3 she unexpectedly encounters the effect of a surreptitious change in the number on the winner plate. Notice the shift from her exuberant mood to one of puzzlement.

The effect of adding or subtracting an object led to notable surprise reactions (see figure 12.1c). Children did a variety of things such as putting their fingers in their mouths, changing facial expression, starting searching, and even asking for another object ("I need another mouse"). That is, they responded in a way that is consistent with the assumption that addition or subtraction is relevant, and they know how to relate them. When we show two-year-olds 1 vs. 2 to start and then transfer to 3 vs. 4 items, the children transfer greater-than or less-than relationship, whichever they learned about in phase 1. That is, we have behavior that fits predictions that follow from the description of the natural number operations.

In a more recent experiment, Hurewitz and colleagues (2006) asked children ranging in age from almost three to almost four to place a sticker on a two- or four-item frame, in one set of testing trials. In a second set of testing trial, they then placed stickers on a *some* vs. *many* frame. The children had an easier time with the request that used numerals than with the one that used quantifiers. This provides another example of early use of cardinal numerosity. The finding that the word "some" gave them the most difficulties in this task challenges the view that beginning language learners bootstrap their understanding of counting words off their earlier understanding of quantifiers (Carey 2001). Further examples of young children's facility with positive natural number can be found in Gelman (2006).

The Animate-Inanimate Distinction and Related Causal Principles

If young children benefit from available skeletal principles, they should be able to solve novel problems with novel stimuli. This led Massey and Gelman (1988) to show preschool children photographs of novel animates, vertebrates and nonvertebrates; statues selected to look like people and animals; wheeled objects; and inert complex objects such as an electric iron. Examples also included a photograph of an echidna, a large "bug," Chinese statues, and wheeled objects from the turn of the nineteenth century. Graduate students were asked to name the items, and when they could not do so it confirmed our expectation that these objects would be novel for young children.

The question put to three- and four-year-old children was a simple one: Could the depicted item go up and down a hill by itself? They judged that only the novel animates could do this. A wheeled object might go down a hill "by itself," given a push, but not up. And the complex inert objects would not be able to move in either direction. Children this age are not especially good at explaining their responses, but when they did so, their explanations were extremely informative. For example, one child said that a statue did not have feet, even though it did. We pointed this out and learned that the feet were "not real." Some children told us that the echidna could move itself because it had feet, even though we pointed out that none were visible. The rejoinder? The echnida was sitting on its feet. These kinds of responses have led us to find ways to show that young children yoke biologically relevant data with the capacity to move on one's own.

A different line of relevant work comes from the extensive collection of findings about infants' ability to assign animate agency to actors in videotapes (see Kulhmeier et al. 2003). The explosion of research like this is directly due to a number of investigators' commitment to a domain-specific theoretical agenda.

There will be many a debate about the findings, but one thing is certain: The domain-specific view has prompted researchers to design studies regarding the possible abstract levels of data interpretations on the part of the very young children.

The Nature of Noncore Domains

Noncore domains have six primary features.

1. Noncore domains are *not universal*; there is no representation of the targeted learning domain, and therefore an individual does not start with any understanding of the data of the domain.

2. Noncore domains involve the *mounting of new mental structures* for understanding and require considerable effort over an extended period time, typically about ten years.

3. Noncore domains are *not processes*, such as discrimination learning, attention, inhibition, and other terms that often serve as chapter headings in textbooks. These task or processe terms do not capture the notion of a body of organized, structured knowledge.

4. The number of noncore domains is *not restricted*. This is related to the fact that individuals make different commitments regarding the extensive effort needed to build a coherent domain of knowledge and related skills. Success at achieving the chosen learning goals depends extensively on individuals' abilities to stick with their chosen learning problem, their talents, and the quality of relevant inputs, be these text materials, cultural values, demonstrations, or the skills of a teacher or tutor. Some examples of masters of noncore domains include: CEO of a Fortune 500 company, chess master, dog show judge,

linguist, army general, composer, master chef, theoretical physicist, yacht racer, string theorist, sushi chef, and so on.

5. Learning about a noncore domain almost always depends on *extensive help from a teacher or master* of the domain—an individual who selects and structures input and provides feedback. Still, no matter how well-prepared the teacher might be, the learner often has a major problem if she is unable to detect or pick up relationships or at least parts of relationships that eventually will relate to other relevant inputs, for example, what characterizes a musical interval of a third, no matter what the key. The task can be even more demanding if one has to acquire a new notational system—for example, learn a new alphabet—which can be challenging in its own right.

6. Early talent in noncore domains *does not guarantee acquisition* of expertise. It takes around ten years of dedicated work to reach the level of expert for the domain in question, whether the domain is in the arts, athletics, academics, or a host of other areas (see Ericsson 2006 for a review and theoretical discussion).

Comparison of a Core Domain to a Noncore Domain

I will conclude by comparing two contrasting numerical concepts, one of which is part of a core domain and one of which is part of a noncore domain.

Successor Principle Is Easy; Rational Numbers Are Hard

Every natural number has a unique "next" number, and it is always possible to add one to a given very large number. The more formal way to put this is to say that the successor principle belongs to the core domain of natural number. By way of contrast, there is no successor principle for the rational numbers. There is an infinite number of rational numbers between any pair of rationals. Rational numbers are not the same as natural numbers, Each is obtained by dividing one natural number by another and therefore do not belong to the same domain.

Assuming that young children know that adding one to a given cardinal number produces a new higher one, we predicted that children in the early elementary grades would readily achieve an explicit induction of the successor principle. As expected, when Hartnett and Gelman (1998) asked children ranging in age from about six years to eight years of age if they could keep adding 1 to the biggest number that they could or were thinking about, a surprising number indicated that they could. Even when we suggested that a googol or some other very large cardinal number was the biggest number there could be, the children resisted and noted it was possible to add another to our number.

The successor principle is seldom taught in elementary school, even though children can easily comprehend it. Notions about rational numbers (also known as fractions) are, on the other hand, taught in elementary school. Still, it is well known that students have a very hard time coming to understand rational numbers (Hartnett and Gelman 1998). The fact that children benefit from a short overview about the successor principle but do not benefit from formal instruction about fractions and division contribute to my conclusion that the rational numbers constitute a noncore domain.

The problem with rational numbers might well be that the principles involved both contradict and are different from those for the domain of natural numbers. The successor principle does not apply. Further, the formal definition of a rational number introduces a new operation, this being division. The answer to a division problem need not be a third cardinal number. The odds are that there will be a remainder. Still, people have a clear tendency to throw away the remainder—that is, to turn a rational number into a cardinal number. This begins to give one the flavor of why I propose that the domain of rational numbers is a noncore domain that involves conceptual change. That is, one has to learn that there is a new kind of number and then assimilate the natural numbers to the rationals (100/100 = 1; 200/100 = 2, etc.).

To continue with the problem of rationals, I illustrate the kind of errorful but systematic patterns of responses we have obtained from school-aged children asked to place in order, from left to right, a series of number symbols, each one of which is on a separate card. The children were given pretest practice at placing sticks of different lengths on an ordering cloth. They also were told that it was acceptable to put sticks there of the same length but different colors and to move sticks. Then the test cards followed, until they were happy with their placement order. Careful inspection of the placements reveals that the children invented natural number solutions. For example, an eight-year-old started by placing each of three cards left to right as follows: 1/2, 2/2, 2-1/2, etc. What the child is doing is taking the first pair of numbers and adding them, and getting 3; the second and adding them, etc. The following interpretation captures these and all of his further placements. A bit of thought reveals that the child took the cards as an opportunity to treat the problem as a novel opportunity to apply his knowledge of natural number addition:

$(1 + 2 = 3), (2 + 2 = 4), (2 + 1 + 2 = 5)$

Other children invented different patterns, but all invented some kind of interpretation that was based on natural numbers.

One might think that students would master the placement of fractions and rational numbers well before they enter college. Unfortunately, this is not the case. When Obrecht and colleagues (2007) asked whether undergraduates made use of the law of large numbers when asked to reason intuitively about statistics, they determined that students who could simply solve percentage and decimal problems were reliably more able to do so. Those who made a lot of errors preferred to use the few examples they encountered that violated the trend achieved by a very large number of instances (Obrecht et al. 2007). This continues into college. If you want to know now why your students are horrified and gasp when they are faced with a graph, it is probably because a nontrivial percentage does not understand rational numbers and measurement.

Other Noncore Domains

Although young children rapidly learn a great deal about the difference between animate and inanimate objects as well as factors that are encompassed by these, it does not follow that it will be just as easy to learn Newton's laws. In fact, it is well known that many a college student who has taken physics comes away with her pre-Newtonian beliefs intact. It is hard to grasp that velocity and acceleration are different concepts, let alone that something at its resting place has zero velocity. These difficulties persist, despite the fact that Newtonian physics has been part of Western culture for several centuries. Similar comments apply to the task of learning modern biology. Conceptual changes do not come easily, a fact that needs to be taken into account in light of the persistent calls for upgrading the scientific and mathematical literacy of the citizens of the world.

Summary

Domains are bodies of knowledge that are organized by a set of principles or rules. They are not information processing operations such as attention, discrimination, inhibition, etc. Core domains constitute a small domain-specific, group of skeletal domains that are part of our endowment and support learning on the fly, all over the world. Of course, the relevant data must be part of the child's everyday environment, and preferably in multiple contexts. Absence of samples from the relevant equivalence class of supporting data might be akin to deprivation. Noncore domains differ by virtue of the fact that their acquisition requires the mounting of new mental structures as well as the body of evidence that the structures organize. Further, teachers or tutors create the relevant inputs and oversee the learning, while learners—even those with definite talents—do serious, concentrated work for many years.

Acknowledgments

This chapter was enriched by the author's participation in a meeting entitled "Dialogues with Chomsky" that took place in San Sebastian, Spain, July, 2006. The talks dealt with the topic of how to characterize domains and distinguish between core and noncore domains. Partial support for this paper was provided by NSF ROLE Grant REC-0529579 and research funds from Rutgers University.

Note

1. A parallel distinction applies to objects attached to the ground. Now it is between things that grow and inanimate structures such as buildings, bridges, etc. These are not discussed here save to point out that the distinction living-inert embraces both separably movable and stationary object kinds. The higher-order classification is biological vs. inert.

References

Bransford JD, Brown AL, Cocking RR, eds (1999) How people learn: Brain, mind, experience and school. Washington, DC: National Academy of Sciences.

Carey S (2001) On the very possibility of discontinuities in conceptual development. In: Language, brain, and cognitive development (Dupoux E, ed), 304–324. Cambridge, MA: MIT Press.

Cordes S, Gallistel CR, Gelman R, Latham P (2007) Nonverbal arithmetic in arithmetic: Light from noise. Percept Psychophys 69: 1185–1203.

Ericsson KA (2006) The influence of experience and deliberate practice on the development of superior expert performance. In: Cambridge handbook of expertise and expert performance (Ericsson KA, Charness N, Feltovich P, Hoffman RR, eds), 685–706. Cambridge: Cambridge University Press.

Gelman R (1972) Logical capacity of very young children: Number invariance rules. Child Dev 43: 74–90.

Gelman R (1990) First principles organize attention to relevant data and the acquisition of numerical and causal concepts. Cognitive Sci 14: 79–106.

Gelman R (2002) Animates and other worldly things. In: Representation, memory, and development: Essays in honor of Jean Mandler (Stein N, Bauer P, Rabinowitz M, eds), 75–87. Mahwah, NJ: Lawrence Erlbaum.

Gelman R (2006) The young child as natural-number arithmetician. Curr Dir Psychol Sci 15: 193–197.

Gelman R, Brenneman K (2004) Relevant pathways for preschool science learning. Early Child Q Rev 19: 150–158.

Gelman R, Brenneman K, Macdonald G, Roman M (in press). Preschool pathways to science. Baltimore: Brookes.

Gelman R, Durgin F, Kaufman L (1995) Distinguishing between animates and inanimates: Not by motion alone. In: Causality and culture (Sperber D, Premack D, Premack A, eds), 150–184. Oxford: Plenum Press.

Gelman R, Lucariello J (2002). Learning in cognitive development. In: Stevens' handbook of experimental psychology, volume 3. 3rd ed. (Pashler H, Gallistel CR, eds). New York: Wiley.

Gelman R, Williams E (1998) Enabling constraints for cognitive development and learning: Domain specificity and epigenesis. In: Handbook of child psychology, 5th ed. (Kuhn D, Siegler R, eds), volume 2: Cognition, perception and language, 575–630. New York: Wiley.

Hartnett PM, Gelman R (1998). Early understanding of numbers: Paths or barriers to the construction of new understanding? Learn Instr 8: 341–374.

Hurewitz F, Papafragou A, Gleitman LR, Gelman R (2006) Asymmetries in the acquisition of numbers and quantifiers. Lang Learn Dev 2: 77–96.

Macario J (1991) Young children's use of color in classification: Foods and canonically colored objects. Cognitive Dev 6: 17–46.

Massey C, Gelman R (1988) Preschoolers' ability to decide whether a photographed unfamiliar object can move itself. Dev Psychol 24: 307–317.

Mix KS, Levine SC, Huttenlocher J (1997) Numerical abstraction in infants: Another look. Dev Psychol 33: 423–428.

Obrecht N, Chapman G, Gelman R (2007) Intuitive t-tests: Lay use of statistical information. Psychon B Rev 14: 1147–1152.

Saxe R, Tenenbaum J, Carey S (2005) Secret agents: Inferences about hidden causes by 10- and 12-month-old infants. Psychol Sci 16: 995–1001.

Spelke ES (2000) Core domains. Am Psychol 55: 1233–1243.

Waxman S, Medin D, Ross N (2007) Folkbiological reasoning from a cross-cultural developmental perspective: Early essentialist notions are shaped by cultural beliefs. Dev Psychol 43: 294–308.

13 Neuroscience, Psychology, and Economic Behavior: The Emerging Field of Neuroeconomics

Paul W. Glimcher

The history of the study of judgment and decision making has been marked by an iterative tension between what are known as *prescriptive* and *descriptive* advances. Prescriptive theories, which typically have their roots in economics, seek to define efficient or optimal decision making. Descriptive empirical advances, with roots typically in psychology, then invariably suggest that these prescriptive theories do not accurately describe human behavior. The neoclassical revolution in economics during the first half of the twentieth century and the period that followed it were no exception to this general paradigm. Working from the theoretically powerful assumption that all of human behavior could be described as a rational effort to maximize a theoretical quantity known as *utility*, the neoclassical theorists largely succeeded in developing a coherent basic mathematical framework for understanding what people *should* choose. They hypothesized that there had to be some sense in which humans could be described as logically consistent, and that given this hypothesis all of the powerful tools of deductive logical mathematics could be brought to bear on the study of human decision making. This conclusion was followed, however, by a series of descriptive insights that indicated that the initial round of neoclassic theories were not consistent with human choice behavior. This meant either that humans could not be described as logically consistent in *any* sense, that the specific models developed during the neoclassical revolution were flawed, or both. The social result of this set of observations was a growing divergence between economics and psychology. In psychological circles the conviction grew that a truly logical mathematical framework for the study of decision making was not possible, while in economic circles the search for such a framework continued unabated.

One recent trend in the study of decision making may, however, reconcile this tension between the now very divergent psychological and economic approaches: a growing interest in the physical mechanisms by which decisions are made within the human brain. Neuroeconomic scholars operating at the interface of the economic, psychological, and neurobiological domains argue that a study of the brain architecture for human decision making will reveal the actual mathematical computations that the brain performs during economic behavior. If this is true, then neurobiological studies that seek to bridge the gap between economics and psychology may succeed in providing a methodology for reconciling prescriptive and descriptive studies of choice. These studies may produce a highly predictive and parsimonious mathematical model of individual decision making that is based on the actual computations performed by the human brain.

Closing the Gap between Economics and Psychology

The revolution engendered by the advent of rational choice modeling in economics had two profound effects during the second half of the twentieth century: at a mathematical-economic level, it succeeded in defining a set of tools that could describe how an individual who wished to maximize anything (whether happiness, money, or progeny) should behave to achieve that maximization. At a behavioral-psychological level it essentially proved that humans did not reliably behave in the way predicted by the existing corpus of theory. This insight led a number of scholars at the borders of psychology and economics, perhaps most notably Herbert Simon (1947, 1983, 1997), to conclude that human decision makers could be viewed as rational utility maximizers in only a limited, or bounded, sense.[1] Conditions under which humans behave in accord with existing theory do occur, but there are also conditions under which humans behave in a way that contradicts existing theory. One result of this insight has been a growing conviction in some segments of the economic and psychological communities that human decision making can often be viewed as the product of two underlying processes: a bounded rational process well described by prescriptive economic theory and an irrational process which is best described empirically and which irreducibly defies formal mathematical analysis with traditional economic tools.

In response to this growing conviction, a number of scholars have recently initiated a revival of the (previously discredited) neo-Freudian neurobiological approach that dominated physiological circles in the 1950s (Freud 1923/1927; MacLean 1952). This approach suggests that two processes, the rational and irrational, are instantiated within the human brain as two anatomically discrete mechanisms. In most of these theories, like those of the 1950s, the irrational module is associated with evolutionarily ancient brain structures presumed to be irrational because of their presence in less complicated animals than ourselves. The rational module, viewed as uniquely well developed in humans, is presumed to reside in the cerebral cortex, often in frontal regions particularly highly developed in humans (McClure et al. 2004; Camerer et al. 2005). Indeed, many have suggested that irrational behavior should be uniquely attributed to limitations intrinsic to the more evolutionarily ancient portions of the brain, whereas rational behavior, when it occurs, may be viewed as the product of a conscious verbal faculty that somehow transcends this biological limitation through the use of the frontal cortex.

At the same time that this neo-Freudian approach has been revived in economic (and to a lesser extent psychological) circles, neuroscientists interested in human decision making have begun to head in a surprisingly different direction as they seek to reconcile prescriptive and descriptive approaches. The revolution that gave birth to modern neuroscience in the early part of the twentieth century also argued that all human behavior could be conceived of as the product of two fundamentally distinct mechanisms: a sophisticated faculty that governed complex behavior, and a simpler, cruder mechanism that could produce reliable, but unavoidably simplistic (and hence implicitly irrational), behaviors (see, for example, Descartes 1664/1972; Hall 1833; Sherrington 1906). This simpler mechanism, which came to be identified with the notion of automated or reflexive responding, was widely believed to be tractable to neurophysiological analysis and formed the core of our understanding of brain function during the first half of that century.

During the last several decades, however, ongoing empirical work has begun to suggest to many neuroscientists that this view of the neural architecture is no longer tenable (Damasio 1995; LeDoux 1996; Glimcher 2003a). Biological evidence now suggests to neuroscientists a more unitary view of the neural architecture that is much more deeply rooted in evolutionary theory than this original dualistic conception. What is emerging in neuroscientific circles is the view that a surprisingly holistic (though clearly multicomponent) decision-making process governs behavior (Parker and Newsome 1998; Schall and Thompson 1999; Glimcher 2003b). The interdependent and varied inputs to this decision-making process, it is argued, have all been shaped by evolution in order to yield a unified pattern of behavior that maximizes the reproductive fitness of organisms (a rather precise and tractable definition of utility) in the environments in which they operate (Maynard Smith 1982; Stephens and Krebs 1986; Krebs and Davies 1991). Evolution makes animals fitness maximizers in a fully defined mathematical sense that has its roots in economic theory. But critically, evolution performs this role on all parts of the organism simultaneously. It yields a single whole organism, the global rationality of which is bounded not by the limits of the Freudian animal-id, but rather by the requirements of the environment within which it evolved.

This unified view stands in contrast to the neo-Freudian view, which argues that the powerful general-purpose decision-making capabilities of humans make us fundamentally different from other animals. When rationality is observed in our behavior, these scholars argue, this rationality can be attributed to a distinct and uniquely human mechanism. Quite compelling empirical data, however, argue against this conclusion. First, it now seems clear that even animals with very small brains can behave in a surprisingly rational manner under a broad range of conditions (Stephens and Krebs 1986; Krebs and Davies 1991). This argues against the idea that in order to behave rationally humans would have needed to evolve some unique facility. Second, there is growing evidence that we share with our nearest relatives not just the ability to behave rationally but also common boundaries to our rationality (Barkow et al. 1992; Hauser 2000). If this is true, then it is both the rational and irrational that we share with our nearest relatives, again challenging the assumption that any of these aspects of behavior involve some uniquely human process. These data argue, in essence, that we differ more in degree than in nature from our nearest living relatives.

In summary, these observations argue for three main points that will be developed below. First, a deep and successful effort to account for decision making will only be possible if scholars employ the rigorous quantitative approaches to decision making that have begun to be developed in economic circles. These models rest on mathematical logic, which is the only starting point for truly scientific studies of decision making and truly mechanistic studies of brain function. Second, although humans are unique organisms, there is growing evidence that we are far less unique in the production of decision-making behavior than many scholars at the boundary of economics and psychology suggest. For example, monkeys can play repeated mixed-strategy equilibrium games of the types Von Neumann and Morgenstern (1944) and Nash (1951) described with the same efficiency as do humans (Dorris and Glimcher 2004). Birds, to take another example, can systematically alter the shape of their utility functions to adopt risk preferences appropriate for their environments (Caraco et al. 1980). This may be the most critical point made here, because it calls into question the pervasive assumption held by many neo-Freudian economists and psychologists that our decision-making process is both a uniquely human faculty and a broadly rational faculty. Third and finally, it is absolutely critical that the economic and psychological communities recognize that neurobiological studies of decision making can be much more than efforts to locate a brain region associated with some hypothetical human faculty such as "cooperation." Such studies are valuable starting points, but have troubled many scholars because they provide no predictive power with regard to behavior. Really useful neuroeconomic studies, from the perspective of working scientists, will have to fully describe the mechanisms by which economic computations yield observed behavior. It is an understanding of these mechanisms in that sense that will yield real predictive power in the mathematical and logical sense.

The Neuroscience of Choice

Modern *utility theory*, the foundation of modern economics, has its origins in the theory of expected value first proposed by Pascal. He argued that the value of any course of action could be determined by multiplying the gain that could be realized from that action by the likelihood of receiving that gain. This product, which we now call *expected value*, represents the average gain or loss associated with any action. Pascal argued that when making any decision one should simply compare the expected values of the available courses of action and then select the action having the highest expected value. The most famous example of this is probably the line of reasoning from his Christian apologia, the *Pensées*, known as Pascal's Wager. Here, Pascal (1670/1966) reasons that a belief in God is normatively rational as long as there is any uncertainty about God's existence because the gain for believing in God is infinitely positive. Since the possible gain of eternal salvation has infinite value, that value times any non-zero probability yields an infinite expected value, making a belief in God a rational decision.

Although Pascal and his colleagues recognized that not all human decision making could be accurately described as being guided by this concept of expected value, they argued that all rational decision making should follow this prescriptive theory (see Arnauld and Nicole 1662/1996; Pascal 1670/1966). By the early 1700s, however, it was clear that the Pascalian approach did an extremely poor job of predicting human choice behavior under conditions of significant risk.

The early psychological evidence for this conclusion arose from empirical observations about a casino game popular in St. Petersburg in the 1700s. In this game, players were asked to pay a fixed sum to participate in a single round. What they won during this round was determined by a series of coin flips. The game begins with the flip of a single coin. If that coin lands heads-up the player wins two coins. If the coin lands tails-up the coin is flipped again. If this second flip lands heads-up the player wins four coins. Otherwise, the flip repeats with the win doubling for each subsequent flip until the coin lands heads-up. Of course, the expected value for the first flip is one coin: a 50 percent chance of a heads-up times two coins. The same, however, is true for every sequential flip: for example, the a priori probability of winning in the second flip is 25 percent and the gain is four coins; of winning on the third flip 12.5 percent; and the gain is eight coins . . . From this one must conclude that the expected value of a single round of this game is infinite, although in practice players are unwilling to pay more than about forty coins per round (making this a highly unprofitable game for the casinos).

To explain this early mismatch between the prescriptive and descriptive domains the Swiss mathematician Daniel Bernoulli (1738/1954) argued for a model of rational decision making in which the likelihood of a gain was multiplied not by the objective number of coins that the chooser stood to gain, but rather by a psychological construct, later called utility, that was related to but distinct from value. His notion was that gains were represented in the psychological decision-making process by a roughly logarithmic function of value that also incorporated a representation of the chooser's wealth. Modern utility theory built on this foundation by developing a more rigorous mathematical foundation for Bernoulli's model and by explicit recognizing that the relationship between value and utility, a relationship known as the *preference function*, is fundamentally subjective and empirical rather than being part of the prescriptively rational choice process.

Even utility theory, however, has been often challenged. Critiques of modern utility theory have tended to fall into one of two domains. The first of these classes of critiques empirically identifies failures of a specific utility-theoretic model like the ones proposed by von Neumann and Morgenstern (1944) or by Savage (1954). The second identifies behaviors for which, in principle, no truly rational model (a model that rests on basic mathematical principles) of any kind could ever account. An example of the first of these classes of failures is Kahneman and Tversky's (1979) famous observation that choosers are more sensitive to losses than to gains. Human decision makers consider a loss of $100 a much more negative event than they consider a gain of $100 positive. Although this observation does challenge von Neumann and Morgenstern's (1944) model for rational choice, it does not challenge the rational framework upon which they hoped future theories would be built (although this is a point rarely made outside of economic circles). Indeed, subsequent prescriptive models that account for loss aversion, for example, have been generated by rational choice economists such as Milton Friedman and Leonard Savage (1948). The second of these classes of critique is more troubling. These critiques rest on the identification of behaviors for which no completely logical theory could account. Consider this central feature of rational choice: if I truly prefer apples to oranges then there should be no circumstances in which I can be led to voluntarily select oranges over apples in a decision-making task. Were I to prefer apples to pears and prefer pears to oranges, then I must prefer apples to oranges. The alternative, that I prefer apples to pears, pears to oranges, but oranges to apples, leads to a logical circularity (formally, a violation of the mathematical principle of transitivity) that would constitute a challenge for which no rational model could hope to account. Unfortunately, a number of these classes of behaviors have been identified by experimentalists, and it is the observation of these "preference reversals" that poses the greatest challenge for traditional economic models of choice.

An excellent example of this kind of challenge to utility theory arises in the study of choices made as a function of time, a class of behavior known as temporal discounting. In the most clear-cut example of this kind of behavior, most subjects can be shown to prefer a hypothetical gain of $22 in thirteen months over a gain of $20 in twelve months. There is nothing irrational about this; it simply expresses a preference for the larger gain despite the additional delay. But if the same subject is asked the same question 365 days later, if he is asked whether he prefers $20 today or $22 in a month, changing his preference represents an inconsistency (Loewenstein and Thaler 1989). This, in a nutshell, is a critical problem for rational-choice theories because there is no way to make this pair of choices anything but logically contradictory in the mathematical sense. The contradiction arises, in a sense, because we need only to choose *when* to ask our subjects to pick in order to control their choices. Put another way, this subject's choice is inconsistent in the same way that the example of apples and oranges is inconsistent because for a subject who behaves this way we can control the subjects' preference for apples simply by adjusting the order in which we present them with fruit.

In summary, then, rational-choice models from economics provide a powerful framework for understanding and modeling choice behavior—a framework that is more extensible than most scholars realize. But that framework also has clearly identifiable limits to its applicability. How, then, one might ask, should scholars interested in choice proceed? Should they discard formal models rooted in economic theory in favor of loosely defined psychological systems rooted in Freudian theory, or should they use more rigorous models, with a clear knowledge of their limitations, as a starting point for building a new mechanistic understanding of decision making? Recent evidence suggests that the latter approach may prove the more fruitful.

Neurobiological studies conducted over the past decade have revealed that the brains of both human and nonhuman primates represent a complex variable which under many circumstances closely parallels von Neumann and Savage's notion of classical expected utility (see Platt and Glimcher 1999; Gold and Shadlen 2000; Breiter et al. 2001; Knutson et al. 2001; Paulus et al. 2001). For example, the rate at which nerve cells in the posterior parietal cortex generate action potentials is very precisely correlated with theoretically derived estimates of expected utility under many conditions (Glimcher et al. 2005). Further, some of these studies even suggest that in the final stages of the decision-making process, the neural architecture selects a course of action by mechanistically generating the response associated with the greatest activity in the posterior parietal cortex. All of these studies suggest that, despite their limitations, traditional economic theories provide tremendous descriptive power for understanding the nervous system.

Identifying the Neurobiological Representation of "Expected Utility"

One of the first studies to make the suggestion that something like expected utility is actually instantiated within the nervous system was Platt and Glimcher (1999). In their experiments, trained rhesus monkeys were allowed to participate in repeated rounds of a simple lottery while the activity of nerve cells in the posterior parietal cortex was monitored. At the beginning of each round a red spot and a green spot were illuminated on a screen directly in front of the monkey. This began the lottery phase of the round, a period during which the monkey did not know whether the red or green light would be linked with a prize at the end of that round. At the end of this phase, a third light changed color to red or green, indicating which of the two initial lights had been randomly selected to yield a fruit juice reward on that particular round. The monkey then received the fruit juice if he simply made visual contact with the selected light at the end of the round. While monkeys played hundreds of rounds of this game, Platt and Glimcher systematically varied either the size of the reward associated with each light, the *value* of that light, or the relative probabilities that the red or green lights would be selected at the end of the round—the *likelihood* that each light would yield a reward.

These two variables were selected for manipulation because essentially all utility theories are based on the assumption that rational decision makers assess the desirability of any course of action by combining the value and likelihood of gain, as originally suggested by Pascal and Bernoulli. Even though in this experiment the monkeys did not need to monitor these values in order to behave efficiently, Platt and Glimcher hoped to determine whether these economic variables were encoded in the nervous system while monkeys observed these repeated lotteries, just as we might expect them to be in human players.

Platt and Glimcher found that a discrete group of nerve cells in the posterior parietal cortex encoded, separately for each light, a combination of the value and likelihood of reinforcement associated with that button during the lottery phase of each round. It appeared from this result that under these conditions the brains of their monkeys explicitly encoded something very much like the economically defined expected value or expected utility of each light in this simple lottery task.

Game-Playing Monkeys

Dorris and Glimcher (2004) extended this finding when they examined the activity of this same brain region while a new group of rhesus monkeys engaged in a strategic conflict known as the *inspection game*. In the human version of that game, two opponents face each other, an *employer* and an *employee*. On each round of the game the employee must decide whether to *go to work*, in which case he earns a fixed wage, or whether to *shirk*, in hopes of earning his wage plus a bonus (in the human version of the game, the free time gained by shirking is itself conceived of as the bonus). The goal of the employee is simply to maximize his gain in terms of salary and bonus. The employer, on the other hand, must decide between trusting his employee to arrive for work or spending money to hire an inspector who can actually check and see whether the employee arrived for work that day. The goal of the employer is to spend as little as possible on inspections while maximizing the employee's incentive to work.

The inspection game is of particular interest to game theorists and economists because rational strategies for utility maximization during strategic conflict lead to predictable outcomes, according to the equilibrium theory originally developed by John Nash in the 1950s. Nash (1951) equilibrium theory describes how, when the cost of inspection to the employer is set high, the efficient strategy for both players converges on a solution in which the employee manages to shirk fairly often. Conversely, a low inspection cost to the employer defines a theoretical equilibrium solution in which shirk rates are low.

Dorris and Glimcher examined the behavior of both humans and monkeys during a version of the inspection game in an effort to determine whether the posterior parietal cortex really encoded something like expected utility, the theoretically defined decision variable, even under these conditions of voluntary choice. In their game, both human and monkey contestants played the role of the employee against a standardized and strategically sophisticated computer employer. Each round began with the illumination of two lights, one for working and one for shirking. At the end of each round, players selected one light and the computer employer simultaneously decided whether or not to pay for an inspection on that round. These responses were then compared by a second computer arbiter that paid both players off according to a fixed payoff matrix (paying off in juice for monkeys, real currency for humans, and virtual currency for the computer employer, as shown in figure 13.1). As in the earlier lottery task, players faced fixed conditions for a hundred or more rounds, after which the payoff matrix was changed by altering the cost of an inspection.

Inspection Game Earnings

Computer Employer			Human Employee			Human Employee		
Employer Action			Employer Action			Employer Action		
	Inspect	No Inspect		Inspect	No Inspect		Inspect	No Inspect
Work	$1.70	$2.00	Work	$1.00	$1.00	Work	1 oz	1 oz
Shirk	–$0.30	–$2.00	Shirk	$0.00	$2.00	Shirk	0 oz	2 oz

(Employee Action rows: Work / Shirk for each table)

Figure 13.1
Payoffs to human and monkey employees during the inspection game (after Dorris and Glimcher 2004).

This permitted Dorris and Glimcher to examine the behavior of human and monkey players under five different sets of conditions, each of which required a slightly different strategy.

Dorris and Glimcher found that the probability a human playing the inspection game for money would choose to shirk was well predicted by the prescriptive Nash equilibrium computations whenever those computations predicted shirking rates of 40 percent or more. When, however, this particular prescriptive theory predicted shirking rates below approximately 40 percent, human subjects were observed to shirk more frequently than was predicted. This descriptive assessment of humans seemed to differ from the prescriptive assessment provided by the Nash equilibrium equations.

When Dorris and Glimcher analyzed the behavior of their monkeys, they found that the behavior of the monkeys was surprisingly similar, even essentially identical, to the behavior of their human employees. Just like humans, the monkeys seemed to precisely track the Nash equilibrium solutions and deviated from those solutions only when shirking rates of less than 40 percent were prescribed during the inspection game (figure 13.2). This was a critical advance because it allowed Dorris and Glimcher to examine the role of the posterior parietal cortex during a voluntary strategic game during which monkeys and humans seemed to employ similar, or identical, strategies.

One of Nash's (1951) fundamental insights was that at a *mixed-strategy equilibrium*, a situation in which a strategic player should distribute her actions among two or more alternatives in an unpredictable fashion, the desirability of the two or more actions in equilibrium must be equivalent. This means that during the inspection game, the expected utilities of working and shirking must be equal, regardless of how frequently the equilibrium solution requires that the player works. The Nash approach argues, essentially, that a behavioral equilibrium occurs when the desirability of working and shirking are rendered equal by the behavior of one's opponent, irrespective of how often that equilibrium

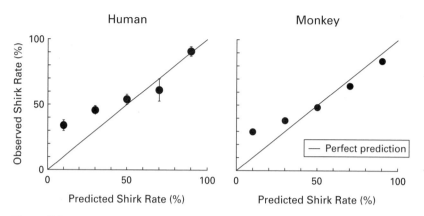

Figure 13.2
Nash Equilibrium Theory predicts human and monkey behavior equally well (after Dorris and Glimcher 2004).

requires that one work. The Nash equations themselves go a step further, defining the precise rates of working and shirking that are prescriptively rational.

Dorris and Glimcher hypothesized from the Nash approach that the desirabilities of working and shirking, rational or not, must be equivalent whenever strategic competition yields a mixed-strategy behavior in players, and thus that mixed-strategy behaviors must be associated with the equal desirability of working and shirking as represented in the nervous system. If the desirability of an action is encoded by the activity of neurons in the posterior parietal cortex not just for some categories of behavior, rational or irrational, but for behavior in general, then during strategic conflict of this type the neural activity for working and shirking should, paradoxically, always be equal. Put another way, if the economic approach is sound, then at behavioral equilibrium the desirability of working and shirking should be equivalent. If the neurobiological approach is sound, then at behavioral equilibrium the level of nerve cell activity in parietal cortex associated with working and shirking should also have been equivalent.

When Dorris and Glimcher examined the activity of neurons in the posterior parietal cortex while monkeys played the inspection game, they found that the posterior parietal cortex carried a signal essentially identical to the one expected. When the monkeys' behavior was well predicted by the Nash equations, neural activity was equivalent to the expected utility of economic theory. When the monkeys deviated from those prescriptive predictions, for example, by over shirking, then Dorris and Glimcher found that the activity in this area seemed to correspond to the subjective desirabilities that should have been guiding the monkeys. The neurons seemed to encode a *physiological expected utility*.

Humans Playing Lotteries

These studies of monkeys are of importance for two reasons. First, they demonstrate the surprising similarities in the economic behavior of humans and our nearest relatives. Second, they employ highly precise brain measurement technologies that cannot be used in humans. Recently, however, the less precise brain scanning technologies that can be employed in humans have also begun to yield significant insights into the neural basis of economic behavior (McCabe et al. 2001; Montague and Berns 2002). One of the first and most compelling of these studies examined the behavior of humans during a lottery similar to the one employed by Platt and Glimcher for the study of monkeys (Breiter et al. 2001). In that experiment, human subjects were presented, on sequential rounds, with one of three possible lotteries (see figure 13.3).

In lottery 1, the *good lottery*, they faced equal chances of winning $10, $2.50, or $0. In lottery 2 they faced an equal chance of winning $2.50, winning $0, or losing $1.50. In lottery 3 they faced an equal chance of winning $0, losing $1.50, or losing $6.

At the beginning of each round the subjects were told which lottery they would be playing, and the average activity in many brain areas was simultaneously measured. After that measurement was complete, the lottery was actually played and the humans were then told how much real money they had earned on that round. This design was particularly interesting because of an important and well-described deviation of human behavior from prescriptive theory (Kahneman and Tversky 1979; Kahneman et al. 1982). All three of these particular lotteries present a one-third possibility of winning $0, but they do so under different conditions. In the first lottery winning $0 is the worst possible outcome whereas in the third lottery it is the best. Kahneman and Tversky noted that although humans rationally prefer lottery 1 to lottery 3, once they enter a lottery their perceptions of outcomes change. Once in lottery 1, winning $0 is experienced as intensely negative while once in lottery 3 winning $0 is experienced as positive. What Breiter and colleagues hoped to determine was whether the activity of some brain area might track both of these human responses.

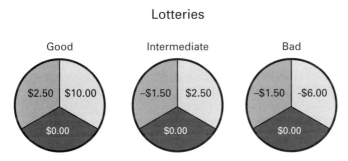

Figure 13.3
The three lotteries used in Breiter's experiment (after Breiter et al. 2001).

What they found was that the activity of a brain region called the sublenticular extended amygdala did behave in essentially this manner. When humans were first presented with the lottery they would face on that round, activity in this brain area was closely related to the overall expected utility of the lottery. After the lottery ran, however, they found that the activity of this area was a rough function of the subjective response of the human to the outcome rather than a function of the actual dollar amount won. Activity in this area was higher when the subjects won $0 in lottery 3 than when they won $0 in lottery 1.

Once again the neural results lead to an interesting and perhaps unexpected result. When human behavior is rational, as defined by prescriptive economic theory, we can find evidence that some brain areas encode expected utility. When, however, human behavior deviates from prescriptive theory, the brain seems to encode something more like the subjective desirability of an outcome rather than the objective economic value of that outcome.

Together, these observations raise an intriguing possibility: the neural architecture may indeed compute and represent something like the expected utility of many possible courses of action, much like that which neoclassical utility theory proposes. When choosers are efficient in the economic sense, that architecture accurately represents the objective expected utility of available choices. When economic and psychological utility differ, however, the neural architecture seems to reflect the psychological utilities that guide choice. Although it may be counterintuitive to economists to believe that subjective, or irrational, decision making reflects the principled output of highly developed neural circuits, this may simply reflect the fact that evolution shaped our neural architecture to perform efficiently under many, but not all, environmental circumstances. In some cases, inefficiencies of these types may simply arise when the most complicated cortical mechanisms inside our skulls encounter problems that they did not evolve to solve. It is these biologically based inefficiencies that therefore place boundaries on the circumstances in which we might be expected to produce economically rational behavior. The available evidence thus suggests a synthesis of modern economic and neuroscientific approaches. By biologically defining the mechanisms that compute physiological expected utility we should be able to derive a mechanistically accurate economic theory that is, by necessity, predictive.

Using Neuroscience to Develop New Economic–Psychological Theories

Bayer and Glimcher (2005) have been attempting to extend this approach by studying how the brain computes, or learns, the expected utilities that guide choice behavior in an effort to combine economic and psychological approaches around a neurobiological framework. They have attempted to do this by studying the activity of a group of nerve cells in the substantia nigra pars compacta that use the neurochemical dopamine to communicate with other nerve cells. These cells are widely believed to compute the difference between the gains that a human or animal expects to receive and the gains that they actually receive (see Schultz et al. 1997; Schultz 2002), and a growing body of evidence now suggests that this is the substrate from which expected utilities, in the economic sense, may be calculated. Of particular interest from an economic point of view is the observation that this particular calculation can be shown to be prescriptively rational under some limited conditions. Of particular interest from a psychological point of view is that this particular calculation would lead to some classes of empirically observed errors under conditions where it is suboptimal. Thus, demonstrating a neural substrate that performs this calculation both when it is rational and when it is not would mechanistically unify prescriptive and descriptive studies of learning behavior. Bayer and Glimcher therefore examined these dopamine neurons during a simple choice task in an effort to derive the precise economic equation that they compute. They then used this equation to predict the behavior of monkeys during the classic psychological matching law task of Herrnstein (see Herrnstein 1961, 1997). In that task, which was studied by Lau and Glimcher (2005), monkeys were faced with two choices reinforced on a discrete trial variable ratio schedule almost identical to the one Herrnstein studied in pigeons. On each round the monkeys could select either a red or green light placed in front of them. Before each trial began there was a fixed probability that each of the two lights would be *armed* with a reward. For example, there might be a 10 percent chance that the red light would be armed before each round and a 20 percent chance that the green light would be armed before each round, and the lights were always armed with the same amount of fruit juice. Critically, once a light was armed it remained armed until chosen by the monkey in a subsequent round.

The accompanying figure (figure 13.4) shows the free choices made by a monkey while performing as a thick gray line.

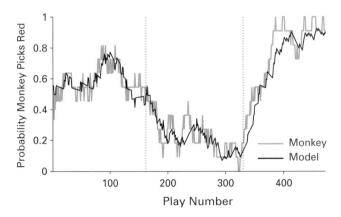

Figure 13.4
Predicting the choices monkeys make with a neuroeconomic model (after Lau and Glimcher 2005).

One can see that the behavior of the animal is chaotic, fluctuating from red to green. The thin black line shows the prediction of the neuroeconomic model derived from a study of the dopamine neurons. What is critical is that the model does a remarkably good job of predicting the behavior of the animal on a step-by-step basis. The model, which is neither truly prescriptive nor truly descriptive, is highly constrained by neurobiological observations and makes clear behavioral predictions. Of course the model is making predictions about a very simple behavior, but it seems likely at this point in time that more sophisticated models of this type will soon be developed. And it is these forthcoming models that will either validate or invalidate the promise of the developing neuroeconomic approach.

Summary

One of the critical and persistent issues in economics has been our inability to reconcile the rational-choice model at the core of modern theory with the fact that humans are the product of a 600-million-year evolutionary lineage. We all recognize that nonhuman animals have limited mechanical and neural capacity. Fish that live in total darkness have neither eyes nor the neural architecture for vision. We all accept that even our closest living relatives, the great apes, face fundamental conceptual limitations that are probably not apparent to them. But it has long been the central premise of economic thought that humans are different from all of these other organisms. That humans rely on a more fundamentally rational neural machinery and that this machinery, which economists presume is subjectively experienced as consciousness and which they often assume is mechanistically located within the cerebral cortex, endows us with nearly perfect rationality.

In the last half century, however, a number of influential psychologists have identified conditions where humans simply do not achieve this prescriptively defined rational behavior. One conclusion that can be drawn from this is that scholars interested in understanding choice must begin to recognize that our biological-evolutionary heritage influences our actions. Many of the decisions that we make may be inefficient today because of that evolutionary history. Surprisingly, however, a group of the same economists have used this insight to argue that an accurate model of human behavior will therefore have to be two-tiered. These economists accept from classical economic theory that there is a fundamentally rational conscious decision maker within our skulls. This is, they presume, an evolutionary development unique to our species that has arisen within the very recent past. But there is also a second more ancient and mechanistic system, and when inefficient decision making occurs it can be attributed to the activity of this evolutionarily ancient mechanism.

For many neurobiologists and psychologists studying the mechanisms by which choice is accomplished, this seems to be an oddly dualist and Freudian approach to the physiology of mind. In the seventeenth century, Descartes proposed that all of human behavior could be divided into two principle classes and that each of these categories of behavior could be viewed as the product of distinct processes. The first of those classes Descartes defined as the simple and predictable behaviors that both humans and animals could express, behaviors that predictably linked sensory stimuli with motor responses. Their simple deterministic nature suggested to him that for these behaviors the sensory-to-motor connection lay within the material body, making those simple connections amenable to physiological study. For the second class—behaviors in which no deterministic connection between sensation and action was obvious—he followed Aristotle's lead, identifying the source of these actions as the rational, but nonmaterial, soul.

Over the last several decades neurobiologists have begun to broadly reject this dualistic formulation for several reasons. First, because there seems to be no physiological evidence that such a view can be supported, and second, because it seems to fly in the face of evolutionary theory, which forms the basis of modern biology. Instead, what seems to be emerging is a much more synthetic view in which economic theory can serve as the core for a monist approach to understanding the behavior not just of simple organisms that survive in narrowly defined environments but also for understanding the most complex and generalist of extant species, *Homo sapiens*.

In sum, neuroeconomics seeks to unify the prescriptive and descriptive approaches by relating evolutionary efficiencies to underlying mechanisms. Neoclassical economics and the utility theory on which it is based provide the ultimate set of tools for describing these efficient solutions; evolutionary theory defines the field within which these mechanisms are optimized by neoclassical constraints; psychology, the empirical tools for the study of behavior; and neurobiology, the tools for elucidating those mechanisms.

Over the past decade a number of researchers in neuroscience, psychology, and economics have begun to apply this approach to the study of decision making by humans and animals. What seems to be emerging from these early studies is a basically economic view of the primate brain: the final stages of decision making seem to reflect something very much like a utility calculation. The desirability, or physiological expected utility, of all available courses of action seem to be represented in parallel, and neural maps of these physiological expected utilities seem to be the substrate upon which decisions are actually made (Glimcher 2003a).

These representations, in turn, seem to be the product of many highly coordinated brain circuits. Some of these brain circuits, such as the dopamine neurons of the substantia nigra pars compacta, are already beginning to be described. The algorithms by which these circuits compute the economic variables from which physiological expected utilities are derived are now under intensive study. Indeed, several of these mechanistic studies are even now being used to make economic predictions about the behavior of human and nonhuman primates, both when that behavior follows and when it deviates from the prescriptive neoclassical model. Studies like these seem to be elucidating the mechanisms by which economic behavior is accomplished, and a critical advantage of this approach to irrational behaviors is that once these mechanisms are understood, all behavior should become broadly predictable. In essence, neuroeconomics argues that it is these mechanism that can serve as the logical and mathematical bridge between the prescriptive and descriptive approaches that dominate economics and psychology, respectively.

As early as 1898 the economist Thorstein Veblen made this point in an essay entitled "Why Is Economics Not an Evolutionary Science?" He suggested that in order to understand the economic behavior of humans one would have to understand the mechanisms by which those behaviors were produced. More recently the biologist E. O. Wilson (1998) has made a similar point. Arguing that a fusion of the social and natural sciences is both inevitable and desirable, Wilson has suggested that this fusion will begin with a widespread recognition that economics and biology are two disciplines addressing a single subject matter. Ultimately, economics and psychology are biological sciences. They are the study of how humans behave. That behavior is inescapably a biological process. Truly understanding how and why humans make the choices that they do will undoubtedly require a neuroeconomic science.

Note

1. The term "utility" has often been the subject of profound misconceptions. When von Neumann and Morgenstern (1944), and Savage (1954) defined utility they meant it to be a theoretical variable associated with any possible event in the outside world that guided decision making. Love, social status, and of course money were all meant to be the subjects of utility theories. Their goal was simply to describe how choosers, given an individual-specific mapping between events in the world and utility, should have to maximize that utility. Subsequent theorists have tended to focus on the maximization of monetary wealth because of the importance of wealth to the economy. One unfortunate side effect of this focus, however, has been a misunderstanding of utility theory and its goals. Utility theory is not about maximizing money. The observation that humans care about quality, will forego money to protect their children, or make different decisions as they age, poses no particular problems for utility theory. Utility theory simply asks whether or not there is a conceptual framework under which the mathematical tools of deductive logic can be applied to the study of choice.

References

Arnauld A, Nicole P (1662/1996) Logic, or the art of thinking (Buroker JV, ed) Cambridge: Cambridge University Press.

Barkow J, Cosmides L, Tooby J, eds (1992) The adapted mind: Evolutionary psychology and the generation of culture. New York: Oxford University Press.

Bayer HM, Glimcher PW (2005) Midbrain dopamine neurons encode a quantitative reward prediction error signal. Neuron 47: 129–141.

Bernoulli D (1738/1954) Exposition of a new theory on the measurement of risk. Econometrica 22: 23–36.

Breiter HC, Aharon I, Kahneman D, Dale A, Shizgal P (2001) Functional imaging of neural responses to expectancy and experience of monetary gains and losses. Neuron 30: 619–639.

Camerer C, Loewenstein G, Prelec D (2005) Neuroeconomics: How neuroscience can inform economics. J Econ Lit 43: 9–64.

Caraco T, Martindale S, Whittam TS (1980) An empirical demonstration of risk-sensitive foraging preferences. Anim Behav 28: 820–830.

Damasio AR (1995) Descartes's error: Emotion, reason and the human brain. London: Pan Macmillan.

Descartes R (1664/1972) L'Homme (Hall TS, trans). Cambridge, MA: Harvard University Press.

Dorris MC, Glimcher PW (2004) Activity in posterior parietal cortex is correlated with the subjective desirability of an action. Neuron 44: 365–378.

Freud S (1923/1927) The ego and the id. London. Hogarth Press.

Friedman M, Savage L (1948) The utility analysis of choices involving risk. J Polit Econ 56: 279–304.

Glimcher PW (2003a) Decisions, uncertainty and the brain: The science of neuroeconomics. Cambridge, MA: MIT Press.

Glimcher PW (2003b) Neural correlates of primate decision making. Annu Rev Neurosci 25: 133–179.

Glimcher PW, Dorris MC, Bayer HM (2005) Physiological utility theory and the neuroeconomics of choice. Games Econ Behav 52: 213–256.

Gold JI, Shadlen MN (2000) Representation of a perceptual decision in developing oculomotor commands. Nature 404: 390–394.

Hall M (1833) On the reflex function of the medulla oblongata and medulla spinalis. Philos T Roy Soc 123: 635–665.

Hauser M (2000) Wild minds: What animals really think. New York: Henry Holt.

Herrnstein RJ (1961) Relative and absolute strength of response as a function of frequency of reinforcement. J Exp Anal Behav 4: 267–272.

Herrnstein RJ (1997) The matching law (Rachlin H, Laibson DI, eds). Cambridge, MA: Harvard University Press.

Kahneman D, Tversky A (1979) Prospect theory: An analysis of decision under risk. Econometrica 47: 263–291.

Kahneman D, Slovic P, Tversky A (1982) Judgment under uncertainty: Heuristics and biases. Cambridge: Cambridge University Press.

Knutson B, Adams CM, Fong GW, Hommer D (2001) Anticipation of increasing monetary reward selectively recruits nucleus accumbens. J Neurosci 21: RC159.

Krebs JR, Davies NB, eds (1991) Behavioural ecology. Oxford: Blackwell Scientific Publications.

Lau B, Glimcher PW (2005) Dynamic response-by-response models of matching behavior in rhesus monkeys. J Exp Anal Behav 84: 555–579.

LeDoux J (1996) The Emotional Brain: The Mysterious Underpinnings of Emotional Life. New York: Simon and Schuster.

Loewenstein G, Thaler R (1989) Anomalies: Intertemporal choice. Journal Econ Perspect 3: 181–193.

MacLean PD (1952) Some psychiatric implications of physiological studies on frontotemporal portion of limbic system (visceral brain). Electroen Clin Neuro Suppl 4: 407–418.

Maynard Smith J (1982) Evolution and the theory of games. Cambridge: Cambridge University Press.

McCabe K, Houser D, Ryan L, Smith V, Trouard T (2001) A functional imaging study of cooperation in two-person reciprocal exchange. P Natl Acad Sci USA 98: 11832–11835.

McClure SM, Laibson DI, Loewenstein G, Cohen JD (2004) Separate neural systems value immediate and delayed monetary rewards. Science 306: 503–507.

Montague PR, Berns GS (2002) Neural economics and the biological substrates of valuation. Neuron 36: 265–284.

Nash JF (1951) Non-cooperative games. Ann Math 54: 286–295.

Parker AJ, Newsome WT (1998) Sense and the single neuron: Probing the physiology of perception. Annu Rev Neurosci 21: 227–77.

Pascal B (1670/1966) Pensées (Krailsheimer AJ, trans). London: Penguin Books.

Paulus MP, Hozack N, Zauscher B, McDowell JE, Frank L, Brown GG, Braff DL (2001) Prefrontal, parietal, and temporal cortex networks underlie decision making in the presence of uncertainty. Neuroimage 13: 91–100.

Platt ML, Glimcher PW (1999) Neural correlates of decision variables in parietal cortex. Nature 400: 233–238.

Savage L (1954) The foundations of statistics. New York: Wiley.

Schall JD, Thompson KG (1999) Neural selection and control of visually guided eye movements. Annu Rev Neurosci 22: 241–59.

Schultz W (2002) Getting formal with dopamine and reward. Neuron 36: 241–263.

Schultz W, Dayan P, Montague PR (1997) A neural substrate of prediction and reward. Science 275: 1593–1599.

Sherrington CS (1906) The integrative action of the nervous system. New York: Charles Scribner's Sons.

Simon HA (1947) Administrative behavior. New York: Free Press.

Simon HA (1983) Reason in human affairs. Palo Alto: Stanford University Press.

Simon HA (1997) Models of bounded rationality: Empirically grounded economic reason. Cambridge, MA: MIT Press.

Stephens DW, Krebs JR (1986) Foraging theory. Princeton: Princeton University Press.

Veblen T (1898) Why is economics not an evolutionary science? Q J Econ 12: 373–397.

Von Neumann JV, Morgenstern O (1944) Theory of games and economic behavior. Princeton: Princeton University Press.

Wilson EO (1998) Consilience. New York: Knopf.

V SOCIAL ENTITIES

The final section of this volume deals with the cognitive biology of social entities, broadly conceived as other conspecifics in an organism's environment. Some of the questions investigated are "How are conspecifics attended, perceived, and represented?" and "What cues reveal important aspects in inter-individual exchange (from social cues of intentionality to language)?" This is another cognitive science subject that has been advanced substantially by converging data cutting across the domains of human adult and developmental psychology, comparative psychology, the neurosciences, and primatology and anthropology. The topics of interest range from the understanding of face processing to the complex issues of social referencing, gaze following, and theory of mind, abilities that are foundational for engaging in dynamic social interactions and for establishing a moral sense. And of course social behavior must have had a profound impact on the evolution of more basic cognitive functions, as Jacobs shows in chapter 2.

In chapter 14, Stephen Shepherd and Michael Platt describe research that combines ethological and psychophysical approaches in an attempt to develop a unified, evolutionarily motivated theory of attention, with an emphasis on how social cues, such as the direction of gaze of other individuals, rapidly guide attention in both human and nonhuman primates such as macaques and ring-tailed lemurs. They examine gaze in both natural and laboratory settings. Shepherd and Platt inferred animals' goals by examining where they look naturally rather than where they look in the service of a task artificially imposed by the experimenters. To do so, they used noninvasive, noncumbersome gaze-tracking devices. They found that social entities, rather than physically salient stimuli, were often the focus of attention, and that conspecifics' gaze direction was a powerful determinant of gaze, although factors such as gender, testosterone levels, and task also had an effect. Shepherd and Platt complement their naturalistic eye movement studies with a psychophysical choice task that allows them to examine the value of looking at social entities. Shepherd and Platt also review research (their own and others') showing that looking behavior can drive preferences and social affiliation. They end their chapter with a proposal regarding the neural substrate for social attention; they take a two-systems approach, advocating a ventral cortical system and a subcortical-to-frontal-lobe system. Although some theorists claim that social attention is a separate module from nonsocial attention, Shepherd and Platt review research inconsistent with a modular interpretation. Much remains to be done in this exciting area of research. This chapter sets the stage, and integrates well with the next chapter, by Mark Johnson.

In chapter 15, Johnson presents an account of the universal role of development in constructing what has come to be known as the "social brain" by comparing two dominant views in developmental cognitive neuroscience: that positing a fully prespecified cortical module and that positing a major role of maturation and epigenetic factors in establishing cortical specialization. Johnson advocates a theoretical position, interactive specialization, that cuts across these two views: he suggests that the interplay of activations of one region and all those connected to it in the implementation of specific behaviors and faculties during development ends up giving organisms the potential for establishing specializations in many cortical regions. Johnson considers the "fusiform face area" as an example of how specialization can arise through development given the interaction of two brain systems: a subcortical system, which predisposes infants to look at or attend to their caregiver's face, and a cortical system, which acquires information about the objects to which the infants attend. Johnson shows how similar constraints can produce imprinting behavior and neural specialization in chicks, albeit mediated by different neural tissue. Given its focus on attention, modularity, and development, chapter 15 integrates well with many chapters in this book. Notably, cortical development is taken as a successful example of approaching the issue of evolutionary and developmental interactions by means of the careful comparative analysis of neural and cognitive development.

In chapter 16, the last chapter in this section and the last chapter of the book, Sylvain Sirois and Annette Karmiloff-Smith present a critical overview on cognition and its ontogenesis, targeting nativist positions at their deep roots. The authors challenge the idea that cognitive abilities are prespecified in the genetic code and argue instead for an essentially plastic organism with some behavioral biases that allow abilities to emerge through development. The discussion grows into a critique of the canonical (read: modular) interpretation of atypical development (genetic disorders) that is paralleled by a close examination of the neural bases of face processing and how they can be altered in atypical development. Thus, in chapter 16 (as in chapter 15) it is argued that behavioral biases, experience, and neural interactions all play a role in normal and abnormal development. On the view espoused in chapter 16, abnormally developing children cannot be easily classified into types with different spared vs. impaired cognitive abilities. Instead, unique ensembles of impairments can arise because of different experiences during development. Chapter 16 ends with a discussion of the value of computational approaches to development in that they can examine the constructive nature of development and can avoid purely taxonomic approaches.

Thus, the three chapters in this section explore major issues in cognitive science from a comparative evolutionary-developmental approach, and thus provide an excellent coda for the preceding chapters.

14 Neuroethology of Attention in Primates

Stephen V. Shepherd and Michael L. Platt

Mobile animals orient to salient features of their environment. In primates, orienting can be covert or overt; covert orienting of attention appears to have evolved as a flexible mechanism for monitoring potentially important locations or stimuli in the absence of overt orienting. Psychophysical, electrophysiological, and neuroimaging studies conducted in the laboratory have extensively probed attention in both human and nonhuman primates trained to discriminate simple stimuli whose salience or behavioral significance has been arbitrarily assigned, typically through verbal instruction or association with rewards (Posner 1980). Such studies suggest the operation of two distinct systems for orienting attention (James 1890; Jonides 1981; Posner and Cohen 1984)—one fast and involuntary (exogenous) and the other slow and voluntary (endogenous), each one associated with partially distinct neural circuitry (Mangun 1995; Eget and Yantis 1997; Corbetta and Shulman 2002).

In contrast, observational studies conducted in natural settings suggest that social stimuli are intrinsically salient and attract attention (Keverne et al. 1978; Caine and Marra 1988; McNelis and Boatright-Horowitz 1998). Moreover, recent laboratory studies indicate that social cues, such as the direction of gaze of other individuals, access a privileged information channel that rapidly guides attention in both human and nonhuman primates (Friesen and Kingstone 1998; Deaner and Platt 2003). These studies imply that at least some mechanisms of attention have evolved in primates to be sensitive to cues predicting the goals and intentions of other individuals, but the precise identity of these social cues and the specific neural systems by which they are processed remain somewhat obscure. Adding to uncertainty regarding the neural substrates of attention, socially cued attention appears to have unique properties that map poorly onto existing models, which emphasize dichotomous exogenous and endogenous attention systems.

To explore these issues, we have investigated the visual orienting behavior of several different primate species in response to social stimuli in both field and laboratory settings. A complete understanding of visual attention in primates must account not only for gross patterns of visual orienting in natural environments but also for the fine spatiotemporal details of visual orienting measured in controlled laboratory settings. These ethological and psychophysical goals are often approached separately, using different animal models and highly divergent techniques, reflecting in part the fact that the demands of naturalistic observation generally preclude precise recording of visual orienting behavior. Likewise, psychophysical experiments have typically failed to replicate the behavioral contexts in which visual orienting behavior normally operates. Nonetheless, it is our contention that these divisions are not insurmountable and that combining ethological and psychophysical approaches will foster the development of a unified, evolutionarily motivated theory of attention. Here we consider the impact of social contexts on visual attention, outlining some of what has been learned from each tradition. In particular, we describe our own efforts to bridge these approaches, and to sketch a tentative model of primate attention for further study.

Evolution of Visual Specializations in Primates

Primates are unusual among mammals in their strong reliance on vision (Allman 1999). Initially, visual specializations probably evolved in primates to support movement through upper tree branches (Robert Martin's "fine-branch niche hypothesis"; Martin 1990), to facilitate hunting for insects (Matt Cartmill's "visual predator hypothesis"; Cartmil 1972), or both. Nonhuman primates might thus be expected to use vision primarily for locomotion and food acquisition, and perhaps also, like many other mammals, for predator avoidance.

Over the course of primate evolution, however, visual processing appears to have become increasingly specialized for guiding social interaction. Many primates make extensive use of vision to localize, monitor, and interact with conspecifics, and likewise devote a large portion of their brains to visual processing; the parallel expansion of the primate brain has been accompanied by a corresponding increase in the flexibility and complexity of primate social groups (Allman 1999). Whereas prosimian primates rely heavily on olfactory and pheromone-mediated modes of communication, these ancestral sensory modalities have been supplanted in more derived primates by visually mediated signals, including coloration, posture, movements, facial expressions, and gaze (de Waal 2003; note also Gilad et al. 2004), as well as affective and referential vocalizations (Cheney and Seyfarth 1990; Seyfarth and Cheney 2003). Researchers have long recognized the importance of studying primate visual attention in the laboratory, but we have all too often neglected the ecological and social role attention plays in natural behavior.

Behavioral Goals Drive Orienting in Natural Settings

The Russian psychologist Alfred Yarbus investigated overt visual orienting behavior in humans (Yarbus 1967) by recording visual fixation patterns during free and instructed scanning of pictures. Recording conditions were decidedly non-naturalistic: light-reflecting mirrors were suction-cupped to the eyes of volunteers. However, the visual stimuli consisted of photographs and paintings of humans and human artifacts, thus representing a significant enhancement in naturalism over contemporary psychophysical studies of attention. Yarbus's seminal work demonstrated the intrinsic salience of social stimuli as well as the strong influence of behavioral goals on visual orienting. For example, when subjects were shown the painting *An Unexpected Visitor*, fixation patterns focused on the people in the scene but were also heavily influenced by verbal instructions (figure 14.1).

Recently, Land and Hayhoe (2001), using noninvasive video gaze-tracking, have reported similar context-dependence in visual orienting. They report that fixations are almost completely specified by task demands, at least during performance of simple actions such as making a sandwich or preparing tea, and that very few fixations are made to task-irrelevant regions of space. These data suggest that visual fixation priorities not only are shaped by evolutionary pressures but also can serve as an external indicator of shifting internal goals that govern an animal's moment-to-moment behavior (Shepherd and Platt 2008).

Social Orienting Bias in Natural Settings

Observational data support the idea that visual orienting in nonhuman primates is also biased toward social stimuli (Keverne et al. 1978; Caine and Marra 1988; McNelis and Boatright-Horowitz 1998). Furthermore, these biases are not uniform; instead, some social stimuli attract more attention than others. For example, monkeys spend more time looking at pictures of faces gazing toward them than at faces with averted gaze (Keating and Keating 1982) and also look more often toward higher-ranking animals than lower-ranking animals (Keverne et al. 1978; McNelis and Boatright-Horowitz 1998). When viewing images of faces, nonhuman primates look preferentially toward the eyes and mouth (Keating and Keating 1982; Kyes and Candland 1987; Guo et al. 2003). Such data have been limited, however, to observations at distance in natural settings or, in the laboratory, to qualitative analysis of fixation patterns within still photographs.

Given the various limitations of previous studies, one goal of our research has been to quantitatively measure visual orienting by nonhuman primates in naturalistic social and physical settings. To do this, we recorded gaze behavior in socially housed ringtailed lemurs (*Lemur catta*) freely moving and interacting in large three dimensional environments. We used a lightweight telemetric optical gaze-tracking device (figure 14.2) (Shepherd and Platt 2006) operating at 0.22 degrees × 33 ms resolution—a degree of precision comparable to eye-tracking methods used in the laboratory.

Our approach differed, however, in that we did not provide any task or instruction, but instead attempted to infer the goals guiding visual orienting in natural behavioral contexts from the observed patterns of visual behavior (Shepherd and Platt 2008). Ringtailed

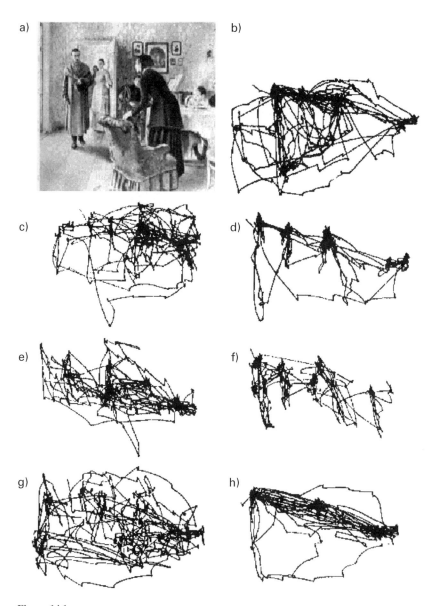

Figure 14.1
Social context and behavioral goals alter fixation patterns during free viewing. Panels b-h show the different gaze patterns of viewers when asked different questions about the illustration, Ilya Rjepin's *Unexpected Visitor*, shown at upper left. Viewers scanned the photographs in very different ways when asked to estimate the family's wealth (c), estimate their ages (d), memorize the position of people and objects (g), or estimate how long the "unexpected visitor" had been away (h). After Yarbus (1957).

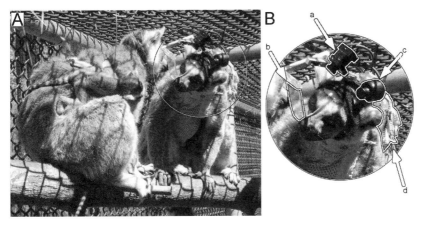

Figure 14.2
Equipment for tracking gaze during the natural behavior of freely moving animals. We tracked gaze during spontaneous and natural interactions with cohabitant conspecifics (A) using a telemetric optical gaze-tracking system developed by Iscan, Inc. The system (B) was composed of an infrared camera and LED (a) imaging the lemur's right eye through a dichroic mirror (b), an optical camera (c) viewing the scene in front the lemur's head, and a telemetry system housed in a primate vest (d), which broadcast to a remote monitoring station, where the subject's recorded gaze direction was analyzed and projected onto locations in the recorded visual scene. After Shepherd and Platt (2006).

lemurs, prosimian primates that diverged from the ancestors of "higher" primates some 60 million years ago, were chosen as subjects for their tolerance of handling and their availability at the Duke University Lemur Center. Ringtailed lemur social groups are similar to those of many higher primates, comprising ten to twenty individuals of both sexes, organized in well-defined social hierarchies, and communicating through auditory, olfactory, and visual modalities (Jolly 1966; Sauther et al. 1999).

We found that male ringtailed lemurs fixated their human handlers, as would be expected, given we had just suited them temporarily into recording equipment. More important, they also fixated their social companions, and did so more often than they fixated small food rewards (figure 14.3a).

Each of these three categories—human handlers, conspecifics, and food rewards—were fixated significantly more often than chance; furthermore, they were fixated significantly more often than high-contrast environmental features (e.g. dark branches in foreground with light-colored ground behind), stimuli we naively expected to attract attention based on their low-level visual salience. Elevating contrast is one of the simplest and most traditional means of driving bottom-up attention, and environmental features were selected partly on the basis of strong visual contrast between them and the local background. These data suggest that animals and food rewards were identified and localized and that this information was used to guide visual orienting during natural behaviors. Social orienting bias was not inflexible, however, and in fact was reversed during periods of active

a)   b)

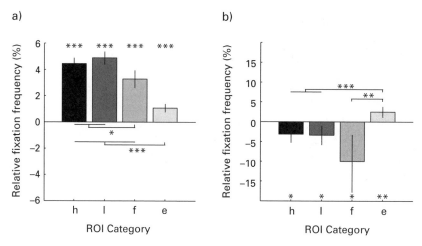

Figure 14.3
Fixation priorities in stationary and moving lemurs. (A) Lemurs fixated humans (h), lemurs (l), food (f), and high-contrast environmental features (e) significantly more than chance expectation; fixated humans and lemurs significantly more than food rewards; and all three significantly more than environmental features. (B) Lemurs fixated environmental features significantly more often when moving than when stationary, seemingly at the cost of fixations toward animals and rewards. After Shepherd and Platt (2008). *** $P < 0.0005$; ** $P < 0.001$; * $P < 0.01$.

locomotion (figure 14.3b). While moving, lemurs instead fixated environmental features that served as potential surfaces across which the lemur could travel toward their subsequent destination. Together with earlier research (Yarbus 1967; Land and Hayhoe 2001), these findings validate the use of quantitative gaze measurements as an externally observable indicator of otherwise unobservable mental states—the specific current behavioral goals of a given animal—and further reveal that the typical behavioral context for a stationary lemur involves not only monitoring environmental threats, such as predators, and rewards, such as food, but also other members of the social group.

Dominance, Sex, and Social Salience

Our ongoing field studies of orienting in ringtailed lemurs support the idea that early primates possessed neural specializations for orienting toward and extracting relevant information from other animals. The sheer variety and complexity of possible stimuli and contexts available in the field, however, has challenged our ability to draw definitive conclusions regarding the specific social stimuli that guide visual orienting during any specific behavior—an endeavor that is ongoing in our laboratory. Moreover, despite the evident similarity between human visual orienting priorities and those we observed in lemurs, the brains, genomes, and social systems of these two species differ dramatically. Finally, ringtailed lemurs do not serve as a model species for any particular neurological or psychological behavior or disorder, and thus little is known about brain function in these animals.

To deal with these limitations we have conducted parallel investigations of the visual orienting behavior of another primate, whose visual abilities, social structure, environmental niche, and physiology more closely mirror our own. Rhesus macaques (*Macaca mulatta*) are an actively studied anthropoid primate with relatively well-understood biology, and like humans, they live in large, hierarchical social groups with extensive repertoires of visual, auditory, and tactile behavioral interaction.

Although rhesus monkeys have been widely used to study visual attention, most of these studies have used arbitrary stimuli with little or no intrinsic behavioral relevance. We know, however, that in the wild, monkeys visually monitor one another (Keverne et al. 1978; Caine and Marra 1988; McNelis and Boatright-Horowitz 1998), and in the laboratory, will preferentially seek out visual stimuli with social content (Butler 1954; Sackett 1966). To precisely quantify how rhesus monkeys prioritize specific classes of social stimuli for orienting, we developed a choice task designed to balance fluid rewards against the potential reward value of seeing images of other monkeys. Specifically, monkeys chose between orienting to either of two targets, one associated with a juice reward and another associated with an alternative juice reward and a photograph of a monkey. By determining the value of differential reward at which monkeys were equally likely to choose the social or control image, we were able to quantify the reward value of different classes of social stimuli (Deaner et al. 2005). We found that male monkeys consistently "overvalued" seeing potential mating cues (female hindquarters) and faces of dominant males, but "undervalued" seeing the faces of low-ranking males (figure 14.4).

The attraction of gaze to high-ranking males is somewhat counterintuitive, since under natural conditions direct staring serves as a threat gesture in many primate species (van Hoof 1967). Analysis of dwell times—the duration of looking at social stimuli once foveated—provides a potential explanation for this paradox: potential mating cues evoked prolonged stares, whereas faces evoked fixations of shorter duration. Frequent, furtive glances toward high-ranked males may serve to maximize acquisition of important social information while simultaneously minimizing risk of conflict.

Evolutionary Biology of Social Gaze Attraction

Thus, both for freely moving lemurs and for macaques performing attention tasks in the laboratory, visual inspection of conspecifics seems to be an important goal of visual orienting. Ethological studies of primate behavior suggest that this behavioral bias may serve at least two important biological functions. Vision has long been known to play a role in hunting and foraging, affecting both predators, where selection pressures favor narrowed,

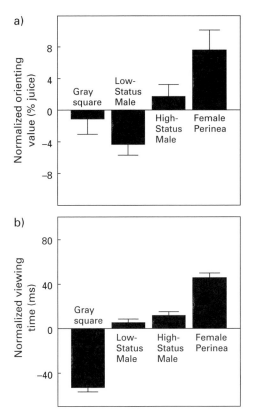

Figure 14.4
Monkeys sacrifice juice to view important social stimuli. (a) When monkeys were offered different juice rewards to fixate two targets, only one of which also yielded an image reward, they chose each option equally when the intrinsic value of viewing an image offset the amount of juice sacrificed. Monkeys paid the highest amount of juice to see female perinea and a lower amount to see high-ranking male faces, but required extra juice to look at low-ranking male faces or, to a lesser extent, uniform gray squares. (b) A similar pattern is evident in the amount of time per presentation that monkeys fixated each category of image. This measure differs, however, in that monkeys dwell for similar lengths of time on low- and high-status faces. After Deaner et al. (2005).

binocular fields of view (such as in carnivores) and prey, where selection favors widened, monocular visual fields (such as in ungulates). Primates have largely binocular visual fields, but this does not free them from the need to be vigilant for hungry predators or for hostile competitors. Primate social groups are often characterized by a certain baseline level of aggression, and individuals thus need to spend some of their time surveying conspecifics, both from within and outside the social group, for possible threats. In fact, many primates may have to actively balance centrifugal surveillance (against external predation or rival social groups) and centripetal surveillance (against bullying from within the social group; Caine and Marra 1988).

Centripetal surveillance, however, implies that there is a social group in the first place. From this we infer a second, more subtle role for social attention, first articulated by Chance and Jolly (1970). Cohesion of social groups requires, as a principal element, the coordination of movements so as to regulate spacing between each individual and its cohort. For this reason, Chance and Jolly (1970) suggested that "the social attention of individuals within a cohort . . . must be directed exclusively at the other members of it" and went on to note that "even when they are an integral part of the complete society, the distinct coherence of a cohort . . . may depend on their maintaining a predominant degree of attention toward themselves." Chance and Jolly proposed that the key mechanism of dominance is not the threat of violence from the strongest member of the troop but rather the ability of these individuals to capture the attention of other group members. In short, Chance and Jolly argued that primate societies are bound together by centripetal attention —specifically, in hierarchical societies, by attention toward high-ranking animals.

Although dominance may be structured by the threat of violence and by the need for coalitional defense against such threats (Keverne et al. 1978; Cheney and Seyfarth 1990), status-based saliency seems to be largely prosocial, and in some sense positively valenced, in that it promotes proximity to the group. For example, Chance and Jolly (1970) describe a behavior called "reflected escape" in which a subordinate animal, threatened, runs in a looping arch, first away from the challenger and then back toward the central members of the group—even if these were the same dominant individuals who initiated the threat. These ideas seem to be supported by findings that gaze (Keverne et al. 1978), allegiances, and grooming (Cheney and Seyfarth 1990) are allocated preferentially to dominant individuals of the group, independent of those individuals' aggressiveness, and also by our finding that macaques sacrifice more juice to view dominant animals than subordinate animals. It currently remains unclear whether the privileged saliency of the social cohort, and particularly the most dominant individuals, is driven by neural systems governing vigilance (such as the amygdala) or those driving pursuit of rewards (such as the ventral striatum).

Our initial assumption was that fixating high-value social targets reflects some sort of intrinsic reward, as suggested by the increased juice premiums paid by monkeys given an opportunity to see these categories of stimuli. However, enhanced salience may in fact be *driving* reward, rather than deriving from it: several strands of research suggest that the mere act of attending to a stimulus may enhance its desirability. Zajonc first described these effects in 1968 when he found that brief presentation of unfamiliar visual stimuli caused human subjects to subsequently rate those stimuli more aesthetically pleasing, even when they could not recall having seen them (Zajonc 1968; reviewed in Bornstein 1989). More recently, two studies have generalized this effect from "mere exposure" to attentional state. Raymond and colleagues (2003) found that stimuli that were presented but ignored accrued negative associations in a variety of task conditions, a finding that confirmed attention could mediate "mere-exposure"-like effects. Shimojo and colleagues (2003) made a complementary discovery, using simple preference judgments. They found that prior to selecting the more attractive of two faces, subjects looked increasingly long and often at the face they subsequently chose; importantly, when subjects were forced to look at a particular face, they were also more likely to select it as the most desirable. Together, these findings suggest that differential orienting may drive changes in affective judgments, and furthermore, that these "mere exposure" effects may mediate social cohesion in primates by encouraging approach behavior toward salient targets. In this way, social saliency could play a critical role in patterning the spacing behavior of animals in a group, making the most often fixated animals most desirable for approach.

A fascinating illustration of this process might be the tendency for both human and nonhuman animals to increase their visual salience during the mating season. Both humans and other animals either maintain sexually selected ornamentation year-round or acquire ornamentation when interest in mating peaks (von Schantz et al. 1999; Haselton et al. 2007). Whether or not these bright, high-contrast ornaments serve to signal reproductive fitness, they may operate by enhancing saliency, and thus the likelihood the ornamented individual will be approached by potential mates.

Socially Cued Attention: Following the Gaze of Another Individual

In 1876, Ralph Waldo Emerson wrote: "The eyes of men converse as much as their tongues, with the advantage, [sic] that the ocular dialect needs no dictionary, but is understood all the world over" (p. 173). As Emerson intimated, where we look often betrays our interests, intentions, and desires. Thus, we use visual orienting not only to localize other individuals but also to interpret their relationships, attitudes, and intentions. Nonhuman primates also appear to use orienting by conspecifics to infer the location of important stimuli and events, to predict behavior, and perhaps even to interpret social relationships among others (Cheney and Seyfarth 1990). Subtler still, humans (and perhaps other primates, particularly apes; de Waal 2003) use and recognize a number of deictic gestures, varying from discreet (a quick flick of the eyes) to overt (pointing), that signal important perceptions and plans. Furthermore, we use these signals in competitive contexts to read intent and predict action (watching someone's eyes during chess) and to confound such predictions by others (the "no look pass" of soccer and basketball, in which a player looks toward a different teammate than the one to whom she intends to pass the ball).

Despite the obvious importance of social cues for guiding attention in natural behavior, this process has remained, until recently, relatively unexplored by psychologists or neurobiologists. One typical laboratory approach to visual attention asks subjects to stare at a fixation point, which is followed by either a central cue or peripheral stimulus directing attention to a peripheral location (Posner 1980). Studies using this technique have revealed that central cues that validly predict the location of a future peripheral target shift attention in a voluntary ("endogenous" or "top-down") manner toward the likely location of the target, whereas abrupt peripheral cues, even when nonpredictive, automatically attract attention ("exogenous", "reflexive", "bottom-up" attention). These attention shifts are evidenced by changes in sensory discrimination performance and reaction time, and have distinct time courses (Muller and Rabbitt 1989): exogenous attention operates more quickly and generates a subsequent orienting deficit ("inhibition of return"), whereas endogenous attention is slower and more sustained. Despite the utility of this paradigm, its generality remains limited because of a failure to study orienting by human and nonhuman primates in the natural world.

To explore this issue, Friesen and Kingstone (1998) modified the Posner paradigm to investigate socially cued attention. In their experiments, subjects were instructed to fixate a central point, where a face briefly appeared with eyes cast either rightward or leftward. A split second after face presentation, a target appeared randomly on the right or left of this cue, irrespective of gaze direction in the face. Subjects were faster to respond to targets appearing in the direction of the observed gaze, even for cue-to-target delays as brief as 105 ms (stimulus onset asynchronies, or SOA). Thus, they discovered that viewing a face that has an averted gaze rapidly and reflexively shifts the viewer's attention in the same direction, even when gaze direction does not predict the eventual location of the target. Subsequent studies reported these effects were both general (viewing a head turned to the side also shifts attention in that direction; Langton and Bruce 1999) and involuntary (social cuing persists even when the target was 80 percent likely to appear in the direction *opposite* viewed gaze; Driver et al. 1999). Attention shifts associated with observed gaze thus appear categorically distinct from both responses to explicit cues (Friesen et al. 2004) and to abstract spatial associations (Galfano et al. 2006).

Results like these supported the argument that humans had evolved a dedicated gaze-following module specialized for rapid and reflexive sharing of attention in social groups (Baron-Cohen 1994; Perrett and Emery 1994). We tested this hypothesis explicitly by measuring visual orienting responses to social gaze cues in monkeys and humans (Deaner and Platt 2003). Surprisingly, we found that both monkeys and humans responded more quickly to an unpredictable target when it appeared where a monkey presented at fixation had been looking. Furthermore, fixation position in both species drifted in the direction of gaze, likely reflecting cumulative microsaccades (Hafed and Clark 2002; Engbert and Kliegl 2003). The magnitude and time course of the gaze-following response was highly similar in the two species (figure 14.5), suggesting shared underlying neural circuitry.

Our results strongly support the conclusion that social gaze following is not unique to humans, and may in fact rely on neural substrates that are widespread among primates and possibly other animals. Though gaze following by nonhuman primates may differ, in both strength and kind, from that evinced by humans (Okamoto-Barth et al. 2007; Tomonaga 2007), it appears that many animals are able to shift attention in response to observed social cues. Consistent with this argument, Tomasello and colleagues, along with a number of other research groups, have amassed a large body of work showing that many

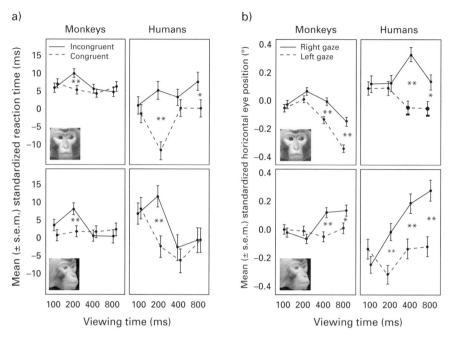

Figure 14.5
Gaze following by monkeys and humans shares psychophysical features. Monkeys and humans show similar magnitude and time course of gaze following in response to nonpredictive monkey gaze cues presented continuously for 100, 200, 400, or 800 ms prior to target presentation. (a) These attention shifts were evident both by decreases in normalized reaction times to congruent (dashed) vs. incongruent (solid) stimuli and (b) by microsaccades in the direction of observed gaze during cue presentation. After Deaner and Platt (2003). ** $P < 0.001$; * $P < 0.05$.

animals, including apes (Brauer et al. 2005), dogs (Agnetta et al. 2000), monkeys (Tomasello et al. 1998), goats (Kaminski et al. 2005), dolphins (Tschudin et al. 2001), and ravens (Bugnyar et al. 2004), can use gaze cues to find hidden food or retrieve objects (reviewed in Emery 2000; Itakura 2004).

This conclusion is supported by our work tracking visual orienting patterns among freely interacting lemurs. Uniquely among studies of gaze following, we quantitatively and precisely monitored gaze during spontaneous interaction with conspecifics. We found that lemurs tended to orient their eyes in the same direction that observed lemurs oriented their bodies and heads (figures 14.6a, 14.6b).

This gaze alignment, however, could reflect simultaneous orienting to the same salient events in a shared environment rather than active gaze following. In order to explore this question we examined the temporal sequence of gaze alignment when the subject oriented to an observed lemur. We found that prior to fixating the observed lemur, there was no alignment between the two animals' gaze. After fixating the observed lemur, however,

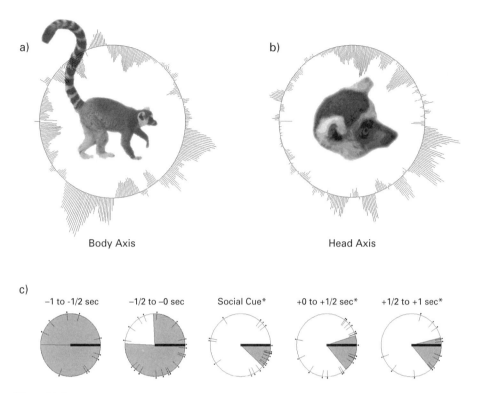

Figure 14.6
Spontaneous gaze-following in lemurs. Lemurs spontaneously follow the gaze direction of their conspecifics in natural interaction. Lemurs not only co-orient with the body (a) and head (b) axes of observed lemurs, but selectively increase gaze alignment with those individuals they have recently attended (c). In panels (a) and (b), outward lines are gaze offsets that are overrepresented with respect to chance, whereas inward lines are gaze offsets that are underrepresented. In panel (c), tick marks occur at mean gaze offsets recorded in half-second periods prior to fixation, in the period during which the lemur is fixated, and for half-second periods after fixation. Shaded regions in panel (c) reflect the dispersion of gaze alignments. Starred intervals are significantly aligned with gaze (chi^2 test $P < 0.05$). After Shepherd and Platt (2008).

gaze alignment increased significantly (figure 14.6c). The temporal sequence of gaze alignment supports the conclusion that lemurs actively follow the gaze of other individuals (Shepherd and Platt 2007). Our results stand in sharp contrast to at least two prior observational studies (Itakura 1996; Anderson and Mitchell 1999) that concluded that prosimian primates cannot follow the gaze of human observers.

Modulation of the Social-Gaze Module

Because both monkeys and humans shift their attention in response to social gaze cues, even when such cues fail to predict the location of a behavioral goal, it has been argued that social gaze following is a strictly reflexive behavior generated by a dedicated neural module (Driver et al. 1999; Deaner and Platt 2003). Recent studies, however, challenge the notion that gaze cueing is purely reflexive, instead indicating that social context can influence gaze-following behavior in both humans and monkeys. Specifically, several lines of evidence suggest that neural systems contributing to social gaze following are regulated by the social milieu as well as by intrinsic factors, including sex hormones such as testosterone or neuromodulators such as serotonin. In humans, for example, females show much stronger attention shifts in response to gaze cues than do males (figure 14.7; Bayliss et al. 2005; Deaner et al. 2007); moreover, our lab has found that gaze following in females, but not in males, is influenced by the familiarity of the observed face (Deaner et al. 2007).

These observations suggest the possibility that sex hormones may play an important role in regulating social attention. Supporting this idea, the amygdala, orbitofrontal cortex (OFC), and hippocampus form a functional circuit important for associating emotional and social salience with mnemonic and perceptual information (Vuilleumier 2002; Sabbagh 2004; Smith et al. 2006), and actively contribute to perception of faces (Ishai et al. 2005). Each of these brain structures is sexually dimorphic (Goldstein et al. 2001), suggesting that sexual differentiation in these areas may directly pattern responses to social cues.

Intriguingly, patients with anxiety disorders show heightened following of a fearful gaze relative to other emotional expressions (Mathews et al. 2003; Hori et al. 2005; Holmes

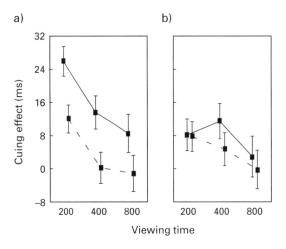

Figure 14.7
Sex differences in gaze following in humans. Human females exhibit stronger gaze following than males and, furthermore, discriminate between familiar and unfamiliar individuals when following another's gaze. Females (solid lines) have greater reaction-time savings for gaze-congruent than gaze-incongruent targets when gaze cues were from familiar (a) rather than unfamiliar (b) individuals (at 200 ms, P < 0.003). Males (dashed lines) did not distinguish significantly between these conditions (at 200 ms, P > 0.4). After Deaner et al. (2007).

et al. 2006; note also Hietanen and Leppanen 2003; Putman et al. 2006). This contextual effect probably reflects the tendency for patients with anxiety to more strongly attend negatively valenced social stimuli, whereas normal subjects dwell less on them (e.g., Bradley et al. 1997; Bar-Haim et al. 2005). These studies imply that focused attention on a social target naturally extends to the objects it attends and the tasks in which it is engaged.

We have found similar evidence that social context and biological factors regulate gaze following in rhesus macaques (Shepherd et al. 2006). Specifically, we probed gaze-following behavior by seven male rhesus macaques in response to four rightward and four leftward gaze cues from each of four familiar monkeys. Importantly, each animal was designated dominant or subordinate on the basis of the direction and frequency of threat and submission gestures during controlled pairwise confrontations (see Deaner et al. 2005; Shepherd et al. 2006). We found that subordinate monkeys rapidly and automatically followed the gaze of all other monkeys (figure 14.8a), while dominant monkeys followed the gaze later, and then only in response to other dominant monkeys' also following it (figure 14.8b).

These differences in gaze-following behavior were weakly correlated with differences in testosterone production (Shepherd et al. 2006), as inferred from measurements of testis volume (Bercovitch and Ziegler 2002). We interpret these data to indicate that biological factors such as testosterone may influence the strength of gaze-following behavior in macaques, and further that the strength of gaze-following behavior in monkeys is modulated by social context, just as it is in humans.

Together, these results demonstrate that gaze following is deeply integrated into the larger social information–processing stream. That gaze following is an inherent component of face perception is indicated by the fact that heightened attention to faces attracts attention centrifugally in the direction of gaze, both in the case of females viewing familiar faces and anxious patients seeing faces with negatively valenced emotional content. At the same time, however, the fact that gaze following is modulated by factors such as familiarity and social dominance suggests that it is not an isolated module sequestered from other aspects of face processing and social knowledge. Finally, sex differences in humans and social rank differences in monkeys both hint at a possible role for sex hormones in shaping social attention systems in the brain. This supposition is strengthened by various results showing that fetal testosterone negatively impacts both social attention and social relationships in human juveniles (Knickmeyer and Baron-Cohen 2006). Together these findings strongly support the idea that social attention contributes strongly to natural primate behavior and cognition, and presents a significant addition to the traditional endogenous/exogenous model of attention control.

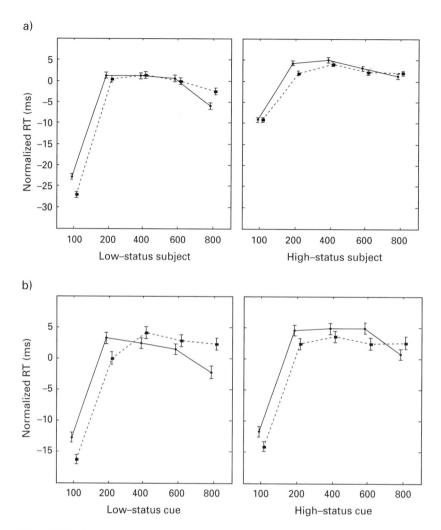

Figure 14.8
Social context influences gaze-following in macaques. (a) Even at the briefest cue durations, subject social status appears to influence gaze-following behavior (P < 0.005). Specifically, low social status makes a monkey more likely to follow gaze within 100 ms of seeing the cue, and also more likely to have strong inhibition of return at the latest time point—a temporal profile consistent with a reflexive attention shift, possibly due to increased anxiety or the modulatory effects of sex- and status-linked hormones such as testosterone on social-processing circuitry in the brain. (b) Cue social status also plays an important role (P < 0.01), leading to prolonged attention in the direction of gaze of a high-status cue and inhibited attention in the direction of gaze of a low-status cue, particularly in high-status subjects. Reaction times for congruent trials are shown in dashed lines and for incongruent trials are shown in solid lines. After Shepherd et al. (2006).

Social Attention and Autism: From the Lab to the Field

Data from the study of autism and other syndromes that disrupt social behavior suggest a gulf between behavioral responses in the laboratory and spontaneous use of social cues in the real world. Contrasting visual behavior in autistic subjects to that of typically developing children, van der Geest and colleagues (2002) showed that the fixation patterns of the two groups could not be distinguished when they viewed simple cartoons that included human figures. In contrast, Pelphrey and colleagues (2002) found substantial differences between these populations when they were inspecting photographs of faces. Similarly, although researchers have often failed to find dysfunctional gaze following in autism using the Posner attention task (Chawarska et al. 2003; Swettenham et al. 2003; Kylliainen and Hietanen 2004; but see Bayliss et al. 2005; Ristic et al. 2005), autistic individuals show severe disruptions of visuosocial orienting in naturalistic contexts. For example, Klin and colleagues (2002a, 2002b) measured gaze patterns in autistic individuals watching the movie *Who's Afraid of Virginia Woolf*, and found that gaze toward social stimuli was disordered—for example, fixations toward the eye regions were seemingly replaced by fixations toward the mouth—and that socially cued locations were severely neglected, as shown by a marked lack of fixations toward gaze- and gesture-cued regions of space. Furthermore, they found that the degree of abnormality in the fixation pattern of individual autistic subjects was strongly predictive of future social impairment.

Outside the laboratory, even high-functioning autistic individuals unaffected by common symptoms, such as seizures or repetitive movements, are nonetheless challenged in responding to the constant exchange of social cues that structures our daily lives. Temple Grandin (1999), an associate professor of animal science at Colorado State University who has autism, reports that she functions in social situations "solely by intellect and visualization skills . . . I did not know that eye movements had meaning until I read *Mindblindness* by Simon Baron-Cohen. I had no idea that people communicated feelings with their eyes. I also did not know that people get all kinds of little emotional signals which transmit feelings. My understanding of this became clearer after I read *Descartes', Error* by Antonio Damasio." Autism frequently involves a marked "lack of spontaneous seeking to share enjoyment, interests, or achievements with other people" or to reciprocate when these experiences and emotions are shared by others (American Psychological Association 1994, p. 66). It may be that the complement of rewards and reflexes evoked by social stimuli in typically developing individuals is disrupted in autism spectrum disorders, and that without these foundational elements, more sophisticated forms of empathy and social reasoning cannot develop.

It is interesting to note that both autism (Wassink et al. 2007) and social anxiety disorder (Skuse 2006) have been associated with dysfunction in the serotonin signaling system. Serotonin has likewise been linked to dominance status, affiliative social interaction, and decreases in antagonistic and impulsive social interactions (Raleigh et al. 1991; Edwards and Kravitz 1997), suggesting that it may also influence socially cued orienting between dominant and subordinate macaques. Together, these findings hint at a role for serotonin in regulating social attention in primates. Determining the impact of biological factors, such as serotonin and testosterone, on social attention may point to possible interventions to improve social functions in common psychopathologies.

Gaze as a Strategic Social Signal

As we have seen, social saliency may play a role not only in guiding attention but also in shaping the physical spacing of social group members and the affective tenor of their social interactions. It may also serve as a starting point for the development of much more advanced cognitive behaviors. David Perrett and Simon Baron-Cohen have argued that detection of eyes and interpretation of gaze are foundational to building a theory of mind, by which we intuitively mirror the attentional and perhaps even intentional states of others. We do this so instinctively that we frequently anthropomorphize even alien and impersonal phenomena, perhaps allowing us to understand complex and dynamic patterns by analogy to human behavioral goals—for example, "The electrons don't like to be near one another and are instead attracted to the positive core of an atom, causing them to settle sequentially into the centermost un-crowded orbitals." Typically developing humans have an intuitive expertise at communicating affect and attentional state, perhaps in part because they have an intrinsic drive to *learn* to do so: from a young age, typically developing humans take pleasure in successfully directing another's attention toward stimuli that we, too, have perceived (Tomasello et al. 2005).

These considerations naturally lead us to consider overt eye movements as an active signaling mechanism that shapes primate social interactions. We have mentioned the role of eye movements in initiating conflict, but monkeys make far more sophisticated use of gaze. For example, eye contact can signal sexual interest (Dixson 1998), aggression (van Hoof 1967), and solicitation for coalition formation in agonistic interactions against third parties (de Waal 2003). Likewise, humans use eye contact as a key aspect of affiliation, courtship, and intimidation (Argyle and Cook 1976), and also during coordination of attention ("triadic" or "joint attention"; Emery 2000). Moreover, gaze acts to structure both verbal and nonverbal human social interactions. To signal rank relationships, for example, people look preferentially toward the most high-ranking person, and when conversing, gaze is used to emphasize spoken arguments, to conclude statements, to emphasize nonverbal reactions to heard statements, and to coordinate taking turns in conversation (Argyle and Cook 1976).

With the evolution of increased visual and social complexity, primates appear to have evolved ever more sophisticated means of structuring social behavior through gaze. Like humans, many animal species are capable of following gaze. Apes are even reported to use deictic gestures (de Waal 2003), though these signals may receive little currency due to the ubiquity of competitive and paucity of cooperative interactions among nonhuman primates (Hare and Tomasello 2004). The importance of gaze cues for facilitating increased cooperation among human ancestors may even have led to somatic adaptations that increase the saliency and specificity of social attention cues, for example, by enhancing the visibility of gaze through increased contrast of the pupil against the sclera (Kobayashi and Koshima 2001; Tomasello et al. 2006). At the same time, however, the continued relevance of competitive interactions between human ancestors may have led to a compensatory enhancement of covert attention abilities in humans relative to those of nonhuman primates and, especially, other mammals.

This manipulative role of gaze is perhaps the least understood aspect of visual orienting behavior, and nothing is known about how the demands of signaling bring their influence to bear on the gaze control system of the brain. Following convention, we have approached macaque orienting toward other macaques in terms of intrinsic reward, and orienting to follow gaze in terms of visuosocial reflex. However, it might be more realistic to assume that initial rapid orienting responses depend upon reflexive processes and that slower orienting behaviors and sustained fixations depend upon reward evaluations. For example, all monkeys in our studies initially looked toward other individuals and followed their gaze, but other behavioral contingencies shaped gaze behavior, as well, such as abbreviating risky glances toward higher-ranked individuals (Haude et al. 1976; Deaner et al. 2005), extinguishing gaze following of lower-ranking animals (Shepherd et al. 2006), and prolonging male visual orienting toward female hindquarters (Deaner et al. 2005).

Toward a Neuroethological Model of Attention in Primates

If we were to develop a biologically plausible, ethologically motivated model of primate gaze, what features must it have? We feel strongly that the bottom-up component of these models must not only reflect what we know about the primate visual system but must also consider the role vision plays in guiding the behavior of primates in realistic ecological and social contexts. For example, Laurent Itti and colleagues, among others, have used visual filters, inspired loosely by the physiology of the primate visual system, to predict human visual attention. Such models can successfully estimate spatial saliency by filtering images through a series of low-level feature maps (Peters et al. 2005; Carmi and Itti 2006). Each map tracks the extent to which a region "pops out" from its surroundings in a particular dimension, such as brightness, orientation, texture, motion, or color, and these maps can be combined to successfully model many aspects of bottom-up attention.

Although these models can accurately identify salient regions of still images and video, they often fail to highlight social stimuli such as faces, or rely heavily on image motion to assign saliency to humans and animals. Without undervaluing either this accomplishment or the importance of motion as a predictor of animacy, we nevertheless note that demands of both sociality and predator avoidance require accurate and fast discrimination of animals, even when those animals are stationary or when dynamic environments such as running water or blowing leaves produce irrelevant image motion. Moreover, whereas identification and tracking of animate objects has proved a challenge for computer vision, these tasks are performed quickly and easily by the primate brain. In laboratory experiments, humans can initiate saccades toward an animal in a novel photograph in as little as 120 ms (Kirchner and Thorpe 2006), and in unconstrained viewing, animate stimuli and especially other humans are quickly targeted for visual inspection.

Serre and colleagues (2007) partially addressed these issues by developing a model that uses biologically inspired filters based on neurons in the ventral visual processing stream (Ungerleider and Mishkin 1982) to quickly identify images containing animals. It is important to note, however, that this model explicitly fails to localize the animals within the images. The processes that link object recognition by the ventral visual processing stream to target localization within the dorsal visual processing stream remain largely unknown, despite the fact that these processes determine how attention selects parts of the visual field for further processing. In fact, Serre and colleagues note that their model "cannot account for our everyday vision which involves eye movements and top-down effects," and that an extension of the model requiring "top-down signals from higher to lower areas . . . limit[ing] visual processing to a 'spotlight of attention' centered around the animal target" results in "significant improvement in the classification performance."

This study illustrates the benefits of considering the natural goals of orienting in social contexts, and likewise of considering evidence from functional imaging and neurophysiological recording studies. Recent fMRI studies have identified human brain areas that are involved in visual analysis of body position and identity (Downing et al. 2001), identification of faces (Haxby et al. 1994), and interpretation of actions and facial expressions (Allison et al. 2000), and are beginning to identify macaque homologs (Logothetis et al. 1999; Tsao et al. 2003). The general conservation of cortical organization across primate species, together with these recent findings, suggests that visual areas specialized for processing social stimuli may be among those primordial visual cortical areas (for example, V1, V2, V5; see Tootell et al. 2003; Rosa and Tweedale 2005) present in stem primates, and perhaps others mammals (Kendrick et al. 2001).

As revealed through behavioral studies, the gaze-control system must recognize and respond appropriately to biological targets. We speculate that two parallel pathways accomplish this goal (Adolphs 2002; Vuilleumier 2002; see figure 14.9). First, a primitive retino-tectal pathway uses crude biological primitives to quickly identify social targets and their gaze direction (Johnson 2005). Just such a relay of social threat signals, from the retina through the superior colliculus (SC) and pulvinar nucleus of the thalamus to the amygdala, has already been identified in humans (Morris et al. 1999), and neurons in the amygdala are sensitive to gaze direction in a viewed face (Kawashima et al. 1999; Hoffman et al. 2007). The amygdala, in turn, sends this first-pass analysis of social targets toward attention control centers and higher visual areas (Vuilleumier 2002).

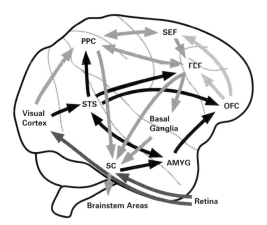

Figure 14.9
Key circuits involved in social attention. Connectivity of social (light), reward (intermediate), and attention (dark) pathways. In addition to the cortical pathway, a fast subcortical pathway connects the superior colliculus to the amygdala via the thalamus (not shown). Note that several social-processing areas lie along the superior temporal sulcus, occupying both the posterior and anterior temporal lobes, and that functional activity in imaging tasks has not yet been systematically related to past anatomical studies. (PPC: posterior parietal cortex, including 7A and LIP; STS: superior temporal sulcus regions; SEF: supplementary eye fields; FEF: frontal eye fields; OFC: orbitofrontal cortex; AMYG: amygdala.)

At longer time scales, information processed in the temporal cortex, in conjunction with contextual signals from the hippocampus and the orbitofrontal cortex (OFC), modulates visual attention via the amygdala (Vuilleumier 2002; Sabbagh 2004; Smith et al. 2006). This pathway may be highly sensitive to biological factors that differentiate circuitry and behavior between the sexes (Goldstein et al. 2001; Bayliss et al. 2005; Deaner et al. 2007) and across psychological conditions (Mathews et al. 2003; Hori et al. 2005; Holmes et al. 2006; Putman et al. 2006), and may, when compromised, contribute to the development of autism (Schultz 2005; though note also Amaral et al. 2003). Ultimately, amygdala-mediated signals pass through the supplementary and frontal eye fields (SEF and FEF), the lateral intraparietal area (LIP), and ultimately to the superior colliculus (SC) as a final common output governing most, if not all, gaze behavior.

Second, and in parallel, a more recently evolved cortical pathway leading from V1 through the ventral pathway to the extrastriate body area (EBA; Downing et al. 2001), the fusiform face area (FFA; Haxby et al. 1994), and the superior temporal sulcus (STS; Allison et al. 2000) identifies biological targets. It remains unclear whether these areas are primarily involved in assessing subordinate-level distinctions between hierarchically classifiable objects; or are more specifically involved in distinguishing the identities and actions of animate objects; or, finally, are areas optimized for visual perception of con-specifics. It seems likely that the development of these areas depends on experience (Gauthier et al. 1999) and may rely upon signals arising in the subcortical pathway for appropriate patterning during development (Schultz 2005).

Ultimately, signals from these ventral ("what") areas must relay social information to dorsal ("where") orienting and attention control systems. Signals from the higher-order areas of the ventral pathway then ramify to multiple targets in the visual orienting system. How exactly this may occur is an open question, since much of the visuosocial cortex (Tsao et al. 2003) is connected in one or two steps to posterior parietal (7A and LIP; Seltzer and Pandya 1991), frontal (SEF and FEF; Seltzer and Pandya 1989), and subcortical orienting areas (pulvinar nucleus; Romanski et al. 1997; superior colliculus; Fries 1984). Some of this ambiguity arises from the inconsistent localization of socially activated cortical domains in terms of previous architectonic and tracing studies, especially along the STS. For example, although particular areas within the STS (Allison et al. 2000; Tsao et al. 2003; Calder et al. 2007) are preferentially activated by particular visuosocial tasks, distinct subregions of the STS appear to have radically different connectivity (Seltzer and Pandya 1989, 1991). It seems likely that whatever pathways are involved, contextual effects on social orienting are implemented by an even more diverse group of cortical areas involved in memory, emotion, and motivation, including the hippocampus, the amygdala, and the OFC. These regions are differentially regulated by sex hormones and make up part of a network of neural populations activated in many visuosocial tasks.

Conclusions

Laboratory research using arbitrary tasks and stimuli have identified two complementary systems for visual orienting—one fast and reflexive, the other slow and deliberative. Neuroethological studies of visual attention, by contrast, have revealed a suite of socially motivated and socially cued orienting behaviors that do not divide neatly along these lines. Specifically, primates and other animals are motivated to look at one another, preferentially orient to high-value social targets such as the faces of dominant males, and follow the orienting movements of others with their own attention. Moreover, these responses are regulated by behavioral context, sex hormones, and serotonin. These observations strongly support the idea that the primate brain is specialized for acquiring useful visual information from the social world and that these adaptations rely on the integration of multiple neural circuits involved in identifying social stimuli and social cues, determining their meaning, and responding appropriately. Despite the commonalities of these systems across primates and even other mammals, the challenge for future neuroethological research is to determine how these mechanisms contribute to adaptive differences in social behavior in different species.

References

Adolphs R (2002) Recognizing emotion from facial expressions: Psychological and neurological mechanisms. Behav Cogn Neurosci Rev 1: 21–61.

Agnetta B, Hare B, Tomasello M (2000) Cues to food location that domestic dogs (*Canis familiaris*) of different ages do and do not use. Anim Cogn 3: 107–112.

Allison T, Puce A, McCarthy G (2000) Social perception from visual cues: Role of the STS region. Trends Cogn Sci 4: 267–278.

Allman JM (1999) Evolving brains. New York: WH Freeman.

Amaral DG, Bauman MD, Mills C (2003) The amygdala and autism: Implications from non-human primate studies. Genes Brain Behav 2: 295–302.

Anderson JR, Mitchell RW (1999) Macaques but not lemurs co-orient visually with humans. Folia Primatol 70: 17–22.

American Psychiatric Association (1994). Autistic disorder. In: Diagnostic and statistical manual of mental disorders. 4th ed. Washington, DC: American Psychiatric Publishing.

Argyle M, Cook M (1976) Gaze and mutual gaze. Cambridge: Cambridge University Press.

Bar-Haim Y, Lamy D, Glickman S (2005) Attentional bias in anxiety: A behavioral and ERP study. Brain Cogn 59: 11–22.

Baron-Cohen S (1994) How to build a baby that can read minds: Cognitive mechanisms in mindreading. Cah Psychol Cogn 13: 513–552.

Bayliss AP, di Pellegrino G, Tipper SP (2005) Sex differences in eye gaze and symbolic cueing of attention. Q J Exp Psychol-A 58: 631–650.

Bercovitch FB, Ziegler TE (2002) Current topics in primate socioendocrinology. Annu Rev Anthropol 31: 45–67.

Bornstein RF (1989) Exposure and affect: Overview and meta-analysis of research, 1968–1987. Psychol Bull 106: 265–289.

Bradley BP, Mogg K, Millar N, Bonham-Carter C, Fergusson E, Jenkins J, Parr M (1997) Attentional biases for emotional faces. Cognition Emotion 11: 25–42.

Brauer J, Call J, Tomasello M (2005) All great ape species follow gaze to distant locations and around barriers. J Comp Psychol 119: 145–154.

Bugnyar T, Stöwe M, Heinrich B (2004) Ravens, *Corvus corax*, follow gaze direction of humans around obstacles. P Roy Soc Lond B Bio 271: 1331–1336.

Butler RA (1954). Incentive conditions which influence visual exploration. J Exp Psychol 48: 19–23.

Caine NG, Marra SL (1988) Vigilance and social organization in two species of primates. Animal Behav 36: 897–904.

Calder AJ, Beaver JD, Winston JS (2007) Separate coding of different gaze directions in the superior temporal sulcus and inferior parietal lobule. Curr Biol 17: 20–25.

Carmi R, Itti L (2006) Visual causes versus correlates of attentional selection in dynamic scenes. Vision Res 46: 4333–4345.

Cartmil M (1972) Arboreal adaptations and the origin of the order primates. In: The functional and evolutionary biology of primates (Tuttle, ed), 97–212. Chicago: Aldine-Atherton Press.

Chance M, Jolly C (1970) Social groups of monkeys, apes and men. New York: Dutton.

Chawarska K, Klin A, Volkmar F (2003) Automatic attention cueing through eye movement in 2-year-old children with autism. Child Dev 74: 1108–1122.

Cheney DL, Seyfarth RM (1990) How monkeys see the world: Inside the mind of another species. Chicago: University Of Chicago Press.

Corbetta M, Shulman GL (2002) Control of goal-directed and stimulus-driven attention in the brain. Nat Rev Neurosci 3: 201–215.

de Waal FB (2003) Darwin's legacy and the study of primate visual communication. Ann NY Acad Sci 1000: 7–31.

Deaner RO, Khera AV, Platt ML (2005) Monkeys pay per view: Adaptive valuation of social images by rhesus macaques. Curr Biol 15: 543–548.

Deaner RO, Platt ML (2003) Reflexive social attention in monkeys and humans. Curr Biol 13: 1609–1613.

Deaner RO, Shepherd SV, Platt ML (2007) Familiarity accentuates gaze cuing in women but not men. Biol Lett 3: 64–67.

Dixson AF (1998) Primate sexuality: Comparative studies of the prosimians, monkeys, apes, and human beings. New York: Oxford University Press.

Downing PE, Jiang Y, Shuman M, Kanwisher N (2001) A cortical area selective for visual processing of the human body. Science 293: 2470.

Driver J, Davis G, Ricciardelli P (1999) Gaze perception triggers reflexive visuospatial orienting. Vis Cogn 6: 509–540.

Edwards DH, Kravitz EA (1997) Serotonin, social status and aggression. Curr Opin Neurobiol 7: 812–819.

Eget HE, Yantis S (1997) Visual attention: control, representation, and time course. Annu Rev Psychol 48: 269–297.

Emerson RW (1876) The conduct of life. Boston: James R. Osgood.

Emery NJ (2000) The eyes have it: The neuroethology, function and evolution of social gaze. Neurosci Biobehav R 24: 581–604.

Engbert R, Kliegl R (2003) Microsaccades uncover the orientation of covert attention. Vision Res 43: 1035–1045.

Fries W (1984) Cortical projections to the superior colliculus in the macaque monkey: A retrograde study using horseradish peroxidase. J Comp Neurol 230: 55–76.

Friesen CK, Kingstone A (1998) The eyes have it! Reflexive orienting is triggered by nonpredictive gaze. Psychon B Rev 5: 490–495.

Friesen CK, Ristic J, Kingstone A (2004) Attentional effects of counterpredictive gaze and arrow cues. J Exp Psychol Hum Percept Perform 30: 319–329.

Galfano G, Rusconi E, Umiltà C (2006) Number magnitude orients attention, but not against one's will. Psychon B Rev 13: 869–874.

Gauthier I, Tarr MJ, Anderson AW, Skudlarski P, Gore JC (1999) Activation of the middle fusiform face area increases with expertise in recognizing novel objects. Nat Neurosci 2: 568–573.

Gilad Y, Wiebe V, Przeworski M, Lancet D, Pääbo S (2004) Loss of olfactory receptor genes coincides with the acquisition of full trichromatic vision in primates. PLoS Biol 2: E5.

Goldstein JM, Seidman LJ, Horton NJ, Makris N, Kennedy DN, Caviness VS, Jr, Faraone SV, Tsuang MT (2001) Normal sexual dimorphism of the adult human brain assessed by *in vivo* magnetic resonance imaging. Cereb Cortex 11: 490–497.

Grandin T (1999) Social problems: Understanding emotions and developing talents. Hyperlink: http://www .autism.org/temple/social.html.

Guo K, Robertson RG, Mahmoodi S, Tadmor Y, Young MP (2003) How do monkeys view faces? A study of eye movements. Exp Brain Res 150: 363–374.

Hafed ZM, Clark JJ (2002) Microsaccades as an overt measure of covert attention shifts. Vision Res 42: 2533–2545.

Hare B, Tomasello M (2004) Chimpanzees are more skilful in competitive than in cooperative cognitive tasks. Anim Behav 68: 571–581.

Haselton MG, Mortezaie M, Pillsworth EG, Bleske-Rechek A, Frederick DA (2007) Ovulatory shifts in human female ornamentation: Near ovulation, women dress to impress. Horm Behav 51: 40–45.

Haude RH, Graber JG, Farres AG (1976) Visual observing by rhesus monkeys: Some relationships with social dominance rank. Anim Learn Behav 4: 163–166.

Haxby JV, Horwitz B, Ungerleider LG, Maisog JM, Pietrini P, Grady CL (1994) The functional organization of human extrastriate cortex: A PET-rCBF study of selective attention to faces and locations. J Neurosci 14: 6336–6353.

Hietanen JK, Leppanen JM (2003) Does facial expression affect attention orienting by gaze direction cues? J Exp Psychol Hum Percept Perform 29: 1228–1243.

Hoffman KL, Gothard KM, Scmid MC, Logothetis NK (2007) Facial-expression and gaze-selective responses in the monkey amygdala. Curr Biol 17: 766–772.

Holmes A, Richards A, Green S (2006) Anxiety and sensitivity to eye gaze in emotional faces. Brain Cogn 60: 282–294.

Hori E, Tazumi T, Umeno K, Kamachi M, Kobayashi T, Ono T, Nishijo H (2005) Effects of facial expression on shared attention mechanisms. Physiol Behav 84: 397–405.

Ishai A, Schmidt CF, Boesiger P (2005) Face perception is mediated by a distributed cortical network. Brain Res Bull 67: 87–93.

Itakura S (1996) An exploratory study of gaze monitoring in non-human primates. Jpn Psychol Res 38: 174–180.

Itakura S (2004) Gaze-following and joint visual attention in nonhuman animals. Jpn Psychol Res 46: 216–226.

James W (1890) The principles of psychology. New York: H. Holt and company.

Johnson MH (2005) Subcortical face processing. Nat Rev Neurosci 6: 766–774.

Jolly A (1966) Lemur social behavior and primate intelligence. Science 153: 501–506.

Jonides J (1981) Voluntary versus automatic control over the mind's eye's movement. In: Attention and Performance IX. (Long JB, Baddeley AD, eds), 187–203. Hillsdale, NJ: Lawrence Erlbaum.

Kaminski J, Riedel J, Call J, Tomasello M (2005) Domestic goats, *Capra hircus*, follow gaze direction and use social cues in an object choice task. Anim Behav 69: 11–18.

Kawashima R, Sugiura M, Kato T, Nakamura A, Hatano K, Ito K, Fukuda H, Kojima S, Nakamura K (1999) The human amygdala plays an important role in gaze monitoring: A PET study. Brain 122: 779–783.

Keating CF, Keating EG (1982) Visual scan patterns of rhesus monkeys viewing faces. Perception 11: 211–219.

Kendrick KM, da Costa AP, Leigh AE, Hinton MR, Peirce JW (2001) Sheep don't forget a face. Nature 414: 165–166.

Keverne EB, Leonard RA, Scruton DM, Young SK (1978) Visual monitoring in social groups of Talapoin monkeys. Anim Behav 26: 933–944.

Kirchner H, Thorpe SJ (2006) Ultra-rapid object detection with saccadic eye movements: Visual processing speed revisited. Vision Res 46: 1762–1776.

Klin A, Jones W, Schultz R, Volkmar F, Cohen D (2002a) Defining and quantifying the social phenotype in autism. Am J Psychiat 159: 895–908.

Klin A, Jones W, Schultz R, Volkmar F, Cohen D (2002b) Visual fixation patterns during viewing of naturalistic social situations as predictors of social competence in individuals with autism. Arch Gen Psychiat 59: 809–816.

Knickmeyer RC, Baron-Cohen S (2006) Fetal testosterone and sex differences. Early Hum Dev 82: 755–760.

Kobayashi H, Koshima S (2001) Unique morphology of the human eye and its adaptive meaning: Comparative studies on external morphology of the primate eye. J Hum Evol 40: 419–435.

Kyes RC, Candland DK (1987) Baboon (*Papio hamadryas*) visual preferences for regions of the face. J Comp Psychol 101: 345–348.

Kylliainen A, Hietanen JK (2004) Attention orienting by another's gaze direction in children with autism. J Child Psychol Psychiat 45: 435–444.

Land MF, Hayhoe M (2001) In what ways do eye movements contribute to everyday activities? Vision Res 41: 3559–3565.

Langton SRH, Bruce V (1999) Reflexive visual orienting in response to the social attention of others. Vis Cogn 6: 541–567.

Logothetis NK, Guggenberger H, Peled S, Paul J (1999) Functional imaging of the monkey brain. Nat Neurosci 2: 555–562.

Mangun GR (1995) Neural mechanisms of visual selective attention. Psychophysiology 32: 4–18.

Martin R (1990) Primate origins and evolution: A phylogenetic reconstruction. Princeton, NJ: Princeton University Press.

Mathews A, Fox E, Yiend J, Calder A (2003) The face of fear: Effects of eye gaze and emotion on visual attention. Vis Cogn 10: 823–835.

McNelis NL, Boatright-Horowitz SL (1998) Social monitoring in a primate group: The relationship between visual attention and hierarchical ranks. Anim Cogn 1: 65–69.

Morris JS, Öhman A, Dolan RJ (1999) A subcortical pathway to the right amygdala mediating 'unseen' fear. P Natl Acad Sci USA 96: 1680–1685.

Muller HJ, Rabbitt PM (1989) Reflexive and voluntary orienting of visual attention: Time course of activation and resistance to interruption. J Exp Psychol Hum Percept Perform 15: 315–330.

Okamoto-Barth S, Call J, Tomasello M (2007) Great apes' understanding of other individuals' line of sight. Psychol Sci 18: 462–468.

Pelphrey KA, Sasson NJ, Reznick JS, Paul G, Goldman BD, Piven J (2002) Visual scanning of faces in autism. J Autism Dev Disord 32: 249–261.

Perrett DI, Emery NJ (1994) Understanding the intentions of others from visual signals: Neurophysiological evidence. Cah Psychol Cogn 13: 683–694.

Peters RJ, Iyer A, Itti L, Koch C (2005) Components of bottom-up gaze allocation in natural images. Vision Res 45: 2397–2416.

Posner MI (1980) Orienting of attention. Q J Exp Psychol 3: 3–25.

Posner MI, Cohen Y (1984) Components of visual orienting. In: Attention and Performance X (Bouma H, Bouwhuis D, eds), 531–556. London: Erlbaum.

Putman P, Hermans E, van Honk J (2006) Anxiety meets fear in perception of dynamic expressive gaze. Emotion 6: 94–102.

Raleigh MJ, McGuire MT, Brammer GL, Pollack DB, Yuwiler A (1991) Serotonergic mechanisms promote dominance acquisition in adult male vervet monkeys. Brain Res 559: 181–190.

Raymond JE, Fenske MJ, Tavassoli NT (2003) Selective attention determines emotional responses to novel visual stimuli. Psychol Sci 14: 537–542.

Ristic J, Mottron L, Friesen CK, Iarocci G, Burack JA, Kingstone A (2005) Eyes are special but not for everyone: The case of autism. Cognitive Brain Res 24: 715–718.

Romanski LM, Giguere M, Bates JF, Goldman-Rakic PS (1997) Topographic organization of medial pulvinar connections with the prefrontal cortex in the rhesus monkey. J Comp Neurol 379: 313–332.

Rosa MG, Tweedale R (2005) Brain maps, great and small: lessons from comparative studies of primate visual cortical organization. Philos T Roy Soc B 360: 665–691.

Sabbagh MA (2004) Understanding orbitofrontal contributions to theory-of-mind reasoning: Implications for autism. Brain Cogn 55: 209–219.

Sackett GP (1966) Monkeys reared in isolation with pictures as visual input: Evidence for an innate releasing mechanism. Science 154: 1468–1473.

Sauther M, Sussman R, Gould L (1999) The socioecology of the ringtailed lemur: Thirty-five years of research. Evol Anthropol 8: 120–132.

Schultz RT (2005) Developmental deficits in social perception in autism: The role of the amygdala and fusiform face area. Int J Dev Neurosci 23: 125–141.

Seltzer B, Pandya DN (1989) Frontal lobe connections of the superior temporal sulcus in the rhesus monkey. J Comp Neurol 28: 97–113.

Seltzer B, Pandya DN (1991) Post-rolandic cortical projections of the superior temporal sulcus in the rhesus monkey. J Comp Neurol 312: 625–640.

Serre T, Oliva A, Poggio T (2007) A feedforward architecture accounts for rapid categorization. P Natl Acad Sci USA 104: 6424–6429.

Seyfarth RM, Cheney DL (2003) Signalers and receivers in animal communication. Annu Rev Psychol 54: 145–173.

Shepherd SV, Deaner RO, Platt ML (2006) Social status gates social attention in monkeys. Curr Biol 16: R119–R120.

Shepherd SV, Platt ML (2006) Noninvasive telemetric gaze tracking in freely moving socially housed prosimian primates. Methods 38: 185–194.

Shepherd SV, Platt ML (2008) Spontaneous social orienting and gaze following in ringtailed lemurs (*Lemur catta*). Anim Cogn 11: 13–20.

Shimojo S, Simion C, Shimojo E, Scheier C (2003) Gaze bias both reflects and influences preference. Nat Neurosci 6: 1317–1322.

Skuse D (2006) Genetic influences on the neural basis of social cognition. Philos T Roy Soc B 361: 2129–2141.

Smith APR, Stephan KE, Rugg MD, Dolan RJ (2006) Task and content modulate amygdala-hippocampal connectivity in emotional retrieval. Neuron 49: 631–638.

Swettenham J, Condie S, Campbell R, Milne E, Coleman M (2003) Does the perception of moving eyes trigger reflexive visual orienting in autism? Philos T Roy Soc B 358: 325–334.

Tomasello M, Call J, Hare B (1998) Five primate species follow the visual gaze of conspecifics. Anim Behav 55: 1063–1069.

Tomasello M, Carpenter M, Call J, Behne T, Moll H (2005) Understanding and sharing intentions: The origins of cultural cognition. Behav Brain Sci 28: 675–691.

Tomasello M, Hare B, Lehmann H, Call J (2006) Reliance on head versus eyes in the gaze following of great apes and human infants: The cooperative eye hypothesis. J Hum Evol 52: 314–320. Tomonaga M (2007) Is chimpanzee (*Pan troglodytes*) spatial attention reflexively triggered by gaze cue? J Comp Psychol 121: 156–170.

Tootell RB, Tsao D, Vanduffel W (2003) Neuroimaging weighs in: Humans meet macaques in "primate" visual cortex. J Neurosci 23: 3981–3989.

Tsao DY, Freiwald WA, Knutsen TA, Mandeville JB, Tootell RBH (2003) Faces and objects in macaque cerebral cortex. Nat Neurosci 6: 989–995.

Tschudin A, Call J, Dunbar RIM, Harris G, van der Elst C (2001) Comprehension of signs by dolphins (*Tursiops truncatus*). J Comp Psychol 115: 100–105.

Ungerleider LG, Mishkin M (1982) Two cortical visual systems. In: Analysis of visual behavior (Ingle DJ, Goodale MA, Mansfield RVW, eds), 549–586. Cambridge, MA: MIT Press.

van der Geest JN, Kemner C, Camfferman G, Verbaten MN, van Engeland H (2002) Looking at images with human figures: Comparison between autistic and normal children. J Autism Dev Disord 32: 69–75.

van Hoof JARAM (1967) The facial displays of the catarhine monkeys and apes. In: Primate ethology (Morris D, ed), 7–68. Chicago: Aldine Publishing Company.

von Schantz T, Bensch S, Grahn M, Hasselquist D, Wittzell H (1999) Good genes, oxidative stress and condition-dependent sexual signals. P Roy Soc Lond B Bio 266: 1–12.

Vuilleumier P (2002) Facial expression and selective attention. Curr Opin Psychiatr 15: 291–300.

Wassink TH, Hazlett HC, Epping EA, Arndt S, Dager SR, Schellenberg GD, Dawson G, Piven J (2007) Cerebral cortical gray matter overgrowth and functional variation of the serotonin transporter gene in autism. Arch Gen Psychiat 64: 709–717.

Yarbus A (1967) Eye movements during perception of complex objects. In: Eye movements and vision (Riggs LA, ed), 171–211. New York: Plenum Press.

Zajonc RB (1968) Attitudinal effects of mere exposure. J Pers Soc Psychol 9: 1–27.

15 The Human Social Brain: An "Evo-Devo" Perspective

Mark H. Johnson

All adult humans have a network of cortical and subcortical brain regions specialized for processing and integrating sensory information about the appearance, behavior, and intentions of other humans. How these specialized regions, collectively termed "the social brain" (Adolphs 2003), emerge during development remains largely unknown. This chapter reviews three big questions related to the ontogeny and phylogeny of the human social brain network, questions whose answers also have broader implications for cortical specialization for perceptual, motor, and cognitive functions:

1. What are the origins of cortical specialization in humans, and what are the respective contributions of phylogeny and ontogeny?

2. How can similar behavioral and computational functions arise in different species, where they are supported by neural tissue from different embryological origins?

3. What can we learn about human development from considering the interaction between phylogeny and ontogeny (sometimes called "evo-devo")?

Through the example of the development of the social brain we discover that ontogeny may have a more important interactive role in the specification of functions within cortical areas than some have previously supposed. In contrast to the view that cortical specialization for cognitive functions is "hard-wired," the empirical evidence indicates that each human infant's brain "discovers" the typical patterns of cortical specialization afresh.

A similar general organization of the brains of young vertebrates may result in the appropriate social behavior directed toward the conspecific caregivers. Interestingly, neural tissue from different embryological origins may end up serving similar functions in different species. This suggests that the constraints on adaptive behavior lead to convergent evolution: for example, the processing of both chick forebrain and human cerebral cortex has developed to specialize in recognizing conspecifics.

At the core of the "evo-devo" model of brain evolution (Finlay and Darlington 1995) is different species' overall rate of brain development. This indicates that the long time span of brain development in humans is related to both the relative size of the human brain structure and the greatly increased scope for postnatal environmental influence. Possibly the human brain is uniquely adapted to complete much of its development within a social context.

The Origins of Cortical Specialization

Perhaps the hottest debate in developmental neuroscience over the past decades has been the one concerning the factors that determine the structural and functional subdivisions characteristic of the mammalian (and particularly, primate) cerebral cortex.

Two possibilities have been put forward to account for the division of primate cortex into areas, the *protomap view* and the *protocortex view*.

According to the protomap view (Rakic 1988), differentiation into cortical regions occurs early in the prenatal formation of cortex, and is due to *intrinsic* factors, factors within the cortex or its proliferative zone. The electrical activity of neurons is not required for regional differentiation. Further, the cortex is viewed as a mosaic from the start, such that each cortical area has individually specified features particularly suitable for the input it will receive or the functions it will perform.

According to the protocortex view, differentiation occurs later in the development of the cortex, and depends on *extrinsic* factors such as input from other parts of the brain or sensory systems. The activity of neurons is required to generate regions within an initially undifferentiated protocortex (Killackey 1990; O'Leary and Stanfield 1989). The division of the cortex into areas in the adult brain is influenced by information relayed from the thalamus, and from interactions with other areas of cortex via inter-regional connectivity.

There is a dense and conflicting literature on the differentiation of neocortex into regions (for recent reviews see Pallas 2001; Ragsdale and Grove 2001; Kingsbury and Finlay 2001). Some experiments appear at first sight to be compelling evidence for the protomap view. For example, the newborns of a strain of "knockout" mice that genetically lack connections between the thalamus and the cortex still have normal, well-defined regional gene expression boundaries within their cortices (Miyashita-Lin et al. 1999) and some other characteristics of wild-type mice. This suggests that input to the cortex is not required for establishing the boundaries between cortical regions. In another example, in vitro studies in which cortical tissue is maintained in culture and thus isolated from potential extrinsic patterning cues still show patterns of gene expression consistent with the development of the hippocampus (Tole et al. 2000). Despite these and other studies supporting the idea of genetically specified regionalization of cortex, there are some important caveats, and also a surprising amount of evidence in support of the opposing, protocortex, view. These lines of evidence include the following:

• Most of the patterns of gene expression thought to contribute to the differentiation of the cortex do not show clearly defined boundaries, instead they show graded expression across large portions of the cortex. This suggests that regionalization of the cortex could emerge from a combination of different gradients of gene expression. Kingsbury and Finlay (2001) refer to this as a "hyperdimensional plaid" and contrast this with a "mosaic quilt" (protomap) view.

• At present there are few examples of clear regionalization that map onto functional areas, and there are good reasons to believe that these cases are exceptions to the general rule. For example, comparisons across a large number of species have led several experts to argue that primary sensory areas that receive direct input from the primary sensory thalamic nuclei are more similar across species than most of the rest of the cortex (see, for example, Krubitzer 1998). In particular, the primary visual cortex in primates has unique characteristics that have led some to propose that it is the most recently evolved part of the cortex. In the primary visual cortex, inputs from the visual thalamus may regulate the extent of cell proliferation in the ventricular zone (see Kennedy and Dehay 1993), ensuring that this area of the cortex has a rate of neuron production nearly twice that in neighboring areas. The entorhinal cortex, the region of the cortex most closely associated with the hippocampus, shows some differentiation from surrounding cortex as early as thirteen weeks of gestation (Kostovic 1990). However, for the majority of the cortex in the mouse and for the vast majority in humans, there is currently no evidence for cortical region–specific gene expression (see below).

• Despite the fact that primary sensory regions are the best candidates for genetic pre-specification, even these regions can have their properties significantly changed through experience. Thus, input may be vital for the maintenance of cortical divisions (Sur et al. 1990).

• Evidence for cortical differentiation prior to birth does not allow us to conclude that neuronal activity is not important, since spontaneous neural activity within the brain is known to be important for prenatal differentiation (Shatz 2002).

Thus, so far the evidence converges on a view midway between the protomap and protocortex hypotheses (Kingsbury and Finlay 2001; Pallas 2001; Ragsdale and Grove 2001), whereby graded patterns of gene expression potentially create large-scale regions with combinations of properties that may better give rise to certain computations. Within these large-scale regions smaller-scale functional areas arise through mechanisms associated with the protocortex view. A hypothetical example is that one region may receive particular thalamic input, overlain with a certain pattern of neurotransmitter expression and the presence of certain neuromodulators. This combination of circumstances, combined with neural activity, may then induce further unique features such as particular patterns of short-range or long-range connectivity. Differentiation into smaller areas within the larger regions may occur through the selective pruning of connections.

The Human Social Brain

Given this background, we can now consider the postnatal development of the cortical regions in the human social brain network. At first sight, an obvious view of the developing social brain is that specific genes are expressed in particular parts of the cortex and consequently "code for" patterns of wiring specific for certain computational functions. These regions may then "come online" at different times during development, enabling the child to succeed in social-cognitive tasks that they previously failed at doing. However, as just described, this view is not consistent with a large body of evidence from development neurobiology. This discrepancy has led us to propose an *interactive specialization* (IS) view of postnatal functional brain development. According to this view, in the cerebral cortex functional development involves organizing patterns of inter-regional interactions (Johnson 2001, 2005a). Further, the response properties of a specific region are partly determined by its patterns of connectivity to other regions, and their patterns of activity. During postnatal development changes in the response properties of cortical regions occur as they interact and compete with each other to acquire their role in new computational abilities. From this perspective, some cortical regions may begin with poorly defined functions, and are consequently partially activated in a wide range of different contexts and tasks. During development, activity-dependent interactions between regions sharpens up the functions of regions such that their activity becomes restricted to a narrower set of circumstances (for example, a region originally activated by a wide variety of visual objects may come to confine its response to upright human faces). The onset of new behavioral competencies during infancy will therefore be associated with changes in activity over several regions, and not just by the onset of activity in one or more additional region(s).

As an example of the specialization of a region in the social brain, let us consider the "fusiform face area" (FFA) within the cortex. This area is known to be selectively activated during face-processing tasks in adults (Kanwisher et al. 1997). According to the IS view, the FFA becomes specialized for processing faces as a result of several constraining factors. Within the cortex, the parts of the FFA that become face-sensitive receive visual input from the fovea and are at the "object-level" of visual stimulus processing in the ventral visual pathway (Malach et al. 2004). Thus, appropriate visual inputs migrate to the region. The FFA also receives multimodal input and has strong reciprocal connections with the hippocampus. This makes the region appropriate for involvement in the storage of individual face identities. By this developmental account it is inevitable, barring some disruption to the normal constraints, that parts of the fusiform cortex will be specialized for faces, but this inevitable outcome is achieved without genetically specified domain-specific patterns of connectivity within the FFA.

An important additional constraint on the developmental emergence of the cortical social brain network comes from subcortical biases in processing (Johnson and Morton

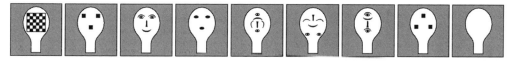

Figure 15.1
Some schematic stimuli that have been used to test newborns' face preferences in several experiments. Some of the stimuli are designed to test the importance of the spatial arrangement of a face (configuration), and others the importance of particular features. Newborns will preferentially attend to patterns that contain the basic configuration of high-contrast areas of a face (for example, the second, third, and fourth stimuli from the left are preferred to those on the right). The mechanisms that underlie this preference are still the focus of debate (figure taken from Johnson 2005a).

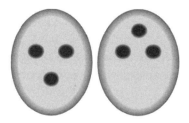

Figure 15.2
Schematic illustration of the stimuli that might be optimal for eliciting a face-related preference in newborns. These hypothetical representations were created by putting together the results of several experiments on newborns' face-related preferences. Conclusions were combined from experiments showing the importance of the number of elements in the upper half of a bounded area or surface (right side), the importance of a face-relevant pattern of phase contrast, and the importance of the basic face configuration as viewed at low spatial frequencies (left-side figure taken from Johnson 2005a).

1991). A recent review of many studies on face-related preferences in human newborn infants revealed that similar stimuli may attract newborns as are found to elicit activation in a subcortical route for face processing in adults (Johnson 2005a). The optimal stimulus could be as simple as dark blobs corresponding to the general location of the eyes and mouth, or a bounded surface with more dark elements in the upper half (see figures 15.1 and 15.2). In either case, the representation is probably close to the minimum sufficient to elicit orienting to faces within the natural environment of the newborn, given the constraints of the newborn visual system.

One purpose of this early bias to fixate on faces may be to elicit bonding from adult caregivers. However, an equally important purpose is to bias the visual input to plastic cortical circuits. This biased sampling of the visual environment over the first weeks of life may ensure the appropriate specialization of later developing cortical circuitry (Johnson and Morton 1991), and thus provide a developmental foundation for the emerging social brain network (Johnson 2005a). In addition, the cortical projection patterns of the subcortical route may enhance activation of specific areas, including the fusiform cortex, when faces are within the visual field of the young infant.

Developing a Simple Social Brain

The idea that a primitive subcortical system selects the appropriate input for still-developing cortical pathways was inspired by earlier work on a species with a much simpler social brain: the domestic chicken. In the laboratory, day-old domestic chicks will imprint onto a variety of objects, such as moving colored balls and cylinders. After even a few hours of exposure to such a stimulus, chicks develop strong and robust social preferences for the training object over novel stimuli. In the absence of a mother hen this learning is relatively unconstrained; virtually any conspicuous moving object larger than a matchbox will serve as an imprinting stimulus, and will come to be preferred over any other.

A particular region of the chick forebrain, the intermediate and medial part of the mesopallium (IMM, formerly called IMHV, for reviews see Horn 1985; Horn and Johnson 1989), thought to correspond to the mammalian cortex, has been shown to be critical for imprinting. Evidence from several vertebrate species supports the suggestion that the forebrain is a site of plasticity and not a location that controls inbuilt, automatic, types of behavior (MacPhail 1982; Ewert 1987).

Figure 15.3 illustrates the location of IMM within the chick brain. The area occupies about 5 percent of total forebrain volume. Like the human FFA, its main inputs come from visual projection areas, and some of its projections go to regions involved in motor control, such as the archistriatum. Thus, the area is well placed to integrate visual inputs and motor outputs.

In the laboratory, a wide range of objects such as moving red boxes and blue balls are as effective for imprinting as more naturalistic stimuli such as a moving stuffed hen. In the wild, however, precocial birds such as chicks invariably imprint on their mother, and

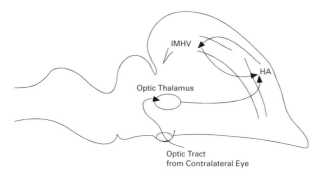

Figure 15.3
Outline sagittal view of the chick brain. Shown here is the main visual pathway to the IMHV, now referred to as the intermediate and medial part of mesopallium (IMM) via the hyperstriatum accessorium (HA), now referred to as the hyperpallium apicale. There are other routes of visual input to the IMHV, which are not shown in this figure (see Horn 1985). The brain of a two-day-old chick is approximately 2 cm long (figure taken from Johnson 2005b).

not on other moving objects. These observations raise the question as to what constraints ensure that the plasticity of some forebrain regions in the chick brain is normally constrained to encode information about conspecifics (the mother hen), rather than other objects in its environment.

An answer to this question became evident from the results of a series of experiments in which stimulus-dependent effects of IMM lesions were observed (Horn and McCabe 1984). Groups of chicks trained on an artificial stimulus such as a rotating red box were severely impaired by IMM lesions placed either before or after training on an object. However, groups of chicks exposed to a stuffed hen were only mildly impaired in their preference. Other neurophysiological manipulations also show differences between the hen-trained and box-trained birds (see Horn 2004 for review).

These results led Johnson and Horn (1988) to seek experimental evidence for an earlier suggestion (Hinde 1961) that naturalistic objects such as hens may be more effective at eliciting attention in young chicks than other objects. A series of experiments was therefore conducted in which dark-reared chicks were presented with a choice between a stuffed hen and a variety of test stimuli created from cutting up and jumbling the pelt of a stuffed hen. Johnson and Horn (1988) concluded from these experiments that chicks have an untrained tendency, or predisposition, to attend to features of the head and neck region of the hen. Although this untrained preference seemed to be specific to the correct arrangement of features of the face and head, it was not specific to the species. For example, the head of a duck was as attractive as that of a hen.

The results of these and several other experiments led to the proposal that there are two independent brain systems that control filial preference in the chick (Horn 1985; Johnson et al. 1985). The first of these controls a specific predisposition that makes newly hatched chicks orient toward objects resembling a mother hen. This predisposition system appears to be specifically tuned to the correct spatial arrangement of elements of the head and neck region, but not to the color or size of the elements. Although the stimulus configuration triggering the predisposition is not species- or genus-specific, it is sufficient to pick out the mother hen from other objects the chick is likely to be exposed to in the first few days after hatching. Although the neural basis for this predisposition is currently unknown, the optic tectum, the homolog of the mammalian superior colliculus, is one likely candidate.

The second brain system acquires information about the objects to which the young chick attends and is supported by the IMM forebrain region. It has been argued that in the natural environment, the first brain system guides the second system to acquire information about the closest mother hen (Horn 1985; Johnson et al. 1985). Biochemical, electrophysiological, and lesion evidence all support the conclusion that these two brain systems have largely independent neural substrates (for review see Horn 1985). For example, although selective lesions to IMM impair preferences acquired through exposure to an object, they do not impair the specific predisposition (Johnson and Horn 1987).

There are, of course, a number of different ways that the predisposition could constrain the information acquired by the IMM system. For example, the information in the predisposition could act as a sensory "filter" or template through which information has to pass before reaching the IMM system. The evidence available at present is consistent with the view that the two systems influence the preference behavior of the chick independently, that is, there is no internal informational exchange between them. Instead, it appears that the input to the IMM system is selected simply as a result of the predisposition biasing the chick to orient toward any hen-like objects in the environment. Given that the species-typical environment of the chick includes a mother hen in close proximity and that the predisposition includes adequate information to pick the hen out from other objects in the early environment, the input to the learning system will be highly selected.

Building a Social Brain: Comparative Questions

The strong surface parallels observed in research on chicks and humans raises the question of homology. Since the thalamus and midbrain are largely preserved across the avian-mammal branches and are derived from a common ancestor, it is possible that the putative subcortical route could also be preserved in some form. Indeed, Sewards and Sewards (2002) report evidence of a social bias in newborns in a wide range of vertebrates. A recent comparison of the tectofugal (subcortical) visual pathway in birds and mammals shows strong parallels with many homologies (Avian Bird Nomenclature Consortium 2005). For example, the putative human subcortical route involves the superior colliculus, the pulvinar, and the amygdala (Johnson 2005a). In the bird tectofugal route the optic tectum (the avian homolog of the mammalian superior colliculus or amygdala may support the predisposition, however, it is difficult to directly test this hypothesis since lesions to the avian optic tectum typically impair a wide range of visuomotor behaviors.

A recent reclassification of the avian brain based on molecular, embryological, and functional grounds has stated that the region of the avian forebrain that contains the IMM should now be classified as a homolog of the mammalian cerebral neocortex, the pallium (Avian Bird Nomenclature Consortium 2005). Although the architectonic structure of the avian pallium is based around nuclei with specific functional properties, and it does not have the characteristic six-layered structure found in the mammalian cortex, the two structures share some common embryological, molecular, and cellular properties (in fact, it is likely that the avian pallium evolved more recently than the mammalian neocortex). It is striking that similar functions can emerge is such different neural tissue, and this emphasizes the importance of converging constraints on the emergence of functions within neural tissue. The FFA and the IMM share common sets of constraints: both receive complex and partially processed visual input, both may have inputs from other sensory modalities, and both are "tutored" early in life by the young animal foveating socially relevant stimuli.

Although there are similarities between the two species, there are some clear differences. First, the primate, and in particular the human, cerebral cortex provides far more extensive tissues for representing and encoding the temporal and spatial properties of social stimuli. There is no question that some of the social cognitive functions mediated by the human prefrontal cortex (sometimes called "theory of mind") will be well beyond the capacity of adult domestic chickens. Second, in the chick it appears that there is no internal interaction between the two systems (Horn 2005). In contrast, evidence reviewed on humans suggests that subcortical route activation modulates the response of cortical structures to social stimuli such as faces. This internal interaction between the two systems may be necessary to further constrain which regions of the more extensive primate cortex become specialized for social stimuli.

"Evo-Devo" and the Social Brain

While evolution and development have been regarded as separate domains of study, a recent thrust in biology, "evo-devo," has been based on the idea that they are inextricably entwined and therefore must be studied together. So far, however, there have been very few examples of an evo-devo approach to brain development. One notable exception is a theory of the evolution of the mammalian brain put forward by Finlay and Darlington (1995). These authors compared data on the size of brain structures from 131 mammalian species, and concluded that the order of neurogenesis is conserved across a wide range of species, and that the general time course of this order predicts not only overall brain size but also the relative enlargement of specific structures. Specifically, disproportionately large growth occurs in the late-generated structures such as the cerebral neocortex. By this analysis, in the relatively slowed neurogenesis of primates the structure most likely to differ in size from that of other mammals is the neocortex. Further, the even greater delayed course of neurogenesis in humans results in a greatly enlarged prefrontal cortex (Clancy et al. 2000).

In this chapter we have seen that despite large architectonic differences between the human neocortex and the bird pallium, strikingly similar interactions between brain pathways generate the emergence of forebrain regions that become specialized for the perception of social stimuli. As is the case with other examples of convergent evolution, such as the wing or the eye, similar adaptive brain functions can be generated from different raw material in different species. Thus, there appear to be different ways for the vertebrate brain to implement specialized processors for social stimuli.

Furthermore, an evo-devo analysis of brain development across many species has demonstrated that most different brain regions cannot be selected for in isolation from the rest of the brain. Rather, the overall course of brain development can be slowed to disproportionately increase the size of different structures. I suggest that the human brain has evolved within a context of the increasing importance of social context and learning from others. This has partly contributed to the general slowing of human brain development when compared to that of other primates and a consequent increase in the relative volume of the cortex, in particular, the prefrontal cortex. This increased quantity of cortex is exploited afresh by each developing child, with regions recruiting functions best suited to their intrinsic and extrinsic patterns of connectivity.

Acknowledgments

I acknowledge financial support from the UK Medical Research Council.

References

Adolphs R (2003) Cognitive neuroscience of human social behaviour. Nat Rev Neurosci 4: 165–178.

Avian Bird Nomenclature Consortium (2005) Avian brains and a new understanding of vertebrate brain evolution. Nat Rev Neurosci 6: 151–159.

Clancy B, Darlington RB, Finlay BL (2000) The course of human events: Predicting the timing of primate neural development. Dev Sci 3: 57–66.

Ewert J-P (1987) Neuroethology of releasing mechanisms: Prey-catching in toads. Behav Brain Sci 10: 337–405.

Finlay BL, Darlington RB (1995) Linked regularities in the development and evolution of mammalian brains. Science 268: 1578–1584.

Hinde RA (1961) The establishment of parent-offspring relations in birds, with some mammalian analogies. In: Current problems in animal behaviour (Thorpe WH, Zangwill OL, eds), 175–193. Cambridge: Cambridge University Press.

Horn G (1985) Memory, imprinting, and the brain: An inquiry into mechanisms. Oxford: Clarendon Press.

Horn G (2004) Pathways of the past: The imprint of memory. Nat Rev Neurosci 5: 108–120.

Horn G, Johnson MH (1989) Memory systems in the chick: Dissociations and neuronal analysis. Neuropsychologia 27: 1–22.

Horn G, McCabe BJ (1984) Predispositions and preferences: Effects on imprinting of lesions to the chick brain. Brain Res 168: 361–373.

Johnson MH (2001) Functional brain development in humans. Nat Rev Neurosci 2: 475–483.

Johnson MH (2005a) Sub-cortical face processing. Nat Rev Neurosci 6: 766–774.

Johnson MH (2005b) Developmental cognitive neuroscience: An introduction (2nd ed). Oxford: Blackwell.

Johnson MH, Bolhuis JJ, Horn G (1985) Interaction between acquired preferences and developing predispositions during imprinting. Anim Behav 33: 1000–1006.

Johnson MH, Horn G (1987) The role of a restricted region of the chick forebrain in the recognition of individual conspecifics. Behav Brain Res 23: 269–275.

Johnson MH, Horn G (1988) The development of filial preferences in the dark-reared chick. Anim Behav 36: 675–683.

Johnson MH, Morton J (1991) Biology and cognitive development: The case of face recognition. Oxford: Blackwell.

Kanwisher N, McDermott J, Chun MM (1997) The fusiform face area: A module in human extrastriate cortex specialized for face perception. J Neurosci 17: 4302–4311.

Kennedy H, Dehay C (1993) The relevance of primate corticogenesis for understanding the emergence of cognitive abilities in man. In: Developmental neurocognition: Speech and face processing in the first year of life (deBoysson-Bardies B, deSchonen S, Jusczyk P, McNeilage P, Morton J, eds), 17–30. Dordrecht: Kluwer Academic/NATO ASI Series.

Killackey HP (1990) Neocortical expansion: An attempt toward relating phylogeny and ontongeny. J Cognitive Neurosci 2: 1–17.

Kingsbury MA, Finlay BL (2001) The cortex in multidimensional space: Where do cortical areas come from? Dev Sci 4: 125–142.

Kostovic I (1990) Structural and histochemical reorganization of the human prefrontal cortex during perinatal and postnatal life. Prog Brain Res 85: 223–239.

Krubitzer LA (1998) What can monotremes tell us about brain evolution? Philos T Roy Soc B 353: 1127–1146.

MacPhail EM (1982) Brain and Intelligence in Vertebrates. Oxford: Clarendon Press.

Malach R, Avidan G, Lerner V, Hasson U, Levy I (2004) The cartography of human visual object areas. In: Attention and performance XX: Functional neuroimaging of visual cognition (Kanwisher N, Duncan J, eds), 195–204. Oxford: Oxford University Press.

Miyashita-Lin EM, Hevner R, Wassarman KM, Martinez S, Rubenstein JL (1999) Early neocortical regionalization in the absence of thalamic innervation. Science 285: 906–909.

O'Leary DDM, Stanfield BB (1989) Selective elimination of axons extended by developing cortical neurons is dependent on regional locale: Experiments utilizing fetal cortical transplants. J Neurosci 9: 2230–2246.

Pallas SL (2001) Intrinsic and extrinsic factors shaping cortical identity. Trends Neurosci 24: 417–423.

Ragsdale CW, Grove EA (2001) Patterning in the mammalian cerebral cortex. Curr Opin Neurobiol 11: 50–58.

Rakic P (1988) Specification of cerebral cortical areas. Science 241: 170–176.

Sewards TV, Sewards MA (2002) Innate visual object recognition in vertebrates: Some proposed pathways and mechanisms. Comp Biochem Phys A 132: 861–891.

Shatz CJ (2002) Emergence of order in visual system development. In: Brain development and cognition: A reader (Johnson MH, Munakata Y, Gilmore R, eds), 231–244. Oxford: Blackwell.

Sur M, Pallas SL, Roe AW (1990) Cross-modal plasticity in cortical development: Differentiation and specification of sensory cortex. Trends Neurosci 13: 227–233.

Tole S, Goudreau G, Assimacopoulos S, Grove EA (2000) Emx2 is required for growth of the hippocampus but not for hippocampal field specification. J Neurosci 20: 2618–2625.

16 Ontogenetic Development Matters

Sylvain Sirois and Annette Karmiloff-Smith

In the seventeenth and eighteenth centuries, preformationism was a common theoretical approach to understanding conception (see Pinto-Correia 1997 for a historical overview). Spermists and their opponents, ovists, believed that sperm and eggs, respectively, contained homunculi, fully formed yet miniature humans. These ideas are now historical footnotes in science, occasionally brought out to provide a good chuckle. Our contention in this chapter is that the homunculi may be gone, replaced by twenty-three chromosomes in both sperm and eggs, but that preformationist ideas continue to pervade the study of both typical cognitive development and of atypical cognitive development with genetic etiology.

There are frequent suggestions, in both the popular and scientific literatures, that a gene (or specific set of genes) for X has been found, where X is some specific cognitive-level function. For example, such claims have been made for spatial cognition (Frangiskakis et al. 1996) and language (Gopnik 1990; Pinker 1994, 1999; Wexler 1996). In our view, the logic behind these suggestions is flawed: the starting point for such logic is the normal adult brain, where cognitive dissociations (ideally, double dissociations) are found between different functions following brain injury. Some take such dissociations to suggest the existence of modular functions (that is, independent and functionally encapsulated). When a genetic anomaly is associated with a seemingly specific impairment of such a modular cognitive function, the conclusion is that the gene or set of genes implicated in the anomaly encode that specific function. A particular genetic mutation damages a module (or a set of modules) and leaves others intact. Because of its prevalence in the 1980s and 1990s we refer to this as the canonical view of atypical development (see discussions in Karmiloff-Smith 1998, 2006a).

We argue that canonical views, which implicitly or explicitly endorse some recent forms of evolutionary psychology (see, for example, Tooby and Cosmides 1990), are analogous to preformationist ideas. Figure 16.1 illustrates this suggestion. DNA is made up of chains of four bases (adenine, guanine, cytosine, and thymine, abbreviated A, G, C, and T, respectively), which encode genes. The genes themselves, through RNA, encode proteins in the construction and maintenance of the organism. According to the canonical view,

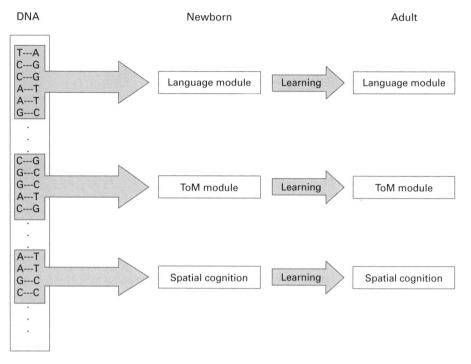

Figure 16.1
The canonical view of genetic disorders. On the left-hand side are DNA base pair sequences that encode particular genes. Such sets of genes encode particular cognitive function that exist, albeit in germinal form, in newborns. Maturation and learning give rise to the adult functions. Deletion of crucial genes would delete or impair specific cognitive functions.

genes or sets of genes are specifically responsible for encoding particular cognitive-level functions. These functions would be present at birth and, save for potential immaturity, would be analogous to those found in adults. Genetic mutations involving the deletion, translocation, or duplication of such genes would therefore be claimed to result in the deletion or mutation of the corresponding cognitive-level functions.

We propose that the canonical view of genetic developmental disorders is actively misleading, its prevalence notwithstanding. In the next section we review the problems it encounters at the biological, cognitive, and behavioral levels. We conclude that the canonical view is untenable, and that the only alternative is a view that puts the very idea of development at the core of the study of developmental disorders (Karmiloff-Smith 1998). In a subsequent section we examine how such a developmental view of atypical development informs our understanding of various syndromes, with a particular focus on Williams syndrome, a neurodevelopmental disorder caused by the deletion of twenty-eight genes on one copy of chromosome 7 (Donnai and Karmiloff-Smith 2000). In the concluding section we discuss the implications of a developmental cognitive neuroscience view of atypical development for research and intervention.

The Case against the Deterministic Role of DNA in Cognitive Function

We argued earlier that the canonical view of atypical development tacitly endorses certain types of evolutionary psychology perspectives (Buss 1995; Pinker 1997; Tooby and Cosmides 1990), one akin to nativism. Unfortunately, despite the inherent biological determinism entailed by such views, proponents of nativism do not typically ground their arguments in molecular biology (Nelson et al. 2006). Moreover, it has been argued that the core findings used to support evolutionary psychology (for example, cheater detection, parental love) are equivocal at best (Buller 2005a, 2005b). In this section we examine the general plausibility of cognitive determinism. We will not tackle the issue of whether or not the brain does symbol manipulation. What we will assume is that whatever the brain does is realized by the activity of neurons.

The human genome consists of about 25,000 to 35,000 genes (Wolfsberg et al. 2001), which is not a particularly large number, considering all that they have to do. In fact, the majority of these genes are likely to be involved in rather more important tasks than expressing cognitive modules for number concepts, object properties, causality, cheater detection, and so forth—namely, keeping the body alive and functioning (Nelson et al. 2006). The human genome also contains a large quantity of transcriptor genes, whose function it is to turn on and off the functions of other genes. Given the scale of complexity of a fully formed brain (over 100 billion neurons, each connected to up to 10,000 others), and the scarcity of genetic material to express it (some fraction of at most 35,000 genes), DNA clearly does not provide a blueprint for the brain but rather provides a loose, good enough solution by using what is known in computer science and information theory as *lossy compression.* If one takes a large, detailed digital image and compresses it to 1 percent of its original size, the compressed image will loose a substantial amount of detail. DNA compression, by necessity, is orders of magnitude far greater than that.

One heuristic (or hack, to continue the computer science analogy) used by DNA in brain development is to start out with higher than necessary connectivity levels within and between cortical regions (Huttenlocher and Dabholkar 1997). Generally, the newborn's cortex doesn't show localization or specialization of function (Goldman-Rakic 1987); rather, these *emerge* as an activity-dependent function of interactions at the cellular, neural, cortical, and environmental levels (Johnson 2001, 2004; Karmiloff-Smith 1998; Kuhl 2004; Majdan and Shatz 2006; Mareschal et al. 2007; Meaney and Szyf 2005). It is becoming increasingly established that near and distant brain areas not only become *co-active* but also become functionally *cooperative,* leading to a dense brain network with functionally connected multiple brain regions (Bhattacharya 2007; Bhattacharya and Petsche

2005). The shift from distributed to localized processing, as well as specialization through progressively restricted inputs, is a developmental process that unfolds over months or years, depending on the function (Johnson 2001, 2004; Karmiloff-Smith 2007). Although substantial pruning takes place—a necessity, since the brain is overly connected at early stages of development—circuit-building activity also occurs (Quinlan 1998). The adult's *modularized* cognitive architecture emerges gradually over time (Karmiloff-Smith 1992), but the starting point is neither predetermined nor fixed (Karmiloff-Smith, 2007).

A common objection one hears when discussing such ideas is something like "Why would all animals but humans have innate knowledge?" This objection is erroneous in two ways. First, one can ask: Is the objection really about knowledge? The observation that most freshly hatched graylag geese follow their mother is both accurate and misleading. The little geese do not *know* that it is their mother. It just so happens that in most cases it is the first moving stimulus that they encounter within a sensitive imprinting window of about thirty-six hours. A myriad of other stimuli are suitable for imprinting, including Austrian ethologists (Lorenz et al. 1996). These are not knowledge states, but rather behavioral biases. Second, the all-or-nothing assumption of the objection is also wrong, as it is more appropriate to talk of degrees of prespecified biases across species. In their excellent review of comparative neuroscience, Quartz and Sejnowski (1997) remark on how the degree of prespecification varies in nonrandom ways across species. It is highest in the most distal animals from humans, and lowest in our closest relatives. Rather than endow us with maximal prespecified knowledge (hyperspecialization), it seems that evolution tended instead toward maximal plasticity for learning. This is entirely consistent with our growing understanding of the newborn brain (Johnson 2001, 2004; Nelson et al. 2006) and of early cognitive development.

The quarter century since the early eighties has seen a flurry of studies into newborn and infant cognition, using procedures based on the habituation research design. These studies have been, explicitly or implicitly, based on the notion that humans are innately endowed with a range of cognitive abilities regarding object properties (Baillargeon 1987; Baillargeon et al. 1985), physics (Spelke et al. 1992), number (Wynn 1992, 1995), and language (Gomez and Gerken 1999; Marcus et al. 1999), to name a few. However, these so-called rich interpretations have been challenged by a number of researchers (Bogartz et al. 1997, 2000; Cashon and Cohen 2000; Cohen 2004; Cohen and Marks 2002; Haith 1998; Houston-Price and Nakai 2004; Roder et al. 2000; Schoner and Thelen 2006), all of whom propose simpler interpretations. These help to resolve the paradox that infants were deemed, through over-interpretation of the data, to be smarter than toddlers (Keen 2003).

Recently, there have been similar claims of early infant competence in goal attribution (Walker et al. 2006; Woodward 1998, 1999) and theory of mind (Onishi and Baillargeon 2005), but these suggestions of precocious social cognitive abilities have also been challenged (Perner and Ruffman 2005; Ruffman and Perner 2005; Sirois and Jackson 2007).

Across the board, we are faced with data about early cognitive competence that are at best equivocal.

It remains the case that newborns do indeed have behavioral biases. One such bias is the newborn preference to look at faces (Johnson and Morton 1991; Morton and Johnson 1991), but not because they have innate knowledge of faces. Rather, they preferentially attend to clusters of three blobs organized in an inverted triangle, and the most reliable source of such clusters in the environment happens to be other people. The purpose of this bias in the infant's perception is to help bootstrap face processing, which provides evolutionary fit. But there is no content specification. There is a bias, and learning and developmental mechanisms capitalize on this bias. Similarly, social smiling appears at about six weeks postpartum in the average infant (Hains and Muir 1996; Watson 1972), but Povinelli and colleagues (2005) argue that early smiling is not a causal precursor of proper social smiling per se. In fact, they propose that it is not social at all, but an imposture that serves to bootstrap the interaction with caregivers who attribute to it a social meaning. Proper social smiling would *emerge* as an outcome of learning and developmental mechanisms trapped in this interaction.

Given that representational nativism (innate knowledge) is implausible, and that there is a strong case in favor of developmental models of cognitive change, we conclude at this stage that human infants are born with a collection of reflexes and biases (and some in utero learning: Hepper 1997) that provide not only a starting point but also an initial trajectory vector in cognitive space, one that will be affected not only by experience (learning and development) but also by interactions within and between levels of causal change (cellular, neural, body, environment; see Mareschal et al. 2007). We thus propose as an alternative to the canonical model shown in figure 16.1 an interactive constructivist model, which is shown in figure 16.2. As the next section illustrates, a developmental perspective on developmental disorders tells a radically different story from the popular canonical one.

Atypical Epigenesis

It follows from the previous discussion that the brains of atypically developing infants should not be conceptualized as normal brains with parts intact and parts impaired. Rather, they should be viewed as brains that have *developed* differently throughout embryogenesis and postnatal development (Karmiloff-Smith 1998). Why, then, has the canonical adult neuropsychological model remained so attractive to many of those studying developmental disorders in children? We believe that it is because the explanatory framework is static and thus leads to simpler types of research strategies. If the researcher considers the normal brain to be composed of prespecified modules and the atypical brain to be a juxtaposition of intact and impaired modules, then the brain can be theoretically represented by a number of independent boxes, suggesting that impairments in one "box" have no effect on other components of the brain. This leads to a mere cursory investigation of the "intact" domains

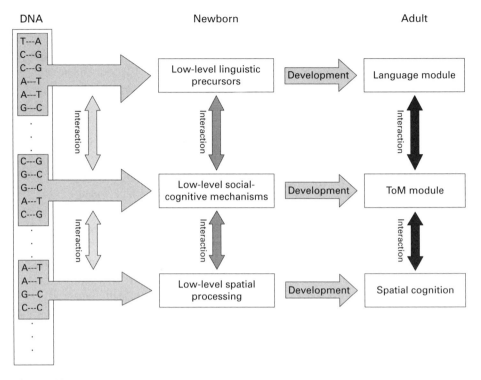

Figure 16.2
Illustration of a constructivist view of genetic disorders. On the left-hand side are DNA base pair sequences that encode particular genes. Such sets of genes encode particular low-level biases that will affect particular cognitive domains. Learning and, crucially, development give rise to emergent adult functions. Deletion of crucial genes would delete or impair domains tapped by particular cognitive functions. Important throughout life are interactions between functions across levels of causal effect (i.e., molecular, cellular, neural, systems, body, environment). The different shadings of the interaction arrows indicate how these interactions may change over time through progressive specialization.

and a focus on the impaired parts. Interestingly, once such a strategy forms the basis of research on children with genetic disorders, relative differences such as that domain X is more impaired than domain Y turn into absolute statements that domain X is deficient and domain Y intact (Clahsen and Almazan 1998; Hoffman et al. 2003; Landau and Hoffman 2005; Piattelli-Palmarini 2001; Pinker 1999; Tager-Flusberg et al. 2003), whereas in fact both are deficient when compared with the levels of healthy controls.

A totally different approach is taken if the researcher considers the initial state of the neonate cortex to be composed of many interconnected parts, implying that a genetic mutation is likely to be widely expressed throughout the brain and affect many emerging cognitive domains. Thus, what may seem like a domain-specific impairment in the phenotypic outcome may simply be due to the fact that the neuronal and biochemical properties of one region are more affected by the mutation than other regions but, crucially, that these other regions are also affected but to a less obvious degree. This means that the neuroconstructivist researcher will pay as much attention to domains where the child displays better outcomes, even scores that fall in the "normal range," as to those where impairment is the most serious. This often leads to the discovery of different cognitive and brain processes that underlie normal behavioral scores (Karmiloff-Smith et al. 2004). Furthermore, the neuroconstructivist researcher will systematically try to trace developmental deficits back to their low-level origins in infancy. Let's examine a concrete example of progressive specialization and localization of function in typical development and how this differs from atypical development.

Progressive Specialization and Brain Localization of Face Processing

Face processing serves as an interesting example, since one might have expected evolution to guarantee that species recognize the faces of their conspecifics by providing innately specified knowledge of faces. But this is not the case. While processing faces during normal infancy, the cortex starts out by being very active over wide brain regions in both the right and left hemispheres (Johnson 2004). After some six months of massive experience with faces and competition between hemispheres, face processing gradually moves more to the right hemisphere, which turns out to possess domain-relevant properties than lend themselves better to the configural processing of faces. By the end of the first year of life, the baby's brain not only shows a pattern of localization for face processing in the right hemisphere, which approaches that of adult face processing, but also displays a restriction of the inputs processed by that particular brain circuit (de Haan et al. 2002; Johnson 2001, 2004). This progressive specialization of function, enabled by the gradual pruning of nonrelevant connections in the brain, continues to refine itself throughout childhood and early adolescence. In summary, children are not born with a dedicated face-processing module. Rather, this *emerges* as a gradual process of modularization from repeated experience with different faces and the processing competition across different cortical regions until the most domain relevant wins out. We call this progressive modularization.

Continuing with our neuroconstructivist approach, we ask what happens with respect to the development of face processing, specifically in the case of the neurodevelopmental disorder known as Williams syndrome? Interestingly, this genetic disorder seemed to suggest that the neuroconstructivist approach was wrong, because despite their low IQs, children and adults with this disorder obtained scores in the normal range on two standardized face-processing tasks, the Benton and the Rivermead (Bellugi et al. 1994, 2000; Udwin and Yule 1991). So if low intelligence doesn't preclude normal scores for face processing, surely the conclusion to be drawn is that face processing must call on an independently functioning module that is innately specified. The neuroconstructivist approach rejects such an automatic conclusion, arguing that before assuming the existence of an intact module, the researcher must first examine the successful behavior in greater depth, in order to uncover underlying cognitive and brain mechanisms.

In a series of experiments, we and others have shown that the Williams syndrome face-processing skills are underpinned by different cognitive processes from those in normal controls (Annaz 2006; Deruelle et al. 1999; Karmiloff-Smith 1997; Karmiloff-Smith et al. 2004). Individuals with Williams syndrome rely more heavily on featural and holistic processing, whereas controls use configural processing—their brains compute all the distances between the features. We further corroborated these cognitive findings by measuring brain processes using high-density event-related potentials (Grice et al. 2001, 2003). Our findings revealed that individuals with Williams syndrome use the same cerebral processes for recognizing both faces and cars, whereas controls displayed a specific brain signature for faces. Moreover, whereas controls showed a strong right-hemisphere specialization for upright faces, the group with Williams syndrome displayed more bilateral processing and no significant difference between upright and inverted faces (Karmiloff-Smith et al. 2004). In other words, despite proficient behavioral scores on some standardized tests, individuals with Williams syndrome fail to demonstrate the gradual specialization and localization of function—that is, the progressive modularization—that we witness over developmental time in the normal case. A neuroconstructivist approach clearly tells a richer and, we believe, developmentally more realistic story than approaches based on the idea of seemingly intact, innate modules.

The Time Course of Development

A lack of specialization and localization of function, which we referred to as a *lack* of progressive modularization (Karmiloff-Smith 1992), leads to the speculation that the brains of individuals with developmental disorders may remain more highly interconnected than the brains of healthy controls, which have undergone progressive pruning over the course of development. The resulting atypical brain would be overly active across multiple brain regions, resulting, for instance, in problems with multitasking (Mackinlay et al. 2006). This certainly holds for individuals with fragile X syndrome, whose brains have been shown to have abnormally high synaptic densities through to adulthood (Comery et al. 1997; and Dabholkar 1997). But the opposite is also possible. In some developmental disorders—for example, autism—the brain may commit too rapidly to specialization and localization of function (Oliver et al. 2000), resulting in less flexibility for processing novel stimuli. Such developmental considerations, in which the time course of development plays a pivotal role, lead us far from the metaphor of static intact and impaired modules, which ignores the importance of ontogenetic development.

The Importance of the Infant Start State

We started this chapter by arguing that the adult neuropsychological model of brain injury was too static for explaining developmental disorders. The corollary of that argument is that researchers must begin their studies of developmental disorders on subjects in early infancy (Karmiloff-Smith 1998, 2006b; Paterson et al. 1999; Scerif and Karmiloff-Smith 2005). A tiny deficit in low-level processes in the visual, auditory, or tactile modalities may cascade on the developing system and subsequently result in a major impairment. We have, for instance, argued that the planning of visual saccades, when impaired, as in Williams syndrome (Brown et al. 2003), may adversely affect the development of triadic interaction (Laing et al. 2002) and the learning of vocabulary (Nazzi et al. 2003) and may also lead to a fascination with detail because of sticky fixation in the absence of rapid saccades. This has strong implications for intervention strategies, which should not only consider seriously impaired domains in the resulting phenotype but also the early precursors that led to that end state.

Concluding Thoughts

We remain puzzled as to why the very idea of development has been discarded from mainstream research into what are, after all, *developmental* disorders. As the chapter illustrates, there is no support for the sort of predeterminism that replaces the notion of development (see also Elman et al. 1996). Not only is such nativism biologically implausible but also the behavioral evidence itself is equivocal. This is not only true of evidence from adults but also from infants, where, if nativism were true, then we should witness *less* effects of experience early on. Yet infant development is experience-dependent from the very start (Johnson 2001). Moreover, neuroconstructivist approaches clearly illustrate how the forced binary distinction between intact and damaged processes is misleading (Karmiloff-Smith et al. 2004). The notions of *specific* impairments and double dissociations are flawed when used in developmental neuroscience (Karmiloff-Smith et al. 2003).

In our view, the field requires a proper theoretical framework about cognitive change (see Mareschal et al. 2007), which would transform research from a taxonomic exercise ("*What* goes wrong?") into a powerful explanatory framework ("*How* does it go wrong?"), with obvious applied implications. The idea of ontogenetic development, once maligned (Fodor 1975; Fodor and Pylyshyn 1988), has become increasingly relevant as our understanding of the developing brain has grown (Nelson et al. 2006). Moreover, we believe that computational developmental cognitive neuroscience (Westermann et al. 2006) offers robust, formal support for such a developmental perspective. Not only does it reject predeterminism on computational grounds (Quartz 1993), but it offers biologically and computationally plausible developmental models that do away with the need for innate knowledge (Shultz 2003; Sirois and Shultz 1999). An important contribution from the computational area shows that development should not be construed as a special form of learning, and erroneously viewing the two as equivalent. Indeed it is a erroneous to consider development and learning as equivalent, a view that has plagued developmental psychology for a long time (Liben 1987). Development is a mechanism distinct from learning, which it supports (Sirois and Shultz 2003).

It is one thing for academics to debate endlessly about the nature or the meaning of abstract concepts. It is an altogether different issue when, as in this case, such debates have real and important implications, for instance, for the welfare and life opportunities of children born with developmental disorders. A case in point is the work of Philip R. Zelazo on pervasive developmental disorders, or PDD (see Zelazo 1986, 1997a, 1997b). PDD is a cluster of severe cognitive impairments that includes autism-like symptoms. Zelazo (1986) proposed methods for assessing cognitive abilities that bypass the need for children to follow verbal instructions, which are features of many psychometric tests that present obstacles for many children. His methods use metrics such as looking time to gain an implicit measure of cognitive abilities. They allow practitioners to carry out differential diagnoses (Zelazo 1997a), which in turn are good predictors of the clinical outcome of lengthy, resource-heavy interventions (Zelazo 1997b). Although Zelazo rests his discussion of the diagnoses on the distinction between intact and impaired cognitive abilities, we would argue that his approach moves in the right direction in that it creates clusters in cognitive space in which to assign different children, based on the variable positions that they occupy along several dimensions. The key point is that if we take seriously the concept of development as trajectories, and atypical development as atypical trajectories, then intervention must take the form of modifying trajectories, which is precisely what Zelazo's methods allow. Our view is that Zelazo's intervention methods precisely illustrate the importance of development in developmental disorders. Uniquely supported by the biological and behavioral sciences, currently they represent the intervention approach most likely to bring about improvements in those born with developmental disorders.

Note

This chapter draws in part on Annette Karmiloff-Smith (2007), "Atypical epigenesis," Developmental Science 10(1): 84–88.

References

Annaz D (2006) The development of visuo-spatial processing in children with autism, Down syndrome and Williams syndrome. PhD thesis, Birkbeck College, University of London.

Baillargeon R (1987) Object permanence in 3-1/2- and 4-1/2-month-old infants. Dev Psychol 23: 655–664.

Baillargeon R, Spelke ES, Wasserman S (1985) Object permanence in five-month-old infants. Cognition 20: 191–208.

Bhattacharya J (2007) Shadows of artistry on the cortical canvas of functional connectivity patterns. Talk delivered at Goldsmiths, University of London, March 2007.

Bhattacharya J, Petsche H (2005) Drawing on mind's canvas: Differences in cortical integration patterns between artists and non-artists. Hum Brain Mapp 261: 1–14.

Bellugi U, Lichtenberger L, Jones W, Lai Z, St George M (2000) The neurocognitive profile of Williams syndrome: A complex pattern of strengths and weaknesses. Journal Cognitive Neurosci 12(Suppl): 7–29.

Bellugi U, Wang PP, Jernigan TL (1994) Williams syndrome: An unusual neuropsychological profile. In: Atypical cognitive deficits in developmental disorders: Implications for brain function (Broman SH, Grafman J, eds), 23–56. Hillsdale, NJ: Lawrence Erlbaum.

Bogartz RS, Shinskey JL, Schilling TH (2000) Object permanence in five-and-a half-month-old infants? Infancy 1: 403–428.

Bogartz RS, Shinskey JL, Speaker CJ (1997) Interpreting infant looking: The event set * event set design. Dev Psychol 33: 408–422.

Brown J, Johnson MH, Paterson S, Gilmore R, Gsödl M, Longhi E, Karmiloff-Smith A (2003) Spatial representation and attention in toddlers with Williams syndrome and Down syndrome. Neuropsychologia 41: 1037–1046.

Buller DJ (2005a) Adapting minds: Evolutionary psychology and the persistent quest for human nature. Cambridge, MA: MIT Press.

Buller DJ (2005b) Evolutionary psychology: The emperor's new paradigm. Trends Cogn Sci 9: 277–283.

Buss DM (1995) Evolutionary psychology: A new paradigm for psychological science. Psychol Inq 6: 1–30.

Cashon CH, Cohen LB (2000) Eight-month-old infants' perceptions of possible and impossible events. Infancy 1: 429–446.

Clahsen H, Almazan M (1998) Syntax and morphology in children with Williams syndrome. Cognition 68: 167–198.

Cohen LB (2004) Uses and misuses of habituation and related preference paradigms. Infant Child Dev 13: 349–352.

Cohen LB, Marks KS (2002) How infants process addition and subtraction events. Dev Sci 5: 186–201.

Comery TA, Harris JB, Willems PJ, Oostra BA, Irvin SA, Weiler IJ, Greenough WT (1997) Abnormal dendritic spines in Fragile-X knockout mice: Maturation and pruning deficits. P Natl Acad Sci USA 94: 5401–5404.

de Haan M, Humphreys K, Johnson MH (2002) Developing a brain specialized for face perception: A converging methods approach. Dev Psychobiol 40: 200–212.

Deruelle C, Macini J, Livet MO, Casse-Perrot C, de Schonen S (1999) Configural and local processing of faces in children with Williams syndrome. Brain Cognition 41: 276–298.

Donnai D, Karmiloff-Smith A (2000) Williams syndrome: From genotype through to the cognitive phenotype. Am J Med Genet 97: 164–171.

Elman JL, Bates EA, Johnson MH, Karmiloff-Smith A, Parisi D, Plunkett K (1996) Rethinking innateness: A connectionist perspective on development. Cambridge, MA: MIT Press.

Fodor J (1975) The language of thought. New York: Crowell.

Fodor JA, Pylyshyn ZW (1988) Connectionism and cognitive architecture: A critical analysis. Cognition 28: 3–71.

Frangiskakis JM, Ewart AK, Morris CA, Mervis CB, Bertrand J, Robinson BF, Klein BP, Ensing GJ, Everett LA, Green ED, Proschel C, Gutowski NJ, Noble M, Atkinson DL, Odelberg SJ, Keating MT (1996) LIM-kinase1 hemizygosity implicated in impaired visuospatial constructive cognition. Cell 86: 59–69.

Goldman-Rakic PS (1987) Development of cortical circuitry and cognitive function. Child Dev 58: 601–622.

Gomez RL, Gerken L (1999) Artificial grammar learning by 1-year-olds leads to specific and abstract knowledge. Cognition 70: 109–135.

Gopnik M (1990) Feature-blind grammar and dysphasia. Nature 344: 715.

Grice SJ, de Haan M, Halit H, Johnson MH, Csibra G, Grant J, Karmiloff-Smith A (2003) ERP abnormalities of visual perception in Williams syndrome. NeuroReport 14: 1773–1777.

Grice S, Spratling MW, Karmiloff-Smith A, Halit H, Csibra G, de Haan M, Johnson MH (2001) Disordered visual processing and oscillatory brain activity in autism and Williams syndrome. NeuroReport 12: 2697–2700.

Hains SMJ, Muir DW (1996) Infant sensitivity to adult eye direction. Child Dev 67: 1940–1951.

Haith MM (1998) Who put the cog in infant cognition? Is rich interpretation too costly? Infant Behav Dev 21: 167–179.

Hepper PG (1997) Memory in utero? Dev Med Child Neurol 39: 343–346.

Hoffman JE, Landau B, Pagani B (2003) Spatial breakdown in spatial construction: Evidence from eye fixations in children with Williams syndrome. Cognitive Psychol 46: 260–301.

Houston-Price C, Nakai S (2004) Distinguishing novelty and familiarity effects in infant preference procedures. Infant Child Dev 13: 341–348.

Huttenlocher PR, Dabholkar AS (1997) Regional differences in synaptogenesis in human cerebral cortex. J Comp Neurol 387: 167–178.

Johnson MH (2004) Plasticity and functional brain development: The case of face processing. In: Attention and performance XX: Functional imaging of visual cognition (Kanwisher N, Duncan J, eds), 257–265. Oxford: Oxford University Press.

Johnson MH (2001) Functional brain development in humans. Nat Rev Neurosci 2: 475–483.

Johnson MH, Morton J (1991) Biology and cognitive development: The case of face recognition. Oxford: Blackwell.

Karmiloff-Smith A (2007) Atypical epigenesis. Dev Sci 10: 84–88.

Karmiloff-Smith A (2006a) Ontogeny, genetics, and evolution: A perspective from developmental cognitive neuroscience. Biol Theory 1: 44–51.

Karmiloff-Smith A (2006b) Modules, genes and evolution: What have we learned from atypical development? In: Attention and performance XXI: Processes of change in brain and cognitive development (Munakata Y, Johnson MH, eds), 563–583. Oxford: Oxford University Press.

Karmiloff-Smith A (1998) Development itself is the key to understanding developmental disorders. Trends Cogn Sci 2: 389–398.

Karmiloff-Smith A (1997) Crucial differences between developmental cognitive neuroscience and adult neuro-psychology. Dev Neuropsychol 13: 513–524.

Karmiloff-Smith A (1992) Beyond modularity: A developmental perspective on cognitive science. Cambridge, MA: MIT Press.

Karmiloff-Smith A, Scerif G, Ansari D (2003) Double dissociations in developmental disorders? Theoretically misconceived, empirically dubious. Cortex 39: 161–163.

Karmiloff-Smith A, Thomas M, Annaz D, Humphreys K, Ewing S, Brace N, van Duuren M, Pike G, Grice S, Campbell R (2004) Exploring the Williams syndrome face processing debate: The importance of building developmental trajectories. J Child Psychol Psyc 45: 1258–1274.

Keen R (2003) Representation of objects and events: Why do infants look so smart and toddlers look so dumb? Curr Dir Psychol Sci 12: 79–83.

Kuhl PK (2004) Early language acquisition: Cracking the speech code. Nat Rev Neurosci 5: 831–843.

Laing E, Butterworth G, Ansari D, Gsödl M, Longhi E, Panagiotaki G, Paterson S, Karmiloff-Smith A (2002) Atypical development of language and social communication in toddlers with Williams syndrome. Dev Sci 5: 233–246.

Landau B, Hoffman JE (2005) Parallels between spatial cognition and spatial language: Evidence from Williams syndrome. J Mem Lang 53: 163–185.

Liben LS (1987) Approaches to development and learning: Conflict and congruence. In: Development and learning: Conflict or congruence? (Liben LS, ed), 237–252. Hillsdale, NJ: Lawrence Erlbaum.

Lorenz K, von Cranach A, Martin RD (1996) The natural science of the human species: An introduction to comparative behavioral research (The "Russian Manuscript" 1944–1948). Cambridge, MA: The MIT Press.

Mackinlay R, Charman T, Karmiloff-Smith A (2006) High functioning children with Autistic spectrum disorder: A novel test of multi-tasking. Brain Cognition 61: 14–24.

Majdan M, Shatz CJ (2006) Effects of visual experience on activity-dependent gene regulation in cortex. Nat Rev Neurosci 9: 650–659.

Marcus GF, Vijayan S, Rao SB, Vishton PM (1999) Rule learning by seven-month-old infants. Science 283. 77–80.

Mareschal D, Johnson MH, Sirois S, Spratling M, Thomas MSC, Westermann G (2007). Neuroconstructivism: How the brain constructs cognition, volume 1. Oxford: Oxford University Press.

Meaney MJ, Szyf M (2005) Maternal care as a model for experience-dependent chromatin plasticity? Trends Neurosci 28: 456–463.

Morton J, Johnson MH (1991) CONSPEC and CONLERN: A two-process theory of infant face recognition. Psychol Rev 98: 164–181.

Nazzi T, Paterson S, Karmiloff-Smith A (2003) Early word segmentation by infants and toddlers with Williams syndrome. Infancy 4: 251–271.

Nelson CA, De Haan M, Thomas KM (2006) Neuroscience of cognitive development: The role of experience and the developing brain. Hoboken, NJ: Wiley.

Oliver A, Johnson MH, Karmiloff-Smith A, Pennington B (2000) Deviations in the emergence of representations: A neuroconstructivist framework for analysing developmental disorders. Dev Sci 3: 1–23.

Onishi KH, Baillargeon R (2005) Do 15-month-old infants understand false beliefs? Science 308: 255–258.

Paterson SJ, Brown JH, Gsödl MK, Johnson MH, Karmiloff-Smith A (1999) Cognitive modularity and genetic disorders. Science 286: 2355–2358.

Perner J, Ruffman T (2005) Infants' insight into the mind: How deep? Science 308: 214–216.

Piattelli-Palmarini M (2001) Speaking of learning. Nature 411: 887–888.

Pinker S (1994) The language instinct. New York: William Morrow.

Pinker S (1997) How the mind works. New York: Norton.

Pinker S (1999) Words and rules: The ingredients of language. London: Weidenfeld & Nicolson.

Pinto-Correia C (1997) The ovary of Eve: Egg and sperm and preformation. Chicago: University of Chicago Press.

Povinelli DJ, Prince CG, Preuss TM (2005) Parent-offspring conflict and the development of social understanding. In: The innate mind: Structure and contents (Carruthers P, Laurence S, Stich S, eds), 239–253. Oxford: Oxford University Press.

Quartz S, Sejnowski TJ (1997) The neural basis of cognitive development: A constructivist manifesto. Behav Brain Sci 20: 537–596.

Quartz SR (1993) Neural networks, nativism, and the plausibility of construction. Cognition 48: 223–242.

Quinlan PT (1998) Structural change and development in real and artificial neural networks. Neural Networks 11: 577–599.

Roder BJ, Bushnell EW, Sasseville AM (2000) Infants' preferences for familiarity and novelty during the course of visual processing. Infancy 1: 491–507.

Ruffman T, Perner J (2005) Do infants really understand false belief? Trends Cogn Sci 9: 462–463.

Scerif G, Karmiloff-Smith A (2005) The dawn of cognitive genetics? Crucial developmental caveats. Trends Cogn Sci 3: 126–135.

Schoner G, Thelen E (2006) Using dynamic field theory to rethink infant habituation. Psychol Rev 113: 273–299.

Shultz TR (2003) Computational developmental psychology. Cambridge, MA: MIT Press.

Sirois S, Jackson I (2007) Social cognition in infancy: A critical review of research on higher-order abilities. Eur J Dev Psychol 4: 46–64.

Sirois S, Shultz TR (1999) Learning, development, and nativism: Connectionist implications. In: Proceedings of the twenty-first annual conference of the Cognitive Science Society (Hahn M, Stoness SC, eds), 689–694. Mahwah, NJ: Lawrence Erlbaum.

Sirois S, Shultz TR (2003) A connectionist perspective on Piagetian development. In: Connectionist models of development (Quinlan P, ed), 13–41. Hove, UK: Psychology Press.

Spelke ES, Breinlinger K, Macomber J, Jacobson K (1992) Origins of knowledge. Psychol Rev 99: 605–632.

Tager-Flusberg H, Plesa-Skwerer D, Faja S, Joseph RM (2003) People with Williams syndrome process faces holistically. Cognition 89: 11–24.

Tooby J, Cosmides L (1990) The past explains the present: Emotional adaptations and the structure of ancestral environments. Ethol Sociobiol 11: 375–424.

Udwin O, Yule W (1991) A cognitive and behavioural phenotype in Williams syndrome. J Clin Exp Neuropsych 13: 232–244.

Walker P, Bremner JG, Merrick K, Coates S, Cooper E, Lawley R, Sageman R, Simm R (2006) Visual mental representations supporting object drawing: How naming a novel object with a novel count noun impacts on young children's object drawing. Vis Cogn 13: 733–788.

Watson JS (1972) Smiling, cooing, and "the game." Merrill Palmer Quart 18: 323–339.

Westermann G, Sirois S, Shultz TR, Mareschal D (2006) Modeling developmental cognitive neuroscience. Trends Cogn Sci 10: 227–232.

Wexler K (1996) The development of inflection in a biologically based theory of language acquisition. In: Toward a genetics of language (Rice ML, ed), 113–114. Mahwah, NJ: Lawrence Erlbaum.

Wolfsberg TG, McEntyre J, Schuler GD (2001) Guide to the draft human genome. Nature 409: 824–826.

Woodward AL (1998) Infants selectively encode the goal object of an actor's reach. Cognition 69: 1–34.

Woodward AL (1999) Infants' ability to distinguish between purposeful and non-purposeful behaviors. Infant Behav Dev 22: 145–160.

Wynn K (1992) Addition and subtraction by human infants. Nature 358: 749–750.

Wynn K (1995) Infants possess a system of numerical knowledge. Curr Dir Psychol Sci 4: 172–177.

Zelazo PR (1986) An information processing approach to infant-toddler assessment and intervention. In: Theory and research in behavioral pediatrics, volume 3 (Fitzgerald HE, Lester BM, Yogman MW, eds), 1–45. New York: Plenum Press.

Zelazo PR (1997a) Infant-toddler information processing assessment for children with pervasive developmental disorder and autism. Infant Young Child 10(1): 1–14.

Zelazo PR (1997b) Infant-toddler information processing assessment of children with pervasive developmental disorder and autism: Part II. Infant Young Child 10(2): 1–13.

Contributors

Chris M. Bird
Institute of Cognitive Neuroscience
University College London, United
Kingdom

Elizabeth M. Brannon
Department of Psychology and
Neuroscience
Center for Cognitive Neuroscience
Duke University
Durham, North Carolina

Neil Burgess
Institute of Cognitive Neuroscience
University College London, United
Kingdom

Jessica F. Cantlon
Department of Psychology and
Neuroscience
Center for Cognitive Neuroscience
Duke University
Durham, North Carolina

Stanislas Dehaene
INSERM Unit 562 "Cognitive
Neuroimaging"
Gif-Sur-Yvette, and
Collège de France
Paris, France

Christian F. Doeller
Institute of Cognitive Neuroscience
University College London, United
Kingdom

Reuven Dukas
Animal Behaviour Group
Department of Psychology, Neuroscience,
and Behaviour
McMaster University
Hamilton, Ontario, Canada

Rochel Gelman
Rutgers Center for Cognitive Science
Rutgers University
Piscataway, New Jersey

Alexander Gerganov
Center for Cognitive Science
New Bulgarian University
Sofia, Bulgaria

Paul W. Glimcher
Center for Neural Science
New York University, New York,
New York

Robert L. Goldstone
Department of Psychological and Brain
Sciences
Indiana University
Bloomington, Indiana

Edward M. Hubbard
INSERM Unit 562 "Cognitive
Neuroimaging"
Gif-Sur-Yvette, France

Lucia F. Jacobs
Department of Psychology
University of California
Berkeley, California

Mark H. Johnson
Centre for Brain and Cognitive
Development
School of Psychology
Birkbeck, University of London
United Kingdom

Annette Karmiloff-Smith
Developmental Neurocognition Lab
Birkbeck, University of London
United Kingdom

David Landy
Cognitive Science Program
Indiana University
Bloomington, Indiana

Lynn Nadel
Department of Psychology
University of Arizona
Tucson, Arizona

Nora S. Newcombe
Department of Psychology
Temple University
Philadelphia, Pennsylvania

Daniel Osorio
School of Life Sciences
University of Sussex
Falmer, Brighton, United Kingdom

Mary A. Peterson
Department of Psychology
University of Arizona
Tucson, Arizona

Manuela Piazza
Center for Mind/Brain Sciences
University of Trento
Rovereto, Italy

Philippe Pinel
INSERM Unit 562 "Cognitive
Neuroimaging"
Gif-Sur-Yvette, France

Michael L. Platt
Department of Neurobiology
Duke University Medical Center
Durham, North Carolina

Kristin R. Ratliff
University of Chicago
Chicago, Illinois

Michael E. Roberts
Department of Psychology
DePauw University
Greencastle, Indiana

Wendy L. Shallcross
Department of Psychology
Temple University
Philadelphia, Pennsylvania

Stephen V. Shepherd
Department of Neurobiology
Duke University Medical Center
Durham, North Carolina

Sylvain Sirois
School of Psychological Sciences
University of Manchester
Manchester, United Kingdom

Luca Tommasi
Department of Biomedical Sciences
University of Chieti
Chieti, Italy

Alessandro Treves
Cognitive Neuroscience Sector
SISSA
Trieste, Italy, and
Centre for the Biology of Memory
Trondheim, Norway

Alexandra Twyman
Department of Psychology
Temple University
Philadelphia, Pennsylvania

Giorgio Vallortigara
Center for Mind/Brain Sciences
University of Trento
Rovereto, Italy

Index